Modern System of Ophthalmology **MSO** Series

Anatomy and Physiology of Eye

Second Edition

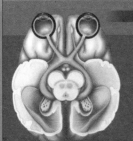

A K Khurana
Indu Khurana

CBS Publishers & Distributors Pvt Ltd

Squint and
Orthoptics

Second Edition

A K Khurana

CBS Publishers & Distributors Pvt Ltd

Modern System of Ophthalmology **MSO** Series

Disorders of Lens and Cataract Surgery

A K Khurana

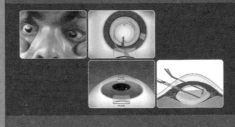

CBS Publishers & Distributors Pvt Ltd

Modern System of Ophthalmology **MSO** Series

Disorders of Retina and Vitreous

Chief Editor
A K Khurana

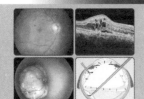

Editors
Sunandan Sood
Atul Kumar

Associate Editors
Subina Narang
Aruj K. Khurana

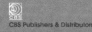
CBS Publishers & Distributors Pvt Ltd

Modern System of Ophthalmology **MSO** Series

Neuroophthalmology

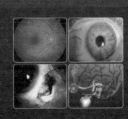

A K Khurana
Rashmin Gandhi

CBS Publishers & Distributors Pvt Ltd

Manual of
Phaco Technique
Text & Atlas

With
Best Compliments
from—:

Manual of
Phaco Technique
Text & Atlas
SECOND EDITION

Dr. HARBANSH LAL MS

- Director, Delhi Eye Centre
- Chairman, Deptt. of CME, Sir Ganga Ram Hospital
- Co-chairman, Deptt. of Ophthalmology, Sir Ganga Ram Hospital
- Treasurer, All India Ophthalmological Society
- Author, Manual of Phaco Technique (Text and Atlas)
- Author, AIOS CME Series
  - A Guide to Phacoemulsification
  - Management of PCT

Positions held in the past
- Immediate Past President, Delhi Ophthalmological Society
- Secretary, Delhi Ophthalmological Society (2005–07)
- Library Officer, Delhi Ophthalmological Society
- Member, Executive Committee, Delhi Ophthalmological Society
- Member, Executive Committee, Indian Implant and Refractive Society
- Member, Scientific Committee, All India Ophthalmological Society
- Joint Secretary, All India Ophthalmological Society
- President, Rotary Club of Delhi, Rajendra Place

Dr. Anita Sethi MD, DNB, FRCS
Nova Medical Centre & Artemis Hospital

Dr. Tinku Bali Razdan MS, FRCS
Consultant, Sir Ganga Ram Hospital

Dr. Ikeda Lal MS, FICO

CBS Publishers & Distributors Pvt Ltd
New Delhi • Bengaluru • Chennai • Kochi • Mumbai • Pune
Hyderabad • Kolkata • Nagpur • Patna • Vijayawada

Manual of
Phaco Technique
Text & Atlas

ISBN: 978-81-239-2433-5

Second Edition: 2014
First Edition: 2002

Published by Satish Kumar Jain for
CBS Publishers & Distributors Pvt Ltd
4819/XI Prahlad Street, 24 Ansari Road, Daryaganj, New Delhi 110 002, India.
Ph: 23289259, 23266861, 23266867   Fax: 011-23243014   Website: www.cbspd.com
                                                                 e-mail: delhi@cbspd.com; cbspubs@airtelmail.in.
Corporate Office: 204 FIE, Industrial Area, Patparganj, Delhi 110 092
Ph: 4934 4934   Fax: 4934 4935   e-mail: publishing@cbspd.com;   publicity@cbspd.com

Branches

- **Bengaluru:** Seema House 2975, 17th Cross, K.R. Road,
  Banasankari 2nd Stage, Bengaluru 560 070, Karnataka
  Ph: +91-80-26771678/79   Fax: +91-80-26771680   e-mail: bangalore@cbspd.com
- **Chennai:** 20, West Park Road, Shenoy Nagar, Chennai 600 030, Tamil Nadu
  Ph: +91-44-26260666, 26208620   Fax: +91-44-42032115   e-mail: chennai@cbspd.com
- **Kochi:** 36/14 Kalluvilakam, Lissie Hospital Road, Kochi 682 018, Kerala
  Ph: +91-484-4059061-65   Fax: +91-484-4059065   e-mail: kochi@cbspd.com
- **Mumbai:** 83-C, Dr E Moses Road, Worli, Mumbai-400018, Maharashtra
  Ph: +91-22-24902340/2341   Fax: +91-22-24902342   e-mail: mumbai@cbspd.com
- **Pune:** Bhuruk Prestige, Sr. No. 52/12/2+1+3/2 Narhe, Haveli
  (Near Katraj-Dehu Road Bypass), Pune 411 041, Maharashtra
  Ph: +91-20-64704058/59, 32392277   Fax: +91-20-24300160   e-mail: pune@cbspd.com

Representatives

- **Hyderabad**   0-9885175004   **Kolkata**   0-9831437309, 0-9051152362
- **Nagpur**   0-9021734563   **Patna**   0-9334159340   **Vijayawada**   0-9000660880

Printed at : Shree Maitrey Printech Pvt. ltd., Noida

Dedicated

To

My loving wife, Jyotsna

and

Lovely daughter, Ikeda

- I would like to make a special mention of **Dr. Bhartendu Kumar Varma** for helping me in completing the second edition of the book.

- I am thankful to **Dr. Lalit Verma** for his contribution in writing PCT Management by Posterior Segment Surgeon along with **Dr. Tinku Bali Razdan**.

- I am thankful to **Dr. Ranjan Dutta** for writing Biometry and IOL Power Calculations.

I would like to make a special mention of two young promising ophthalmologists whom I will always remember fondly:

- **Dr. Jasmita Popli**, Senior Resident, SGRH, for her hard work in putting this book together; and
- **Dr. Saurabh Sawhney**, an ophthalmologist with a keen interest in computer applications, for the time and effort spent in making the diagrams for this book.

My heartfelt wishes for their successful career.

A special mention too for my dear friend, **Ramit Sethi**, for being an understanding husband of my co-author and encouraging her all through the project.

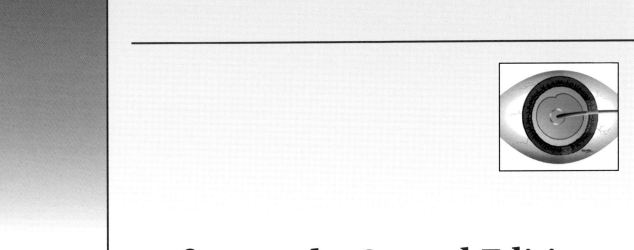

Preface to the Second Edition

The first edition of this book was written twelve years ago and had a very enthusiastic response, as at that time there were very few comprehensive books available for beginners. Being out of print, it was not available in the market for the last seven years. I had initially never planned to revise this book, but then I changed my mind due to repeated phone calls and queries about the book. On many occasions in various conferences, young ophthalmologists have approached me saying that they were reading photocopies of my book.

I realized that the basics of phacoemulsification will always remain the same. There may have been improvements in the microscopes and phacomachines, but still there is a learning curve, albeit smaller than before.

The second edition of the book has been completely revised without changing its basic character. There is an additional chapter on correcting pre-existing astigmatism, which is simple and can be practised by beginners. The chapter on biometry has been revised completely. The most important addition in this book is the management of complications. We hope that this revised edition will help our younger ophthalmologists in performing safe phacosurgery and, in case a complication does take place, they would feel confident in handling it expertly.

Harbansh Lal

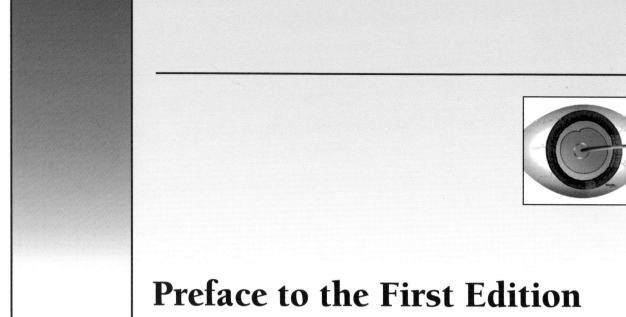

Preface to the First Edition

Being one of the pioneers of phacoemulsification in the country, I have participated in numerous workshops all along the length and breadth of the country. While interacting with participants, the question that I have found most difficult to answer is *'Which is the best book to read for understanding phacoemulsification?'*. Over the years, I have found that though certain topics are discussed well in some books, there is no **ONE** book which describes the basic principles of phaco completely. Many of these books are not accessible to the average ophthalmologist, for the want of availability or price, who then has to depend on conferences and demonstrations for practical learning. Though many surgeons are now routinely performing phaco, there are a large number who are still getting stuck at basic steps, on points which are no longer being addressed in the conferences today as the emphasis seems to have shifted to the more advanced techniques, leaving the beginners still confused.

Thus a void was felt in the existing available literature on phaco, especially in the Indian context. This practical manual on phaco has been written with the aim of elaborating the basic techniques for performing safe and successful phacoemulsification. Through our lectures and demonstrations we have seen that concepts can be clarified better through diagrams and illustrations and, so, we have included as many figures as possible for easy explanation. We have tried to illustrate how to safely do phacoemulsification in all conditions and situations.

We have purposely omitted the more advanced concepts of LRI, multifocal IOLs, etc. and hope to include these in the later editions. With your encouragement, we hope to continue to disseminate information as *six-monthly booklets* and in future editions. Our endeavour is to keep updating the phaco surgeons, especially those in remote areas with not much access to the latest information by the way of modern libraries, workshops or conferences. For this we would request your cooperation by way of *filling out the tear sheet at the back and sending it to us.*

Harbansh Lal

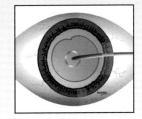

Contents

Preface to the Second Edition vii
Preface to the First Edition viii

1. Preparing for Phacoemulsification 1

2. Setting the Operation Theatre and Sterilization Techniques 3

Design of OT 3
Sterilization technique 3
Formaldehyde fumigation 4
Sterilization by heat 4
• Dry heat 4
• Autoclaving 4

Glutaraldehyde 2% (Cidex) 4
Ethylene oxide (ETO) 5
Formalin chamber 5

3. Phacomachine and Phacodynamics 7

Phacomachine 7
Console 7
Handpiece 7
Foot pedal 7
• Foot gradient 8
• Sidekick functions of foot pedal 9
Phacodynamics 9
Power 9
• Control and delivery of power 10
• Hyperpulse 10
• Utilization of power 11
• Tips 11
Fluidics 12
• Infusion system 12
• Aspiration system 13
• Venturi system 13
• Peristaltic system 13

• Flow rate (FR) 13
• Vacuum 13
• Rise time (RT) 14
• Central safe zone (CSZ) 14
• Peripheral unsafe zone (PUSZ) 14
• Followability 14
  – Zones of followability 15
• Compliance 16
• Surge 16
  – Critical limit 16
  – Role of vacuum and compliance in
    post-occlusion surge 17
  – Relationship between vacuum, surge and
    flow rate 17
• Control of surge 18
  – Surge prevention by the machine 18
  – Surgeon's control of surge 19

4. Choosing the Phacomachine, Instruments and Viscoelastic Substances 21

Phacomachine 21
Instruments 21
Viscoelastic substances (VES).................21
Properties of an ideal viscoelastic substance 24

Usc in the steps of phacoemulsification 24
Choosing the phacomachine 25
Newer modifications.................................26

5. Biometry and IOL Power Calculation 29

Estimation of IOL power 29
IOL calculation formulas 29
• First generation formulas........................29
• Second generation formulas 30
• Third generation formulas 30
• Fourth generation formulas 30
The measurement of axial length 31
• Echography principles 31
• Biometry technique 32
• Manual mode 32
• Automatic mode 32
Echograph 32
• Characteristics of a good A-scan 33
• Selection of the scan 33
• Avoiding errors in biometry 33
• A-scan biometer features 33
Partial coherence laser interferometry 34
Measurement of corneal power 35
• Instrumentation......................................35

Keratometry in eyes with corneal transplant 35
Biometry and IOL power calculation in special
situations 35
• The pseudophakic eye 35
• The aphakic eye 36
• Intumescent cataract 36
• The highly myopic eye with posterior
staphyloma 37
• The very short eye 38
• Silicone-filled eyes 38
• IOL power calculation in eyes after previous
corneal refractive surgery 38
IOL power calculation after radial keratotomy (RK) 41
Scarred corneas, keratoconus 41
Corneal transplantation combined with cataract
surgery 41
• Selecting the appropriate IOL power 41
IOL power selection in children 42
Biometry: Important considerations 42

6. Incisions and Wound Construction 43

Applied anatomy......................................43
• Astigmatic neutral funnel 43
• Self-sealing incision 44
Instruments 45
Pre-requisites 45
Side port incision (SPI)............................45
Scleral tunnel/scleral pocket 45
Technique 46
• Initial groove 46
• Making the tunnel 46
Problems 47

Clear corneal incision 48
Types of corneal incision 48
• Triplanar incision 48
• Hinged incision 48
• Biplanar corneal incision 48
• Uniplanar clear corneal incision 50
Limbal incision 50
Modified temporal incision (corneolimbal/
limboscleral) 50
Problems of corneal and limbal incisions 51

7. Continuous Curvilinear Capsulorrhexis 65

Applied anatomy......................................65
Physics of capsulorrhexis 66
• Types of force 66
• Tangential force 66
Size of CCC 66

Instruments 67
• Cystitome 67
• Forceps 68
Pre-requisites 68
Techniques of CCC 69

Needle CCC 69
• Initiation 69
  – Linear cut 69
  – Raising the flap 69
  – Problems in initiation 69
• Continuation of CCC 70
• Completion of CCC 72
Forceps CCC 72
• Technique 73

Combination CCC 73
Loss of control of CCC 73
• Why we lose control 73
• How to regain control 73
Dyes in CCC 74
Enlargement of CCC 74
CCC in young patients 75
Posterior capsulorrhexis 75
• Technique 75

8. Hydroprocedures 93

Applied anatomy 93
Instruments 93
Hydrodissection 94
• Pre-requisites 94
• Technique 94
• Site for hydrodissection 95
Cortical cleaving hydrodissection 95
Special Situations 96
Hydrodelineation 96
• Pre-requisites 96
• Technique 96

Mini-delineation/mechanical delineation 97
Soft cataracts 97
Partial delineation ring 97
Rotation of the nucleus 97
• Single-handed rotation 97
• Bimanual rotation 97
Non-rotation of nucleus 98
Posterior capsular tear during hydrodissection 98
Dos and Don'ts of hydroprocedures 98

9. Nucleotomy 101

Applied anatomy 101
Instruments 102
• Phaco tip 102
• Choppers 102
Nucleotomy 103
• Entering the eye 103
• Removal of the anterior epinuclear plate 103
Trenching 103
• Settings for trenching 103
• Dimensions of the trench 103
• Length of the trench 104
• Width 104
• Starting the trench 104
• Completing the trench 105
• Assessment of depth 105
Difficulties in trenching 106
• Too wide a trench 106
• Too narrow a trench 106
• Bumps in the depth 106
V-shaped or victory trench 106
Splitting 106
Divide & Conquer 108
• Modified technique of Divide & Conquer 108

Chopping 109
• Stabilization of the nucleus 109
• Creating a platform 109
  – Complete trench 109
  – Partial trenching 109
  – Chopping without a trench 109
• Creation of vacuum seal and vacuum hold 110
  – Steps in vacuum hold 110
  – Settings for vacuum seal 111
Phaco chop 111
• Peripheral chop 111
  – Problems with peripheral chop 111
• Central chop 112
  – Modification 112
  – Problems with central chop 112
• Modified peripheral chop 113
• Direct chop 113
Stop & Chop technique 113
Aspiration phaco 113
• Settings 114
• Types of grips 114
• Procedure 115
• Problems 116

10. Epinuclear Plate Removal 145

Applied anatomy 145
Instruments 146
• Rounded iris repositor/rod-shaped iris repositor 146
• Phaco settings 146
Technique: Flip & Chip method 146
Problems 146

11. Cortical Aspiration 155

Instruments 155
Techniques of irrigation and aspiration 155
• Co-axial irrigation and aspiration 155
  – Problems with co-axial IA 156
• Bimanual irrigation and aspiration 157
• Bimanual modified technique of irrigation and aspiration 157
• Manual irrigation and aspiration 157
• Sub-incisional cortex removal 158
• Removal of cortical matter after IOL insertion 158

Capsular polishing 158
Technique 158
• Central PCC polishing 158
• Polishing beyond the optical zone 158
• Polishing of anterior and equatorial zone 159
• 'Cap vac' mode 159
  – Orifice facing downwards 159
  – Orifice facing upwards 159

12. Insertion of IOL 171

Phaco profile IOLs 171
Foldable IOLs 171
Instruments 171
Pre-requisites 171
• Viscopressurized eyeball 171
• Adequate incision size 172
Technique for single-piece PMMA lenses 172
• Putting the trailing haptic by forceps 173
Foldable IOLs 173
• Holder-folder method 173
  – Technique 173
Injecting systems 175

13. Our Preferred Technique for Phacoemulsification and Settings in Different Situations 191

Assessment of the patient 191
Anaesthesia 191
Draping 191
Betadine cleaning 191
Incision 191
CCC 192
Hydroprocedures 192
Nucleotomy 193
Trenching 193
Splitting 193
Chopping and phacoaspiration 193
Epinuclear plate removal 194
Cortical aspiration 194
Capsular polishing 194
IOL insertion 194
Hydration of the wound 194
IOP at the time of leaving the eye 194

14. Correction of Pre-existing Astigmatism: LRIs, OCCIs & Toric IOLs 197

Incidence of astigmatism 197
Limbal/corneal relaxing incision 197
• Limitations 198
On axis cataract incision and opposite clear corneal incisions 198
• Types of incisions 199
• Site of the incision 200
• Wound construction 200
• Number of incisions 200
• Amount of astigmatism 200
Nomograms 200
Do I need to change IOL power? 201
Toric intraocular lens 201
Surgical pearls 201
Techniques of correction 202
• Treat only corneal astigmatism 202

15. Complications of Phacoemulsification 205

Wound-related complications 205
• Scleral/corneal burn 205
• Descemet's detachment 205
Corneal complications 206
• Endothelial damage 206
Iris complications 206
• Iris chaffing 206
• Iridodialysis 206
Capsular complications 206
• Zonulodialysis 206
 – Cionni's ring fixation in cases of
  zonulodialysis 206
Posterior capsular tear 207
Predisposing factors 207
Surge 210
Control of surge 211
• Surge prevention by the machine 211
• Surgeon's control of surge 211
Mechanism of PCT 211
• Primary RMT 212
• Secondary RMT 213
Types of RMT 213
Signs of a PC rupture during hydrodissection 214
Partial occlusion of tip 214
Diagnosis and goals 216
Converting tear to PCC 216
Confirmation of PCT and hyaloid face rupture
(HFR) 216
• Signs of HFR 216
• Tests 216
Goals of management 217
• Major goals 217
• Important goals 217
Management by Anterior Segment Surgeon 217
• Factors in decision making 217

• Primary management strategies 218
 – Nucleus/nuclear fragments 218
 – Epinucleus 223
 – Cortex 223
 – IOL implantation 224
 – Final vitrectomy and closure 234
Management by Posterior Segment Surgeon 234
• Role of cataract surgeon 234
• Role of Posterior Segment Surgeon 235
• Initial examination 235
• Indications for surgery 235
• Timing of surgery 236
• Operative technique 236
 – Pars plana vitrectomy 236
 – Removal of retained lens matter 237
Conversion to SICS/ECCE 238
Reasons to convert 239
• CCC related problems 239
• Excessive use of phaco and fluids
 (prolonged surgical time) 239
• Wound related problems 239
• Corneal edema 239
• Intraoperative meosis 239
• Improper case selection 239
How to convert? 239
• Conversion of intact CCC to perform
 planned ECCE/small incision (non-phaco)
 cataract extraction 239
• Conversion of superior scleral tunnel 240
• Conversion in a superior clear corneal/limbal
 incision 240
• Conversion in a temporal incision 240
Immediate post-operative endophthalmitis/TASS ...240
Technique of periocular antibiotic-steroid
injection 241

Index 251

Abbreviations Used in the Text

AC	Anterior chamber		PC	Posterior capsule
ACD	Anterior chamber depth		PCC	Posterior continuous capsulorhexis
ACIOL	Anterior chamber intraocular lens		PCIOL	Posterior chamber intraocular lens
CCC	Continuous curvilinear capsulorhexis		PCT	Posterior capsular tear
CCI	Clear corneal incision		PFCL	Perfluorocarbon liquid
CL	Contact lens		PMMA	Polymethylmethacrylate
CME	Cystoid macular edema		PPV	Pars plana vitrectomy
CSZ	Central safe zone		PUSZ	Peripheral unsafe zone
ECCE	Extracapsular cataract extraction		PVD	Posterior vitreous detachment
EPN	Epinuclear plate		RD	Retinal detachment
I/A	Irrigation aspiration		RMT	Rhexis margin tear
IOL	Intraocular lens		RR	Rounded repositor
IOP	Intraocular pressure		SFIOL	Scleral-fixated intraocular lens
IPD	Interpupillary distance		SICS	Small incision cataract surgery
PAL	Posterior-assisted levitation		VES	Viscoelastic substance

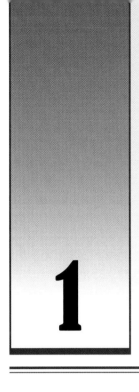

1 Preparing for Phacoemulsification

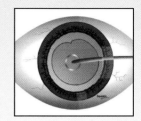

The preparation for phaco must be started *much* before one has even ventured near a phacomachine if you are to achieve success. Mental preparation needs to be commenced before the actual physical preparation. The first step is to **BELIEVE IN YOURSELF** that *you too* can be a successful phaco surgeon. Regardless of the so called 'learning curve', if you apply *both* your mind and hands to the task, you will definitely master phaco.

Having crossed the first hurdle, that of self-belief, you must now equip yourself with all the **knowledge** available regarding phaco. What the mind does not know, the hands can not achieve! This information may either be obtained from books, CDs, videos or by attending courses or workshops. **Observing other phaco surgeons**, those proficient and even those not so proficient can offer some valuable lessons.

Before attempting phaco, one must be **proficient at extracapsular cataract extraction, small incison cataract surgery** and other intraocular surgeries. This surgical experience will stand you in good stead while attempting various manoeuvres with the phaco probe or the second instrument. It is important to be **ambidextrous** during phaco and this can be improved by practising activities with the left hand. One also needs to be able to coordinate the **foot pedal** of the microscope and the machine. The movement of the foot pedal is of paramount importance and you should practise the positions of the foot pedal (i.e. moving between irrigation, irrigation-aspiration and phaco) for at least *10 hours* before even starting phaco.

Even before actually obtaining a phacomachine, one must initiate a few steps while performing planned ECCE. For example, CCC and hydroprocedures may be attempted, taking care to release or extend the CCC in 2–3 places before delivering the nucleus. Alternatively, one may attempt **small incision non-phaco cataract extraction** by Blumenthal technique or any other technique one feels comfortable with. Once you are fairly comfortable at the above, you can then advance to actually using the phacomachine in an experimental OT set-up, if available. Though the animal eyes are very different from the human eyes, it does give you a feel of the machine. If an experimental laboratory is not available, one can take the animal eye in the OT and use the same instruments and machine which one would have used for the human eye and afterwards the instruments can be properly sterilized. Animal eye is to be washed with betadine before taking into the OT. **Understanding the phacomachine** is vital to a successful surgery. You should **read the manual** carefully. It is helpful to observe an experienced surgeon operating on the machine that you plan to use so that you may understand the finer tricks of getting the best of the machine.

How to proceed further will depend on whether you are performing phaco under supervision, or if a senior surgeon is nearby and can be called if required. It is also prudent to have a good understanding with vitreoretinal surgeon. If operating under supervision, you can be a little bolder since the senior surgeon will take over in case of a problem. The toughest part of surgery is trenching and splitting so the supervising surgeon can make the trench and split the nucleus and you can perform phacoaspiration. However, if you are on your own, try not to be complacent. If CCC is not complete, **DON'T HURT YOUR EGO BUT CONVERT**. Similarly, after making a small trench if you find it difficult, then convert. After delivering the nucleus see how deep your trench was so that you can do better trenching next time. After conversion and nucleus delivery, close the section completely. Try to do automated bimanual cortical aspiration. Do not attempt automated aspiration without proper closure of the chamber. Suturing has to be done well either by four to five interrupted or by running sutures, the disadvantage of this being removal of sutures to put the IOL. One can similarly remove the viscoelastic substance in an automated manner. You should watch videos of your own surgery and constantly evaluate yourself.

Phaco surgery is performed in the mind. If you keep thinking about the procedure all the time, your understanding of the machine, mechanisms and instruments will be better and you will be able to master the technique much faster.

"Our Best Wishes for joining the Phaco club."

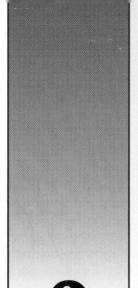

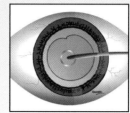

2 Setting the Operation Theatre and Sterilization Techniques

Before embarking on phaco procedure you must take care that the OT is well set. This makes the patient, the surgeon and the assistant more comfortable and confident during the procedure. The surgeon is then able to concentrate entirely on the surgery. Making adjustments during the surgery or having to wait for instruments is cumbersome and disturbs the surgeon's concentration.

Patient is reassured and shifted to the OT. The pulse and blood pressure of the patient should be recorded. Position the patient and check the microscope settings. The operating microscope should be set according to the surgeon's convenience. The OT table height, the chair height and the microscope height should be adjusted to suit the surgeon's comfort allowing sufficient space for movement of the foot pedal under the table. The microscope head should be in the centre to permit full range of up-down and X-Y movements. Correct the eyepiece for your refractive error. The interpupillary distance (IPD) is then set. The eyepieces are pulled apart to the maximum and then the distance is gradually reduced while looking through them. The maximum distance at which a single image is obtained is your IPD. At this point if one eye is closed the image should be central for the other eye.

The assistant and the staff nurse should be familiar with your steps. Check that the tray is set with all the instruments that may be needed, according to your requirements. All the drugs required during the surgery like intracameral adrenaline, intracameral pilocarpine should be ready in their correct concentrations.

Next, the phacomachine should be primed. Check that the tip of your choice is well fit by the assistant. The silicone sleeve should be intact and the system patent. Microscope foot pedal and phacomachine foot pedal should be arranged in position depending on the surgeon's preference.

After the patient has been anaesthetized, the skin is cleaned twice with betadine by the assistant. Gentle application is sufficient. There is no need to scrub the skin. Betadine must be allowed to dry for 5 to 6 minutes to allow for full antiseptic effect to take place. The surgeon can then proceed to the scrub room.

Design of OT

OT should be separate from the general traffic of the hospital or clinic. A sequence of increasingly clear zones from the entrance to the operating area should be developed such that infected/used materials can be disposed of without passing through clean areas. Air flow should be from clean areas to less clean areas.

Sterilization technique

In larger institutions the surgeon may not be directly involved in the sterilization of the OT and instruments. However, in one's own set-up, this is one of the most important aspects of the surgery and should be given due importance. Most cases of post-operative endophthalmitis result from inadequate sterilization techniques.

Formaldehyde fumigation

Formaldehyde is an effective agent commonly used to sterilize the OR. The efficacy of the process is uncertain at temperatures below 20°C and relative humidity below 70%. For optimum OR disinfection, formaldehyde fumigation is recommended fortnightly as a routine, and at the end of an operating session of a grossly infected case.

All apertures in the room should be sealed with adhesive tape prior to fumigation. Formaldehyde can be generated by addition of 150 gm of potassium permanganate to 280 ml of formalin for every 1000 cubic feet of the room volume. As this reaction produces considerable heat, a heat-resistant container should be used. Temperature and humidity should be controlled to a minimum of 18°C and 60% respectively. After formaldehyde vapour is generated, the room is left unopened for 48 hours. Alternatively, 500 ml of 40% formaldehyde in one litre of water is put into an electric boiler or a large bowl placed on a electric hot plate with safety cut-out when boiling dry. Subsequently, ammonium solution may be introduced and left in the room for a few hours to neutralise the formaldehyde (one litre ammonium solution plus one litre of water for every litre of 40% formaldehyde used). Room doors can be opened for a short period or the air-conditioning switched on to replace the formalin with air.

Sterilization by heat

Dry Heat

Hot air by itself is an inefficient sterilizing agent since it is a poor conductor and does not penetrate well. A temperature of 160°C for one hour or 180°C for 20 minutes will sterilize the contents by a destructive oxidation of cell constituents. The one-hour holding period is timed after the temperature reaches 160°C. Its usefulness is limited to some sharp instruments and glass, which would otherwise be damaged by moist heat. The main disadvantage is long cycle time.

Autoclaving

This method is more effective than dry heat and requires lower temperatures in a given time. Autoclaving at 121°C for 15 minutes at 15 psi pressure effectively kills most microorganism. A temperature of 134°C at 34 psi pressure sterilizes instruments within 3 minutes. Sterilization occurs due to the latent heat which is given out when steam condenses to water. Therefore, to sterilize effectively, the steam must come into direct contact with the surfaces to be sterilized.

It is essential to remove all the air from the autoclave. In a bigger hospital, horizontal autoclaves (front loading) are available in which this is ensured by **downward displacement method** in which steam is introduced through the upper end of the chamber. This then descends down pushing the air out through the outlet at the floor of the chamber. Another method used for replacement of air is use of **high vacuum pump**. However, in a smaller set-up, vertical autoclaves (top loading) are used. In this if you close the chamber and put on the weight, air gets trapped and does not allow the steam to come in direct contact with instruments and linen. To avoid this, do not close the chamber till the steam has replaced the air in autoclave completely and starts coming out. Also the drum should not be packed so tightly that the steam cannot percolate. Make sure that the perforated sieve on the sides of the drums is open. For further safety, one can do the autoclaving for 30 minutes and those instruments that are going into the eye can be autoclaved twice. Though the autoclaved instruments can be used upto 48 hours after sterilization, they should be autoclaved as close to the theatre time as possible. Autoclaving is suitable for sterilization of most metallic ophthalmic instruments. Autoclaving irrigating solution bottles may kill heat-labile microorganisms but bacterial spores may still survive, since steam cannot penetrate the bottles. Though autoclaving of bottles is not required, they may be autoclaved so that the outer wall is sterile and they can be kept on the trolley for easy access. Temperature-sensitive detectors must always be used to ensure adequate autoclaving.

I recommend a repeat autoclaving of all instruments after 5–6 hours i.e. **double autoclaving**.

Glutaraldehyde 2% (Cidex)

This is an effective sterilizer for instruments that cannot be autoclaved. It is non-corrosive, does not impair the sharpness of cutting instruments and may be used with plastic, aluminium and rubber. Glutaraldehyde in a 2% aqueous solution is more effective and less irritant. It is stable in acidic solution and does not require activation. However, the sporicidal effect is slow. Alkaline solution such as cidex requires activation. Once activated it is stable for 2–4 weeks. It is effective against vegetative, pathogens in 10 minutes and resistant pathogenic spores in 3 hours. It is very effective against the tubercle bacillus.

The low surface tension allows for easy penetration to inner surfaces and it can be readily removed by rinsing. Thorough rinsing of all sterilized material is mandatory because residual glutaraldehyde is extremely irritating to tissues. Sterilization of lumen-containing instruments such as irrigating cannulae by glutaraldehyde is not recommended as this leads to corneal endothelial cell damage and uveitis.

Sharp instruments must be rinsed serially two to three times in trays filled with Ringer's lactate or normal saline (0.9%) to eliminate the residual chemical from the instruments.

Ethylene oxide (ETO)

ETO is widely used commercially to sterilize single-use items. It is also used in some large hospitals for resterilizing packaged heat-sensitive devices like sharp knives and blades. Gas sterilization using ethylene oxide is effective and safe for heat-labile tubings, vitrectomy cutters, cryoprobes, lightpipes, laser probes, diathermy leads and most disposable items for cost reduction. Sterilization is done by a process known as alkylation in which a hydrogen atom is replaced by a hydroxyl ethyl radical within a protein molecule. When a sufficient number of positrons within molecules of microorganisms have been alkylated, death ensues. The process kills all microorganisms, including tubercle bacilli and spores.

It penetrates very well, is non-corrosive and relatively non-toxic compared to formalin. The easy penetrability allows the article to be pre-packaged. The type of packaging used is important because ETO must be both capable of penetrating it and of being removed from it. Polyethene of 200-gauge thickness satisfactorily wraps equipment for long-term storage and its transparency allows one to see what is in the package. This package should be heat sealed or sealed with tape.

To be effective and safe, several parameters must be considered. For effective sterilization, the minimum concentration required is 400–1000 mg/L (the concentration of ETO is measured in mg of gas per litre of space). Required exposure time can be decreased by increasing the temperature. Most automatic sterilizers employ temperatures of 40–60°C. Moisture enhances the diffusion of the ETO gas. The time required varies with the type of sterilizer depending upon all the above factors, and also the type of load. Sterilization time could vary from 1–12 hours. Blood, pus and other proteinaceous materials act as barriers to ETO. Equipment must therefore be cleaned well before sterilization.

During the typical cycle, air is removed from the load. The chamber is heated to the desired temperature. Steam is introduced to rehumidify the load. Gas is then introduced from a cylinder. Temperature and pressure should be maintained for the sterilization period. The gas is removed and the chamber and its contents are flushed with filtered air.

A thorough aeration is essential for all items sterilized by ETO as ETO and its residues are toxic and irritant. The duration varies and is dependent upon the absorbency of the load and the temperature and air exchange rate of the aeration facility. If higher aeration temperatures are used, for instance 55°C, 12 hours is usually sufficient, but periods of up to one week are usually necessary at room temperature. After aeration, the equipment can be stored sterile for extended periods of time.

Formalin chamber

It was earlier used for cryo probe and retinal lenses. It is not very reliable and is also very toxic and is not used for intraocular instruments. If used, the instruments need to be rinsed well especially those with lumen.

3 Phacomachine and Phacodynamics

PHACOMACHINE

The machine consists of the *console, foot pedal, handpiece* and their connections. Though there are many variations in the models, the basic functions are similar.

CONSOLE

The *console* consists of a computer which controls all the functions of the machine. The setting for the various parameters, i.e. power, vacuum and flow rate are fed in here. These settings represent the maximum level of the parameter that will be achievable: the further linear control is with the foot pedal. Newer machines have a multi-mode panel, where multiple settings of all variables, as is required by different surgeons, can be fed in. The same surgeon may like to change all the variables during the surgery and these parameters can also be fed in and can be recovered by touching the memory button only. Settings for different types of cataract can also be fed into the memory. In some machines the memory can be activated by the foot switch so that the surgeon can continue the surgery without having to look at the console.

HANDPIECE

There are two types of handpieces—*phaco handpiece* and *irrigation aspiration handpiece* (latter is discussed in **Chapter 11: Cortical Aspiration**). The phaco handpiece contains the piezoelectric crystal, which is in contact with the tip. The tip is covered by a silicon sleeve.

The infusion fluid flows between the tip and the sleeve cooling the former. There are two openings on the sleeve for the exit of this fluid, which should be kept perpendicular to the tip bevel. The proximal end of handpiece is connected to the console with an electric cord. There are two more connections: one each for the irrigation tubing and for connecting the aspiration system.

There are various types of tips, the utility and functions of which are discussed in the power system.

FOOT PEDAL (Figs. 3.1 & 3.2)

Foot pedal control is *the* most important aspect of phaco. Control and coordination of the foot pedal is a step that *must* be mastered even before you have put the probe into the patients' eye. In fact at least 10–12 hours of practising the various foot pedal positions in order to familiarize oneself with the feel of dentations of the pedal (*tactile feedback*) and the sounds that the machine makes (*auditory feedback*) is *mandatory* before attempting phacoemulsification.

If you are already using your right foot for controlling the complex functions of the microscope, you may train your left foot for the phaco control. You can, however, use any foot, keeping in mind that both feet need to be well coordinated so that you remain in control of both the phaco and the microscope.

Though the foot pedal of each machine may have a different design, it essentially consists of main **central part** and **sidekicks**. The main part of the foot pedal

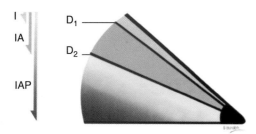

Fig. 3.1. Foot pedal. In phaco mode there are 2 dentations (D_1, D_2) where the resistance is felt. Note the 3 excursions. **I** – irrigation only, **IA** – irrigation-aspiration, and **IAP** or **P** is the phaco mode.

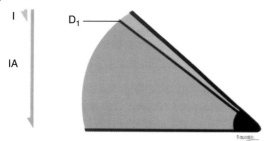

Fig. 3.2. Foot pedal in irrigation-aspiration mode. There is only one dentation and 2 excursions. **I** – irrigation, **IA** – irrigation-aspiration.

controls infusion, aspiration and phaco power. The entire distance that the foot pedal traverses is divided by 2 dentations into 3 excursions—**I** (**irrigation only**), **IA** (**infusion and aspiration**) and **IAP** (**infusion, aspiration and phaco**). The excursion before the first dentation is the I excursion, the excursion between the 1st and the 2nd dentation is the IA excursion and the excursion after the 2nd dentation is the IAP excursion. Resistance is felt at the dentations or position where the mode changes and it is to feel these dentations that one has to train oneself both while depressing and while coming back up. Ability to move quickly from one mode to the other at the correct time is the key to successful chopping, as will be explained later.

The point to remember is that in the *I excursion*, irrigation is fully on. In the *IA excursion* both irrigation and aspiration are on and in the *IAP excursion*, irrigation is on, aspiration is at the maximum preset, and phaco power will depend on the amount of depression.

In the I excursion, the pinch valve opens and irrigation is switched on. There is no gradient in this step and the irrigation is either switched fully on or off. In the absence of gradient, the function of this dentation is to dissociate infusion from irrigation-aspiration. As foot is brought back from IA/IAP excursion, stopping at this dentation will keep the infusion on preventing the collapse of anterior chamber. Many steps like nuclear rotation,

manipulation of nuclear fragments, epinuclear plate etc. require a formed AC without any aspiration.

Dentation 1 to dentation 2 is the aspiration or the **IA** excursion. From dentation 2 to full depression is the phaco or the 'IAP' excursion. At IAP_0 phaco energy delivered will be zero and at IAP_{max} the energy will be maximum preset. The delivery of phaco energy is linear both in the surgeon and the pulse mode. However, in panel or burst mode, as soon as foot clears IAP_0, maximum preset energy is delivered.

Foot gradient (Fig. 3.3)

Foot gradient is the excursion of foot pedal in mm to produce unit power of phaco energy. To give an example—If the total foot excursion, from IAP_0 to IAP_{max} is 10 cm i.e. 100 mm and the maximum preset phaco energy is 100%, then the foot gradient (FG) becomes

$$FG = \frac{100 \text{ mm}}{100} = 1 \text{ unit power per } \textbf{1 mm} \text{ of excursion}$$

Now, if maximum preset phaco power is changed to 50%,

$$FG = \frac{100 \text{ mm}}{50} = 1 \text{ unit power per } \textbf{2 mm} \text{ of excursion}$$

At phaco power 25% maximum,

$$FG = \frac{100 \text{ mm}}{25} = 1 \text{ unit power per } \textbf{4 mm} \text{ of excursion}$$

Decreasing the maximum preset power on console increases the foot gradient and hence the foot control. Therefore, phaco maximum should be set at the minimum power which is required for a particular step in that grade of cataract e.g. phaco maximum is kept between 20–30%

- If P_{max} = 100%, then 1% power = 1 unit footpedal excursion
- If P_{max} = 25%, then 1% power = 4 unit footpedal excursion

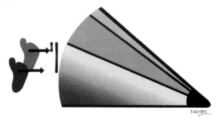

Fig. 3.3. Foot gradient. Note that for the same unit change in power, the excursion of the foot pedal is 4 times more when the maximum power is set at 25% (blue pedal), thus giving better control.

lower in phacoaspiration as compared to trenching and further lowered for epinuclear plate removal. Similarly power settings are lower in a softer cataract.

Sidekick functions of foot pedal

The most important sidekick function of foot pedal is *reflux*. On kicking the side switch, aspiration flow rate is inverted and the material aspirated is expelled into the AC. Since it is not a continuous function, for further reflux, the switch needs to be kicked again. Inadvertent aspiration of wrong tissue (iris, capsule) can be released by this function especially by beginners.

Continuous infusion mode (CIM) can prove to be a boon for an inexperienced surgeon. In this mode, the infusion remains on regardless of the position of the foot pedal (i.e. even if the foot is accidentally lifted *off* the pedal the infusion remains on, and the chamber remains formed). It is started by kicking the side switch and remains on, till kicking the same switch again stops it. While changing modes, the backward tactile feel on the foot pedal is less, so one may not be able to judge when one is in the **Infusion** mode. With **CIM**, the eye remains pressurized even when the pedal is released. Whenever the probe is in the eye the infusion must remain on and in steps like cracking the nucleus, where the probe is inside, but no phaco or aspiration are being used, this mode is especially useful. In machines, which do not have the CIM mode, the assistant can remove the infusion tubing from the pinch valve as soon as the probe is in the eye.

Few machines also have pulse on-off, bottle height adjustments, multi-mode panel, and dual linear control in the foot pedal. In the latter, linear control is in both directions—downwards and sideways.

PHACODYNAMICS

The various functions of the phacomachine and their interrelationship is called phacodynamics. The basic functions of the machine are two, which include *ultrasonic power* for emulsification and *irrigation-aspiration* for safe suction of the emulsified material. Irrigation-aspiration system and the parameters on which it depends together are called *fluidics*.

POWER (Fig. 3.4)

Phaco power is produced by the ultrasonic vibrations of the quartz crystal in the handpiece. There may be 2–4

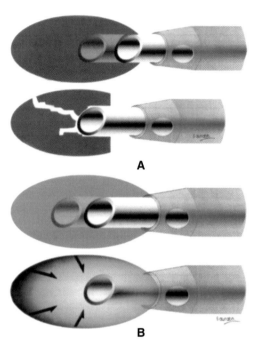

Fig. 3.4. Mechanism of phaco. (A) **Jack-hammer effect:** The rapid to & fro movement of the tip bombards the tissue in front and disintegrates it. (B) **Cavitation phenomenon:** The frequency of oscillation is 40,000/second. The swift backward movement of the tip results in a cavitation phenomenon causing an implosion of surrounding tissue.

crystals, 4 giving more stroke length and more power. The frequency is variable from 29–60 Hz in different machines. Higher frequency ensures a better cutting action but more heat is generated though, practically this does not significantly affect the surgical outcome. However, in each machine, the frequency remains fixed—power is varied by varying the **stroke length** which is the to & fro movement of the tip and varies from 2/1000 – 6/1000 of an inch. The actual mechanism of emulsification is a combination of the bombarding action of the tip (*Jack-hammer*) and *cavitation* phenomenon caused by the high velocity of the tip moving backwards. The *Jack-hammer* action requires that the nucleus should be fixed as during trenching, or the nuclear fragment held by vacuum, during phaco-aspiration, for the bombarding action to be effective. This is the action that is primarily used during trenching. The rapid backward excursion of the tip creates a cavity into the area (as the tip moves faster than fluid) causing the surrounding fluid to fall into this space, virtually generating an '*implosion*' thereby causing disintegration of the nuclear material. The forward movement of the tip also generates an *acoustic wave* of fluid that can disintegrate the softer lens material. This shock wave is also responsible for some emulsification. The disadvantage of this wave is that it may push nuclear pieces away if the hold is not good and thus decrease the ***Jack-hammer*** effect. If the vacuum hold is good, then this action can be synergistic with the ***Jack-hammer*** effect.

Control and delivery of power (Figs. 3.5 & 3.6)

All machines provide 0–100% power and the power required can be chosen from the computer controlled panel. There are various modes—surgeon/linear or panel. In the ***surgeon*** mode, the power delivery varies from 0 to the maximum that one sets on the panel, by varying the foot pedal in phaco mode. At pedal position 2, i.e. at

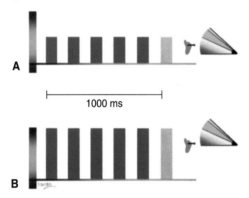

Fig. 3.5. Pulse mode. Note that if there are 5 pulses/second, each pulse has an equal duration (100 msec) of phaco on & off. (A) If the foot pedal is half depressed, power will be **half** of the maximum preset but pulse duration and frequency is unaltered. (B) If foot pedal is fully depressed, the power in each pulse will be the **maximum preset**, pulse duration and frequency remains the same.

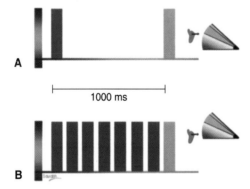

Fig. 3.6. Burst mode phaco power delivery. Note that the power is maximum preset regardless of the foot pedal position. (A) The foot pedal is at P_0—only one burst per second of fixed power and duration. (B) As the foot pedal moves, the duration and power of the pulse remains the same but frequency keeps on increasing so much so that full depression of the pedal (P_{max}) will result in continuous power delivery.

the start of phaco mode (P_0) the power will be 0 and at full depression (P_{max}) power will be the maximum that has been preset. Thus, the excursion of the foot in phaco mode will determine the amount of power being delivered. In the **panel** mode, as soon as you depress the foot pedal into the phaco mode (P_0), you will immediately reach the maximum power that you have set on the panel. Here, there is no variation and full power is delivered. As we know the hardness of the nucleus is not uniform, most surgeons prefer the linear mode so that they can control the power according to the hardness of the cataract. The only probable indication for the use of panel mode is in a very hard cataract where the nucleus is uniformly hard requiring more or less uniformly high power for emulsification.

There are a few other modes of power delivery available in certain machines. In **pulse mode** each pulse of energy is followed by a gap of equal duration. For effective power delivery, the nuclear fragment has to be held, so the interval between the pulses of phaco allow the vacuum to build up and thus a good hold is developed. Pulse mode is a variant of linear phaco mode where the frequency of the pulses is fixed and the phaco energy delivered in each pulse will depend on the amount the pedal is pressed. Thus the power is delivered at preset intervals, the frequency of which is preset and decided by the surgeon. For example, if set at 5 pulses/sec, there will be 5 pulses of energy and each energy burst will be followed by a gap of equal duration, i.e. each pulse and each gap will be of 100 msec duration (1 sec = 1000 msec, 1000 sec/5 pulses + 5 gaps = 100 msec). Most machines have from 0–12 pulses. If the pulses are too many, then it acts as a continuous mode and there is not enough time for adequate vacuum build up. A frequency of 2–6 pulses/second is useful in phacoaspiration; my personal preference is 3 pulses per second. The use of the pulse mode in phacoaspiration almost halves the power use, as the vacuum build up between the pulses ensures efficient emulsification and aspiration. This is especially useful in limiting the energy used by beginners in hard cataracts though it may not be so useful in soft cataracts.

Hyperpulse (Figs. 3.7 & 3.8)

This expands on the traditional pulse technology. In hyperpulse mode we have a bundle of pulses clubbed together, with interwining off periods. The gap between on and off periods within this bundle of pulses is constant

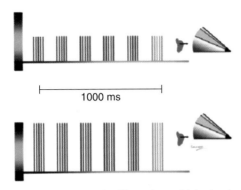

1000 ms

Fig. 3.7. Hyperpulse mode. Note that within the bundle on and off time of energy is same i.e. 10 ms and also note that bundle width is 100 ms and gap between the bundle is also 100 ms. Duty cycle in this case is 100/(100 + 100) = 1/2.

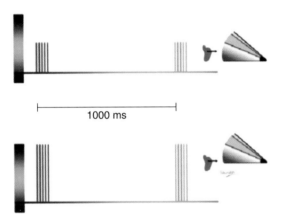

1000 ms

Fig. 3.8. Note that the bundle width is 100 ms while the gap between the two bundles is 900 ms i.e. duty cycle is 100/(100 + 900) = 1/10.

as in the pulse mode. We can have varied duration of on and off periods between the bundle of pulses in this mode. Duty cycle is the ratio of phaco-on time divided by total time (cycle), expressed as a fraction. In other words, phaco-on time/(phaco-on time + phaco-off time). The main benefit being the increased time of phaco-off periods resulting in reduced amount of heat generation. The number and duration of pulses within the bundle and gap between the bundle can be decided by the surgeon and type of machine.

One other mode that is useful in hard cataract is the **burst mode** where maximum power is delivered at intervals which vary with the amount you depress the foot pedal. Burst mode is a variant of panel mode where the energy is fixed and the frequency of phaco bursts will increase with increasing depression of the foot pedal in phaco mode. At P_0 there will be one burst per second and at full depression (P_{max}) the power delivery is

continuous. The duration of the burst can be selected and is usually 100 msec. This mode is only available in the higher end (third generation) machines.

The amount of power to be set depends on the hardness of the cataract and will be discussed in the relevant chapters. Also the surgeon may vary the power setting depending on the stage of the surgery i.e. lower setting for epinuclear plate removal. Though power is most important for emulsification, it has to be used judiciously since the setting of the power is dependent on the surgeon. It has to be kept in mind that both too little power and too much power can cause problems for the surgeons.

Utilization of Power

How the power is delivered depends upon the type of tips.

Tips (Fig. 3.9)

The angulation of the tips may vary from 0–60°. Tips with 60°, 45°, 30°, 15° and 0° angulation are available. More the angulation, the lesser the holding power but the cutting power is more, e.g. 60° tip is a sharper tapered tip making occlusion difficult. Therefore, this tip has a better cutting and less holding power. The **45°** tip has a very good cutting ability and was very popular initially as the emphasis was then on 'Divide and Conquer' in which trenching (thus cutting ability) was more important than occlusion. A 45° tip is recommended for beginners

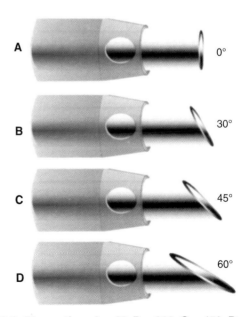

Fig. 3.9. Phaco tips. A = 0°, B = 30°, C = 45°, D = 60°.

as it cuts well and has a larger exposure permitting deeper access. This tip is good for trenching especially in hard cataract, but it must be replaced before chopping.

With the advent of aspiration phaco the most popular tip today is **30°**. This has adequate holding *and* cutting power and is useful both for trenching and in chopping. The 15° and 0° angulated tips are better for holding but have a poorer cutting action. Some people prefer 0° tip for direct chop and hard cataract as it provides for a good hold. However, it is not good for trenching as the area being cut cannot be visualized.

FLUIDICS

The fluidics of the machine refers to the integrated functions performed by infusion and aspiration systems by which a stable AC is maintained. One of the major advantages that phaco has over conventional cataract surgery is the fact that it is performed in a closed chamber. Maintaining a stable chamber depth is vitally important for avoiding damage to all the intraocular structures especially the cornea, iris and PC. Though newer technology has now increased the options available to the surgeon by giving more control in the integrated foot pedal, a better understanding of the fluidics of the machine gives one a safety margin for performing complicated manoeuvres in the eye.

Infusion system (Fig. 3.10)

The infusion system consists of a bottle, the height of which provides the gradient for flow. The tubing from the bottle is run through a pinch valve which is controlled by the foot pedal. The infusion is gravity fed, 2 feet bottle height conforming to approximately 44 mmHg (2 ft =

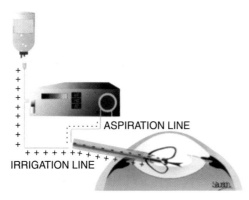

Fig. 3.10. Note the gradient created at the tip by the interplay of the negative pressure due to the aspiration system and the positive pressure of the infusion. This gradient or **followability** is greatest at the tip.

60 cm = 600 mm water column, 600/13.6 = 44 mmHg). This would be the IOP in the eye, presuming that there is no wound leakage.

As the bottle height is increased, the fluid entering the eye increases, though it may not be directly proportionate. The accompanying rise in the IOP is more proportionate and thus is the limiting factor in raising the bottle height. For example, a bottle height of 5 feet will cause an IOP of 110 mmHg. In this situation withdrawal of even a small amount of fluid will lead to a large fluctuation in the IOP which would be detrimental to the eye. However, aspiration and wound leak don't usually allow the IOP to reach such high levels. Raising the bottle height too much can have other undesirable effects due to the fact that the AC has a fixed volume and trying to fill excess fluid results in zonular stress leading to patient discomfort. Also, too much fluid can lead to fluctuation of the lens iris diaphragm resulting in irritation to the iris and miosis. Another problem in raising the bottle height may be repeated iris prolapse, especially if the pupil is small and wound is large and there will be unnecessary lavage of the cornea and iris.

When setting the bottle height, a few points need to be kept in mind. The AC should be maintained so that there is no collapse of the chamber in case there is surge. At the same time the IOP should be at a safe level without putting stress on either the zonules or the lens-iris diaphragm. A bottle height of 3 ± 1 ft maintains a safe IOP with sufficient fluid entering the eye.

There are a *few* indications for raising the bottle height. However, this is in special situations and for a limited duration, e.g. when using high vacuum during chopping or when you are expecting surge after emulsification of a hard piece or when the last piece is being aspirated. In hypermetropes or those with shallow AC, one can deepen the AC by raising the bottle height, provided the wound is tight. The reverse is true for myopes or those with a deep AC where the minimum bottle height is usually adequate.

One technique for increasing the flow is a *positive pressure pump* which increases the amount of fluid but is still of limited use, because for all practical purposes it works in the same way as increasing the bottle height, where one uses pressure created by the pump instead of atmospheric pressure. The occurrence of a vascular occlusion due to sudden increase in the IOP, though rare, must be kept in mind. To prevent this complication various methods have been devised to raise the infusion flow without raising the IOP. One such method is by attaching a *TUR set* which, having a wider tubing, has a lower resistance to flow. In this, the amount of fluid entering the eye increases marginally. However, still better system in use is *Anterior Chamber Maintainer* (*ACM*). This system increases the fluid in the AC without raising the IOP.

An ideal system would perhaps be one in which the irrigation gets totally synchronized with the aspiration such that a constant IOP and chamber depth can be maintained, regardless of the foot pedal position.

Aspiration System

The evolution of the aspiration systems is mainly responsible for propelling phacoemulsification to the level it is now. Lack of basic understanding of the aspiration system with over-emphasis on power made the surgery less safe with a higher incidence of complications. The present computer-assisted aspiration systems together with improved tubing have made phacoemulsification a swift and safe surgery.

The two functions of the aspiration system are lavage of the anterior chamber and creation of a hold for emulsification/crushing of the nucleus. Lavage is governed by the *flow rate* and the hold is a function of the *vacuum* generated by the system. The aspiration systems consist of a pump that is either flow-based or vacuum-based. The common type of flow pump is the **Peristaltic pump**. **Venturi** is the prototype of a vacuum-based machine.

Venturi System

Venturi Effect: The swift movement of a compressed gas creates a negative suction force, i.e. the vacuum, inside a closed chamber. In a venturi system, this principle is used to create vacuum in the cassette (closed chamber). This vacuum is then directly transmitted to the handpiece. The amount and speed of the gas decides the level of vacuum developed in the cassette. This process is controlled by the foot pedal.

In the venturi system only the level of vacuum can be controlled and not the flow rate, which is the amount of fluid withdrawn from the anterior chamber per second. Here the flow rate is a fixed fraction of the vacuum. However, the change in vacuum level doesn't always lead to a proportionate change in the flow rate since port size and resistance in the passage also modify flow rate. The advantage of this system is that the vacuum is directly transmitted to the tip from the system ensuring a better followability.

Peristaltic System

In a peristaltic pump, the rotation of the rollers by the pump pinches the soft, silicon tubing, creating a negative pressure by squeezing the fluid out of the tube. The faster the rollers rotate, more fluid is withdrawn and therefore there is a higher flow rate. In this system, vacuum will be built up only after the tip is occluded. Flow rate and vacuum can be set independently in a peristaltic system.

Flow Rate (FR)

The FR is the amount of fluid removed from the eye per minute. FR is determined by the speed at which the pump rotates—the faster the pump rotates, the higher the FR. The flow rate is usually set for a standard tip, fluids and tubing. The machine cannot sense when any of these are altered and if this is so, the flow rate indicated on the machine may differ from the actual flow rate. For example, the smaller the port size, the more the resistance offered and the lower the flow rate. Similarly, more resistance is offered by viscoelastic materials and lens matter in the AC. These would also effectively decrease the amount of fluid being withdrawn. The flow rate is also decreased when there is partial or complete occlusion of the tip with hard nuclear fragments. The decreased elasticity of tubing (worn out with repeated autoclaving) may also contribute to a reduced flow.

Flow rate determines how fast things will happen in the eye. The higher the flow rate, the lesser the rise time and sooner the debris in the AC is cleared. However, if the flow rate is too high, the events may occur faster than you are able to control them. At a very low flow rate things are painfully slow. Most peristaltic machines work best at an optimum FR of 26–36 cc/min with regular tip and 30–40 cc/min with a microtip.

Flow rate settings are basically for flow-based pumps. In a venturi system, FR cannot be set separately and is a fixed fraction of the vacuum.

Vacuum

Vacuum is generated by the machine and is a measure of the strength of the 'hold' that the handpiece has on the nucleus. Level of vacuum and port size will determine how strong the grip is. The holding power is inversely proportional to the port size. Vacuum is a double-edged sword which must be used/set carefully depending on what needs to be held (nucleus, cortex), for what purpose (chopping, aspiration) and with what instrument (phaco tip, I/A cannula). The setting of vacuum also depends on the machine since each machine has its own capabilities. In the first generation machines vacuum may be set upto 120 mmHg in Phaco mode. In the second-generation machines vacuum levels upto 250 mmHg can be used safely whereas in the newer third generation machines vacuum levels upto 450 mmHg can be used comfortably. While checking the machine, one can pinch the aspiration tube and let the vacuum build upto the maximum one plans to use. On release of the tubing, if the test chamber collapses then post-occlusion surge is inevitable at that vacuum setting and flow rate, so the setting should be lowered.

Rise Time (RT) (Fig. 3.11)

The rise time is the time taken by a machine to reach maximum preset vacuum after occlusion has been achieved. In a Venturi system, the RT is fast, linear and dependent upon the highest preset vacuum, while in a peristaltic pump, RT depends on the FR of the machine. The higher the FR, the lesser the RT though the relationship is not absolutely linear. For a given flow rate, the initial rise time is more till a certain level has been achieved after which the vacuum build up is faster.

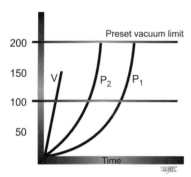

Fig. 3.11. Rise time. Time taken for vacuum to build at the tip. Note that in a venturi system (V) the rise time is linear and fast. In a peristaltic system (P_1, P_2), after initial slow start, vacuum builds up faster. Increasing the flow rate will shorten the rise time, more so for the initial vacuum build up. The curve of P_2 (flow rate 30 cc/min) is steeper than P_1 (flow rate 20 cc/min).

Rise time may be modified by other factors. RT is not dependent on the bore size of the tip since it is calculated after full occlusion. In partial occlusion, preset maximum vacuum may not be achieved at all and even if it is achieved, the time taken is very long. The hold in such a case is very poor especially for chopping though rest of the procedures may still be performed.

Some terms must be understood before proceeding further.

CENTRAL SAFE ZONE (CSZ) (Fig. 3.12)

The *central safe zone* is not an anatomical area but a concept that needs to be understood for performing safe aspiration. This is an area within the CCC margin which is bounded vertically by the cornea on the top and the posterior capsule in opposite direction. This is the area with maximum space in the AC. All aspiration—nuclear, epinuclear or cortical—should be done here as there is maximum safety here. Even if there is AC flutter, the probe will not damage any vital structures. The nuclear pieces and cortical matter can be held in the periphery and then brought to the CSZ for aspiration. This is a dynamic area – as more of the nuclear pieces are removed, the space and thus the safety margin keeps on increasing. **In myopes, zonular stress syndromes and vitrectomized eyes the CSZ is further increased whereas in hypermetropes, small pupil and small CCC the CSZ is smaller.**

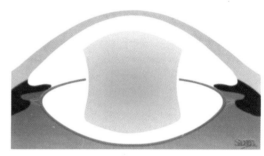

Fig. 3.12. Zone of safety. The green shaded area represents the **Central safe zone**. Phaco aspiration should be done here. The surrounding peripheral anterior chamber and capsular fornices constitute **Peripheral unsafe zone**.

PERIPHERAL UNSAFE ZONE (PUSZ)

Due to the corneal curvature, as one proceeds towards the periphery, one enters an unsafe zone as there is less space for manoeuvring. The capsular fornices and the angle region are thus areas where it is dangerous to do phacoaspiration since the vital structures are extremely close. This constitutes the *Peripheral unsafe zone (PUSZ)*.

FOLLOWABILITY (Fig. 3.10)

The positive pressure due to the infusion and the negative pressure created by the aspiration pump are responsible for the creation of a pressure gradient at the tip. This in turn leads to eddy currents from the infusion orifice to the phaco tip. The area encompassed by these eddy currents is known as the zone of followability. **Follow-**

ability refers to the tendency of the nuclear fragments/ cortical matter to come into the tip.

The positive pressure is governed by the bottle height as has been previously explained. The negative pressure is regulated by the aspiration pump. In a venturi machine, the vacuum is transmitted directly to the tip, even without occlusion. For example, for a bottle height of 3 ft. (3 ft. corresponds to 66 mmHg), if the vacuum is 120 mmHg, then the pressure gradient is approximately 186 mmHg. Due to this high gradient, the followability is good in a venturi system.

In a peristaltic pump, there is no negative pressure at the tip till occlusion, so the gradient is less and so is the followability. At the usual flow rate (20–22 ml/min), the gradient is provided by the positive pressure of the infusion. However, negative pressure at the tip is increased by increasing the flow rate. Though the maximum vacuum will not be achieved till occlusion, increasing the flow rate (28–30 ml/min) will increase the followability as more fluid is withdrawn/unit time. If the flow rate is increased too much, the fluid cannot be withdrawn that fast, the resistance to flow acts like a partial occlusion allowing some vacuum (i.e. negative pressure) to build up at the tip even without occlusion. This increases the gradient at the tip and so, the follow-ability but corresponding increase in the post-occlusion surge is the limiting factor specially in second generation machines. Some third generation machines utilize this feature, and if surge control is good, then at a high flow rate the system will act like a venturi system, e.g. immediate transmission of vacuum with a good gradient at the tip and better followability.

Another important aspect of followability is the size and location of the pieces. It is seen that the smaller pieces tend to come into the eddy currents easier. This highlights the importance of mechanical crushing of pieces to increase the followability. However, if they are lodged in the angle/capsular fornices (PUSZ), it is tougher to suck them into the CSZ and may require mechanical dislodging.

Zones of followability (Fig. 3.13)

The gradient is maximum at the tip and the eddy currents generated ensure a zone of reasonable followability around the tip. The area just in front of the tip is the **area of highest followability**. All the fragments in this area will be attracted towards the tip. Followability decreases as you go further away (both horizontally and vertically) from the tip.

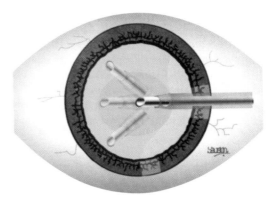

Fig. 3.13. Zones of followability. Area around the tip (shaded green) represents zone of **good followability**. Area around the incisions (shaded gray) represents zones of **no followability**. The remaining area (shaded yellow) represents the area of poor followability. Followability in these areas can be increased by moving the probe in the directions as shown by the shaded probes.

The angle of the anterior chamber and the capsular fornices are the areas of poor followability. As there is no infusion pressure here, these pieces do not get aspirated easily. It is possible to aspirate them by either increasing the gradient (increasing vacuum/flow rate) or taking the probe closer to the pieces making them fall into zone of followability. However, now you are in the peripheral unsafe zone, i.e. you are in the periphery of the anterior chamber where the AC depth is less and both the iris and capsule are dangerously close to the tip. If you want to engage the fragments in that position, avoid holding the iris and bring the piece quickly into the CSZ before aspiration. This is usually easier in a venturi system though the danger to the iris increases. One should not make repeated attempts to engage the piece, it is rather safe to mechanically bring twhe piece into the CSZ.

There are some **areas of no followability**, i.e. fragments here will not come into the tip. These are the areas of the AC from where the fluid is spontaneously leaking out, i.e. the side port and the main wound behind the infusion ports on the handpiece. Here the positive pressure from the infusion pushes the pieces out of the eye. These pieces will not come into the tip even if vacuum is increased to the maximum as the AC will collapse before these can be aspirated. One needs to mechanically bring these pieces into the followability zone either with a second instrument or using viscoelastic material after removing the phaco probe from the eye. Another area of no followability is the dome of the cornea; the eddy currents do not reach here and due to surface tension the pieces tend to get stuck. These need to be dislodged with a VES and then brought into the CSZ. Repeated attempts with the phaco probe can damage the endothelium. Nuclear fragments lying in sub-incisional capsular fornices have to be brought mechanically in front for aspiration.

COMPLIANCE (Figs. 3.14 & 3.15)

A silicon tube connects the aspiration system with the handpiece in both types of pumps. Additionally a thick wide bore tubing is required for the rollers to be effective in a peristaltic pump. While the rollers are rotating, there is no occlusion and no collapse of tubing. When occlusion occurs, vacuum builds up, the rollers stop and negative

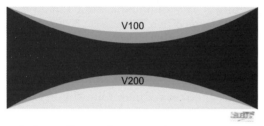

Fig. 3.14. Compliance. Collapse of the tubings developing due to negative pressure inside is called the **compliance of the system**.

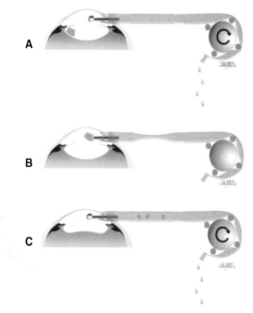

Fig. 3.15. Compliance in a peristaltic system. (A) Rollers are rotating, no occlusion, no collapse of tubing. (B) Occlusion occurs, vacuum builds up, rollers stop, negative pressure generated within the whole system, **tubings collapse**. (C) Occlusion breaks, release of negative pressure, tubing re-expands to the original size (this is what causes surge). **Property of the tubing to collapse (deform under pressure) is the compliance of the tubing.**

pressure is generated within the whole system. This causes the tubings to collapse.

Property of the tubing to collapse (deform under pressure) is the compliance of the tubing.

Once the occlusion breaks, there is a release of negative pressure and the tubing re-expands to the original size. Fluid is drawn from the AC to fill up this extra volume (this is what causes surge).

This extent of collapse of the tubings will depend on the level of vacuum generated, lumen size, hardness and thickness of the tube. The collapse is more at higher vacuum levels and less if the lumen is smaller and the walls are thicker (less compliant tubing). Tubings of these characteristics are known as '*High vacuum*' tubings and these have made it possible to go upto 250 mmHg vacuum in some second generation machines. The tubing which passes over the pulley cannot be made non-compliant so second generation machines will have surge beyond this vacuum setting. In third generation machines, tubings over the pulley have been replaced by a cassette; therefore, it is possible to use a vacuum setting of 300–450 mmHg without surge.

SURGE

Sudden withdrawal of fluid from AC after occlusion breaks is called surge. Beyond a certain limit it may cause collapse of chamber, jeopardizing the vital structures of eyes and making the surgery filled with complications. In fact modifications introduced over a period of time have taken place to manage this surge and thus make phaco surgery free from complications. If there was no surge, any one could have mastered phacoemulsification.

Critical limit (Figs. 3.16 & 3.17)

To maintain a constant volume and IOP of the AC, inflow, i.e. infusion, has to be equal to outflow, which is the sum of aspiration by pump and the wound leakage. For a given bottle height inflow is constant and so is the leakage. The only variable parameters left in the above equation are the aspiration flow rate and the vacuum, i.e. the outflow by aspiration.

For a fixed bottle height and leakage, the upper limit of AFR for which the chamber remains stable can be called the *critical limit*. At a FR higher than this, the chamber will be unstable. Lower the FR, more is the safety margin. This *critical limit* is the value of FR set in an occlusion-free system. In a system with fixed bottle height and leakage, let us presume this critical limit of AFR to be 35 cc/min.

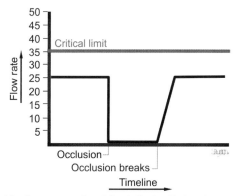

Fig. 3.16. Surge and critical limit. If the bottle height, wound leak and infusion are constant, there is a critical limit of aspiration flow rate beyond which there will be surge and collapse of the chamber. Let us assume the critical limit of flow rate to be 35 cc/min. At flow rate 25 cc/min. if there is no surge there will be no collapse of chamber.

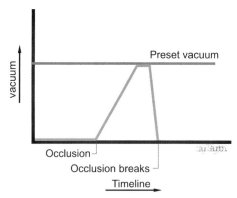

Fig. 3.17. Surge and vacuum. After occlusion, vacuum reaches preset value, the time taken depends on the flow rate.

Role of vacuum and compliance in post-occlusion surge (Fig. 3.18)

Let us take the position of walls of a set of tubings in an occlusion-free system to be 'O', i.e. with no collapse. On occlusion the new positions due to collapse will be X and Y at the vacuum of 100 and 200 respectively. Now when the occlusion is broken, the vacuum goes back to zero. At zero vacuum the walls of the tube also resume their original position 'O'. This increased volume of the tube due to its expansion will be filled with fluid from the AC. More the vacuum, more is the collapse leading to a greater withdrawal of fluid from the chamber.

Though this volume is not much, it is this instantaneous withdrawal of fluid over an extremely short period of time which causes the surge. To give an example—Suppose the preset AFR is 25 cc/min, a preset vacuum of 100 mmHg leads to 0.2 ml of fluid being withdrawn in 1 sec. Then in 60 sec, the fluid withdrawn

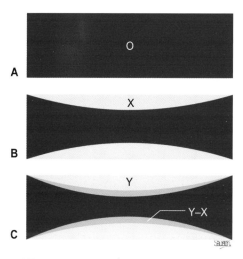

Fig. 3.18. (A) No occlusion, no collapse. (B) Vacuum of 100 mmHg; occlusion and collapse of tubing upto 'X'. (C) Vacuum of 200 mmHg; occlusion and collapse of tubing upto 'Y'.

will be 12 ml, i.e. the FR increase will be 12 ml/min. for that instant over and above the existing AFR.

Similarly, if the preset maximum vacuum is double, i.e. 200 mmHg then the fluid withdrawn will be more but not double of 0.2 ml, say 0.3 ml of fluid will be withdrawn in 1 sec. The momentary increase in FR for that second will be 18 cc/min. over and above the FR in an occlusion-free system. Thus, for a preset AFR at 25 cc/min, which is much lower than the critical limit, in the 1st situation the FR will be 37 cc/min. and in the 2nd it will be 43 cc/min. In the instant following the break of occlusion, the critical limit will be exceeded in both the cases. Though doubling the vacuum will not double the momentary rise in FR, it will still take it much above the critical limit.

Relationship between vacuum, surge and flow rate (Fig. 3.19)

Suppose at 25 cc/min FR and 200 mmHg vacuum setting one is getting the surge beyond acceptable limit. Now he has two options—either reduce the flow rate or the vacuum.

On lowering the FR, all the peaks will go down. If FR is decreased to 1/2, i.e. 12.5 cc/min. then even at 200 vacuum, momentary increase in FR will be only 12.5 + 18 = 30.5 cc/min. This value is well within the safe limit. However, if FR was kept at 25 cc/min. and vacuum decreased to 1/2, i.e. 100 mmHg, then the momentary increase of FR will cross the critical limit, i.e. 25 + 12 = 37 cc/min. From the above it is clear that the surge can

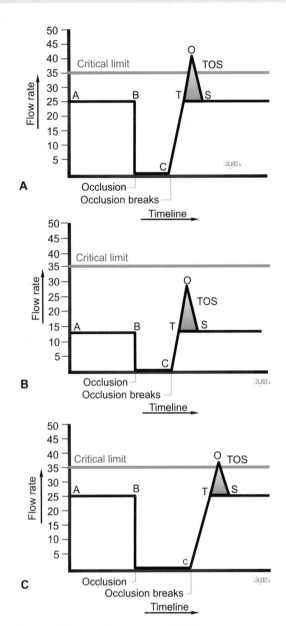

Fig. 3.19. (A) Triangle of surge (TOS). Let us assume a flow rate of 25 cc/mm and vacuum setting of 200 mmHg. Graph AB represents no occlusion, fluid withdrawn is in safe limit. At point B occlusion takes places, no fluid withdrawn, but vacuum builds up to 200 mmHg (maximum preset). At point C occlusion breaks, pump starts and withdraws fluid at the rate of 25 cc/min. At the same moment, the fluid is withdrawn as per the compliance of the system and the vacuum setting resulting in a momentary increase in flow rate exceeding the critical limit represented by triangle of surge (TOS). **(B) Surge and flow rate.** Flow rate is halved (12.5 cc/min), vacuum is kept the same (200 mmHg). In this situation, in spite of surge, the peak flow rate will fall within the critical limit. **(C) Surge and vacuum.** Flow rate remains the same (25 cc/min.), vacuum is halved 100 mmHg. Decreasing the vacuum by half reduces the TOS but it is still above the critical limit.

be reduced either by decreasing the flow rate or decreasing the vacuum. Decreasing the AFR has a direct and linear effect but increases the rise time and makes the procedure slower, which may not be such a disadvantage to a beginner. On the other hand decreasing the vacuum will decrease the holding power which is not desirable in steps like chopping/phacoaspiration of a hard cataract. So, it is better to lower the FR in such a situation to decrease the surge, while maintaining high vacuum. On the other hand, in situations where a firm hold is not so important like *divide and conquer* technique, soft cataracts or epinuclear plate removal, one can lower the vacuum settings to decrease the surge while maintaining the AFR.

In a venturi system, surge is encountered less often. For details, refer to Chapter 4.

CONTROL OF SURGE

There are various methods of controlling the surge. Some are incorporated into the newer machines and there are some measures that the surgeon can apply.

Surge prevention by the machine

In a peristaltic machine, apart from the high vacuum tubings and use of cassettes (to decrease the compliance of the tubings) there are a few more methods of decreasing surge.

1. Venting (Figs. 3.20 & 3.21)

In this, the machine has a sensor which detects occlusion break and releases fluid/air into the system to fill the volume of the re-expanding tubing. This prevents fluid being drawn out of the AC.

Fluid venting is superior to air venting since air is compressible. If it remains in the system, it increases the compliance of the tubing and thus increases the surge.

2. Delay in start of the motor following occlusion break

Here, following occlusion break, there is delay in starting pump by a second or so. Since the pump is not rotating, the AFR is effectively zero. Start of the motor is delayed till the expansion of the tubings is complete. This ensures that the fluid withdrawn by the re-expanding tubes is not added to the flow rate and thus remains within the safe limit.

3. Differential FR/vacuum settings before and after occlusion

Some machines have an option of setting different FR and vacuum settings which the machine can switch to after

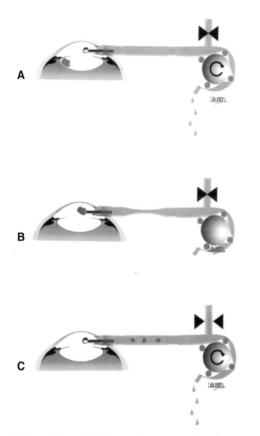

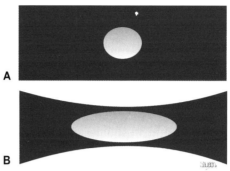

Fig. 3.21. Air in the system increases the compliance as air is elastic. (A) The air bubble is small when there is no occlusion. (B) As the occlusion takes place the negative pressure in the system will increase the size of the air bubble. On occlusion break, air bubble will come back to its original size. This decrease in volume of air bubble will have to be compensated from AC.

Fig. 3.20. Venting. (A) No occlusion, valve closed, tubing normal, pump rotating. (B) Occlusion, valve closed, vacuum build up, tubings collapsed. (C) Occlusion broken, valve opens momentarily, provides fluid/air to overcome collapse of tubing, thus preventing the withdrawal of fluid from AC and surge.

occlusion break. The vacuum and AFR are decreased for a short period of time as soon as the occlusion breaks, to decrease the surge. Once the piece has been aspirated, the settings then revert to whatever had been previously set.

Surgeon's control of surge

1. ***Decreasing the effective flow rate:*** Without changing the actual setting on the machine, the surgeon can decrease the effective FR by using a smaller bore aspiration port, e.g. microflow tip. Due to the greater resistance offered by a smaller port, the effective flow rate will be less and for the same settings, the surge will be less.

2. ***Increasing the infusion*** by raising the bottle height or using a TUR set may be useful in some cases.

3. The use of an ***ACM***, which has already been described, is useful for decreasing surge (especially for beginners).

4. ***Proper wound construction:*** A leaking wound will disturb the equilibrium of the chamber so that even a very small amount of fluid withdrawn can cause it to collapse. This highlights the importance of making a good main wound and side port. The wound construction should be such that it conforms to the tip that you are using, i.e. 2.75 mm is usually good enough for regular tip. For microtip incision size has to be 2.2 mm or 1.8 mm depending upon the machine and tip being used. Premature entry also results in a leaking wound. Distortion of the wound, i.e. with the IA handpiece, may cause a leak too. Too tight a wound or too long a tunnel can also cause a problem by reducing the inflow. Thus either a leaky or too tight a wound can increase the surge. Attention must be paid to the side port incision. Side port is usually made large enough to accommodate the irrigation or aspiration port while doing bimanual I/A, while side port required for chopper is much smaller. It is not a bad option to make a very small side port for chopping and phacoaspiration and increase its size while doing bimanual I/A.

5. ***Increased viscosity of the AC contents:*** The flow rate settings are for clear fluids like BSS/Ringers. A thicker fluid increases the resistance and does not flow out easily. The use of viscoelastic fluids can cause a decrease in the effective FR and thus decrease the surge. The commonly used VES, methyl cellulose does not alter the vacuum or the rise time but decreases the post-occlusion surge. This is particularly useful in hard cataracts where the settings are usually high and while aspirating the

last nuclear fragment. It is wise to inflate the bag with methyl cellulose to avoid post-occlusion surge as the last piece goes in.

6. ***Partial occlusion of the tip:*** Partially occluding the tip with another piece before the occlusion breaks and the occluding fragment gets aspirated ensures that any surge that occurs will be used to draw in the next piece to occlude the tip. This will maintain occlusion and prevent fluid from the AC being aspirated.

7. ***Autoclaving:*** Repeated autoclaving increases the compliance of the silicon tubing. Using disposable tubings or changing the silicon tubing after 50–100 autoclavings is a better idea.

8. ***Foot control:*** Above all, good foot pedal control is of paramount importance in controlling surge and utilizing it to your own advantage. If one can anticipate the events then surge control is not a problem. That is why experienced surgeons can operate on any settings and any machine. In a peristaltic system, the surge will depend on the FR and the collapse of tubing at the time of occlusion break. As soon as the occlusion is about to break (i.e. the piece is about to be aspirated into the tip), the surgeon lifts the FP to IA_0 (or completely in CIM), the piece will go in on its own momentum and without any of surge as the FR will decrease. Thus, fluid withdrawn from the AC will be very little to overcome the compliance of the system. However, if the FP is withdrawn too early and there is not enough momentum then it will take more time to build up vacuum again. This balancing between the AFR, vacuum and momentum of the pieces needs to be done very carefully. It is ideal to bring the FP to a position where the surge is decreased without breaking the momentum.

However, it must be kept in mind that since there are so many variables affecting surge, it may not always be present to the same extent in every case. It may vary from day-to-day depending on the type of cataract and settings being used but good FP control will ensure safe surgery in all circumstances.

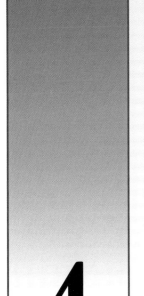

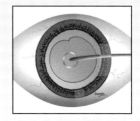

4

Choosing the Phacomachine, Instruments and Viscoelastic Substances

PHACOMACHINE (Fig. 4.1)

The machine consists of the ***console, foot pedal, handpiece*** and their connections. Though there are many variations in the models, the basic functions are similar. The functions of the various parts are discussed in the chapter on phacodynamics.

INSTRUMENTS (Figs. 4.2 to 4.16)

The other relevant instruments are depicted below. The detailed description and uses are in the relevant chapters

VISCOELASTIC SUBSTANCES (VES)

The introduction of VES for ophthalmic intra-ocular procedures has had a significant impact in ophthalmology. Viscoelastic substances possess a unique set of properties based on their chemical structure which enables them to protect the corneal endothelium and epithelium from mechanical trauma and maintain intraocular space even in the face of an open incision. VES can be broadly classified into three groups:

1. Sodium hyaluronate group which have high molecular weight, e.g. Healon, Hyal 2000, Hyvisc Plus.
2. Chondroitin sulphate group with medium molecular weight, Viscoat being its prototype.
3. Hydroxypropyl methyl cellulose (HPMC) with low molecular weight, e.g. Visilon Viscomet.

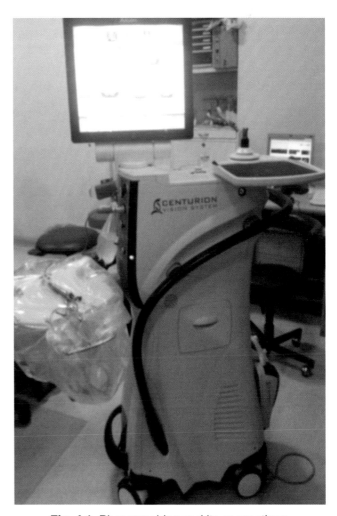

Fig. 4.1. Phacomachine and its connections.

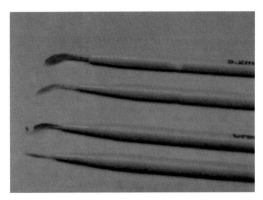

Fig. 4.2. Knives used for making incisions. Note that the knives should always be kept covered to protect the blade.

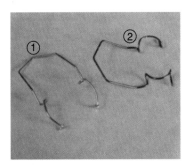

Fig. 4.3. Wire speculum. 1. Nasal, 2. Temporal.

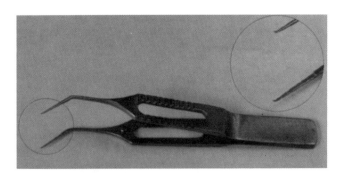

Fig. 4.4. Utrata capsulorrhexis forceps.

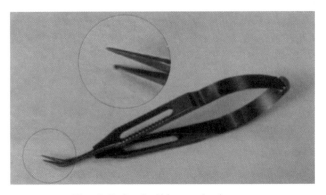

Fig. 4.5. Angled Vannas' scissors.

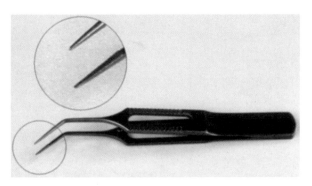

Fig. 4.6. McPherson forceps.

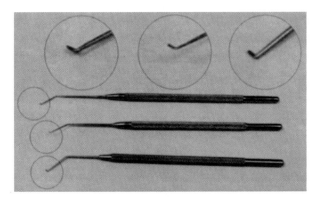

Fig. 4.7. Various types of choppers.

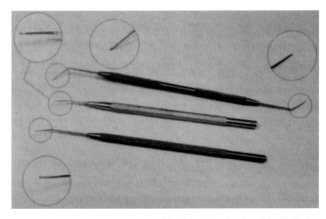

Fig. 4.8. Rounded repositor, Sinskey hook, dumbbell dialer.

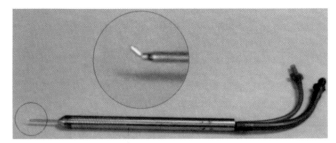

Fig. 4.9. 45° coaxial irrigation-aspiration handpiece with metallic sleeve.

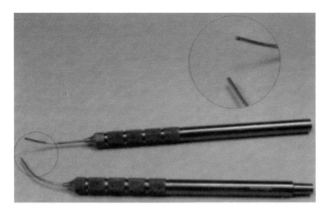

Fig. 4.10. Bimanual irrigation-aspiration infusion and aspiration cannulae with handles.

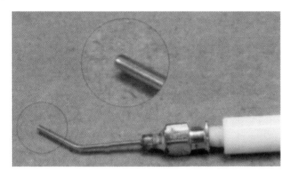

Fig. 4.11. Thick cannula for modified bimanual irrigation-aspiration.

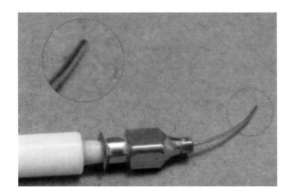

Fig. 4.12. Aspiration cannula without handle for bimanual irrigation-aspiration.

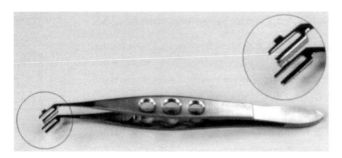

Fig. 4.13. IOL folder.

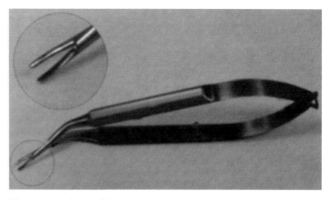

Fig. 4.14. Box IOL folder. Bottom arm folds the IOL. Top arm prevents the IOL from slipping out. Holder is placed between the two arms for an exact fold.

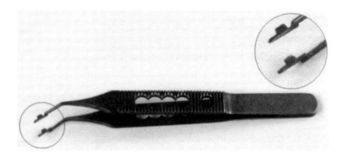

Fig. 4.15. Holder with lock.

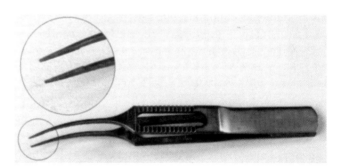

Fig. 4.16. One-toothed forceps.

The following properties are most relevant for use in ophthalmic surgery.

1. Viscoelasticity

Elasticity refers to the ability of a solution to return to its original shape after being stressed. Elasticity allows the anterior chamber to reform after deformation by depression on the cornea when external forces are released. A non-elastic substance like balanced salt solution (BSS) will show no reformation after the release of forces so that anterior chamber volume is lost. Elasticity affords ocular protection against high frequency mechanical insults such as vibrations associated with phacoemulsification or other turbulence induced by rapidly delivered irrigating stream. The amount of elasticity of an elastic compound increases with increasing molecular weight and greater molecular chain length. Sodium hyaluronate is more elastic than chondroitin sulfate or HPMC.

2. Viscosity

Viscosity reflects a solution's resistance to flow. The higher the solution's molecular weight the more it resists flow and so lower the shear rate. Viscosity is best understood by placing a quantity of the viscoelastic substance between two parallel plates and measuring the force required to slide one plate across the other. With a solution of low viscosity the plates slide easily, with high viscosity more energy is required to overcome the internal cohesion of the molecules and to move the plate. Therefore, a high viscosity solution like Healon is difficult to displace from the anterior chamber and helps to maintain space against vitreous pressure.

3. Psuedoplasticity

It refers to a solution's ability to transform under pressure from gel-like substance to a more liquid substance. Therefore, under stress (i.e. at high shear rate) the psuedoplastic solutions can be pushed easily through a small diameter cannula. BSS and air do not transform and are not psuedoplastic. HPMC and chondroitin sulphate are less psuedoplastic, so, it is more difficult to initiate and maintain an injection of HPMC and chondroitin sulphate. Healon can be passed easily through a 30 G needle as it is much more psuedoplastic. It has longer chains of molecules which align parallel to the walls of the cannula and thus can be pushed easily. On the other hand HPMC needs a larger bore usually 23–25 G for injection.

4. Cohesiveness

Cohesiveness, the degree to which a material adheres to itself, is a function of molecular weight and elasticity. Long strand viscoelastic substance molecules with high molecular weight like sodium hyaluronate become entangled and cling together and are more likely to remain as a large mass whereas VES of low molecular weight and shorter chain length substances like HPMC are less entangled and upon aspiration leave the eye in pieces. A disadvantage of more cohesive substances is that it is more likely to plug the trabecular meshwork as a mass and cause raised IOP post-operatively.

5. Surface tension

The coating ability of a viscoelastic material is determined by the surface tension of the VES and by the surface tension of the contact tissue, surgical instrument or IOL. By measuring the angle formed by a drop of VES on a flat surface (the contact angle), the coating ability of a substance can be estimated. Lower contact angle indicates a better ability to coat. HPMC makes lower contact angle compared to sodium hyaluronate. Therefore, these substances are called viscoadhesives. This tendency to coat the cornea and the IOL is protective. The disadvantage is that if HPMC remains in the bag behind the IOL then it is very difficult to remove it.

Properties of an ideal viscoelastic substance

- It should be clear.
- Non-toxic, non-inflammatory and non-antigenic.
- Be easy to inject.
- Be able to retain itself under positive pressure.
- Protect the endothelium.
- Not interfere with instruments or IOL.
- Easily removable.
- Should not obstruct aqueous outflow.
- Inexpensive.

Use in the steps of phacoemulsification

Most of the properties of a VES required during phacoemulsification are present in the sodium hyaluronate derivatives. The steps where this is of special use are:

- While injecting through a small cannula e.g. through the side port.
- For stretching the small pupil.
- In cases where the intralenticular pressure is high e.g. pediatric, hypermature cataracts, especially while doing CCC.
- During CCC, these substances maintain the AC better; repeated injections are not required.
- Decreasing the vitreous upthrust.

   The only situation where chondroitin sulphate and HPMC score over sodium hyaluronate is when they coat the cornea and protect it especially in cases with compromised endothelium. The most important step in which the use of sodium hyaluronate is very useful is CCC and posterior capsulorrhexis, especially CCC under topical anaesthesia. Most of the other steps can easily be done with any of the VES. One must viscopressurise the chamber whenever any manoeuvre or manipulation with instruments is being attempted in the eye. Some of the steps in which VES must be used are:

- Before making the incision.
- During CCC.
- Pupillary stretching.
- Nuclear rotation.
- Completing the splitting.
- IOL implantation.
- In case of a PCT – chondroitin sulphate coats the vitreous too.

CHOOSING THE PHACOMACHINE
(Figs. 4.17 & 4.18)

Which phacomachine to buy is a question often asked by the beginner phaco surgeon. For an experienced surgeon the machine does not matter so much and I am now comfortable with most machines. There has always been a debate about the peristaltic system versus the venturi system especially for the beginners. However, both systems are equally effective and safe if you understand your machine.

As we know, followability depends upon the pressure gradient at the tip. In a peristaltic system this gradient is provided by bottle height while in a venturi system, as the negative pressure is transmitted directly to the tip, e.g. at the bottle height 3 ft. and vacuum 120, the pressure gradient between the infusion port and tip will be 66 mmHg in peristaltic while 186 mmHg (66 + 120) in venturi system. Though increasing the flow rate can increase the pressure gradient in the peristaltic system, it can never match the venturi system. This attraction power of the venturi helps in each and every step of the surgery. For example, while creating vacuum seal, one has to advance the tip in a peristaltic system and one may reach the peripheral unsafe zone. In venturi system, the piece gets attracted to the tip leading to easy occludability. Similar things happen in ENP removal and it is easier to flip the ENP with the venturi system. In cortical aspiration, if the fibres are very thin do not occlude the port completely; the venturi system can still attract them and pull them. In other words, in venturi system even if the tip is kept in the CSZ, the nuclear pieces tend to follow into it due to high followability. The only disadvantage of venturi system is that the flow rate cannot be separated from the vacuum settings.

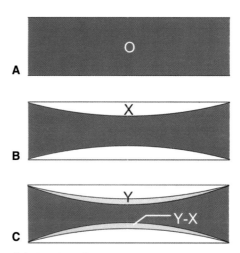

Fig. 4.17. (A) Machine off; no occlusion; no collapse of tubing. (B) Machine on; no occlusion; collapse of tubing upto 'X' as negative pressure in venturi is transmitted into the system without occlusion. (C) Machine on; occlusion takes place; increased collapse of tubing to 'Y'. On occlusion break the tube will come back to 'X' as the machine is on. Fluid withdrawn will be 'X-Y' only.

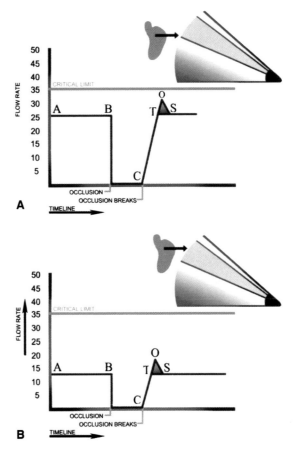

Fig. 4.18. (A) Note the smaller TOS in a venturi system. (B) In a venturi system FR is a fixed fraction of the vacuum, so keeping the foot pedal between positions 1 and 2 decreases the FR and the surge.

Surge in a venturi system is very low. In a venturi system, surge is encountered less often. To understand this, let us go back to the phacodynamics of vacuum-based pump. When foot pedal is at rest the walls of tubings are in their normal positions—say 'O'. On pressing the foot pedal to say 'IA$_x$' most of the vacuum will build up at the probe tip even without occlusion. This will cause collapse of the tubings by a certain volume, say 'X'. When occlusion takes place, the vacuum will rise to maximum preset at 'IA$_{max}$'. As the vacuum increases so will the collapse of tubings. Let us assume the new volume of collapse to be 'Y'. Now when occlusion breaks, the vacuum will decrease and the collapsed walls of tube will go back to 'X' volume and not to their original volume 'O'. The total fluid with-drawn will be Y-X and not Y-O. Since the withdrawn volume of fluid is much less, the height of the triangle of surge (TOS) is less, and so is the surge.

Newer modifications

Ophthalmologists now find themselves weighing the benefits of newer technologies—including torsional and transversal phacomachines—over traditional longitudinal devices.

In longitudinal phaco, the needle tip uses a to & fro motion (Fig. 4.19) to break up the lens material. When the tip moves forwards, the material is not only broken but also pushed away from the tip. Hence, higher fluidic parameters are needed to hold the fragments leading to more surge. When the tip retreats it causes no emulsification. Heat is generated in both forward and backward motion of the tip, thereby increasing the risk of wound burn.

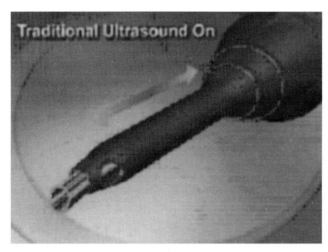

Fig. 4.19. To & fro motion of a traditional handpiece.

The **Ozil** handpiece, developed by Alcon industries, acts on a torsional principle. This handpiece uses a Kelman tip, with downward angulation. The sideways movement created at the base is minimal but gets magnified at the tip (Fig. 4.20) due to the angulation. This increases the cutting efficiency with no repulsion at the tip, and minimal movement at the base leading to very little heat being generated.

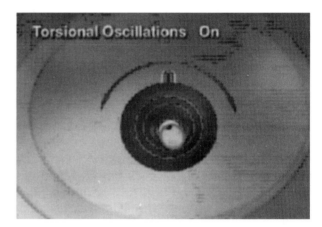

Fig. 4.20. Torsional oscillation of Ozil handpiece.

A newer modification of this tip is the Balanced tip (Fig. 4.21). In this, to counter the downward angulation a forward angulation is created at the base. This has led to a further increase in the amplitude at the tip and the cutting efficiency. The main disadvantage of downward angulation of Kelman tip of causing more PCT has been taken care of.

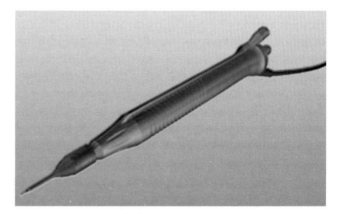

Fig. 4.21. Balance tip and sleeve.

AMO has come out with its own modification of power delivery (Ellips). This is called as transversal cutting. In this the phaco tip moves forwards as well as sideways, i.e. making an elliptical area of cutting (Fig. 4.22), which is much larger than the tip size, thereby

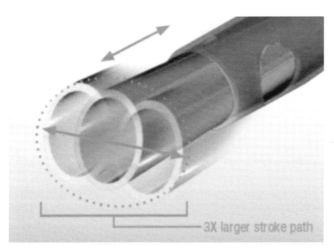

Fig. 4.22. AMO phaco tip with Ellips technology.

increasing its efficiency. This form of motion can use straight tip also. The chances of tip occlusion are less in cases of hard cataract as compared to plane transverse movement.

The other factors that need to be considered while choosing the machine are:

1. **Cost:** There is a wide variation in the cost of these machines starting from around Rs. 3 lakhs for the indigenous machines and going upto more than Rs. 70 lakhs for the higher end machines like the Centurion/Sovereign. The budget would probably depend upon the type and volume of your practice i.e. solitary/group/institutional. One must also keep in mind the associated recovery cost of disposables for phaco e.g. disposable cassettes and also cost of a good operating microscope which is absolutely necessary. The cost of accessories such as various handpieces, vitrectomy attachments, etc. must also be noted. Also, with advancing technology, the option of upgradeable hardware and software is preferable.

2. **Service & Demonstrations:** It is important to choose a machine which is supplied by a company having a good service network and a proven track record. You should discuss all these aspects with those surgeons who have been using the machine to determine user satisfaction both with the machine and the company. One should insist on demonstrations of the machine at least a couple of times. In fact, if the company is not willing or appears reluctant for demonstration, it is perhaps better to look to some other company. All machines will come with some warranty but you should look for a company that also assures future maintenance including standby machines. Some companies also send trained operators to guide the surgeon through the first few surgeries, which is very helpful. One should also watch the surgeries done with various machines at other establishments to determine exactly what parameters the machine can achieve. No matter what the company tells you, the feedback from the surgeon, comfortable with using his machine, is invaluable.

The most important aspect of choosing a machine is, however, still the cost, the service and the personal comfort of the surgeon.

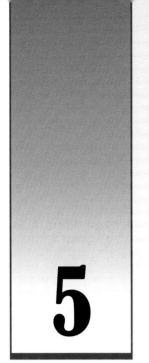

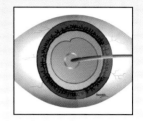

5 Biometry and IOL Power Calculation

Sir Harold Ridley created history in November 1949, when he implanted the first intraocular implant. His first patient however had a post-operative refraction of –18.00/ –6.00 × 120°. Since then intraocular lens power calculation has evolved into a rational discipline to achieve the desired post-operative refraction. In the early days of IOL implantation, the standard practice for IOL power calculation was based on the pre-operative refractive error in diopters before the development of cataract clinical history. Obviously this formula led to large post-operativee errors, one of the reasons being the difficulty in determining the patient's stable refractive error prior to the development of cataract.

Estimation of IOL power

IOL power is obtained by **IOL calculation formulas**, which require the estimation of **axial length** of the eyeball and **refracting power** of the cornea.

IOL calculation formulas

First Generation Formulas

In 1967, Fyodorov developed the first theoretical formula based on principles of geometric optics as applied to schematic eyes utilizing keratometry and A-scan ultrasonography. This was followed by Colenbrander, Thijssen, Van der Heijde and Binkhorst. All these first generation formulas can be algebraically transformed to:

$$P = \frac{n}{L - c} - \frac{nK}{n - cK}$$

where P = emmetropic IOL power, n = aqueous and vitreous refractive index, c = estimated post-operative lens position, L = axial length and K = corneal power. This basic two-lens formula is the basis for all modern IOL power calculation formulas where the lenses under consideration are the cornea and the crystalline lens.

Whereas theoretical formulas were based on principles of thin-lens optics, regression formulas were based on retrospective statistical analysis of post-operative refractions of a large number of patients having undergone intraocular lens implantation. The most popular regression formula was the SRK formula published in 1980 based on results analyzed by Sanders, Retzlaff and Kraff:

$$P = A - 2.5L - 0.9K$$

where P is emmetropic IOL power, L is axial length and K is corneal power and A is A-constant which varies with the IOL style and manufacturer.

The first generation formulas (both theoretical and regression) worked well for eyes with average axial lengths between 22 and 24.5 mm, but were not satisfactory for shorter or longer eyes. The reason for this error was that although axial length and corneal power could be accurately measured pre-operatively, there was no means of predicting where the IOL would finally come to rest in the eye post-operatively. The first generation formulas used a constant value for the estimated lens position (ELP) irrespective of the individual dimensions of a particular eye.

Second Generation Formulas

The second generation formulas attempted to predict post-operative ELP based upon the axial length measurement. Various modified formulas were developed and included Hoffer's formula, Shammas' formula and Binkhorst's Adjusted formula. The rationale was that the ELP was likely to be a smaller value in shorter eyes and a larger value in longer eyes. In other words, the IOL was likely to rest closer to the cornea in shorter eyes, and further away from the cornea and closer to the retina in longer eyes.

Similarly the regression formulas underwent modification to improve their accuracy. The SRK II formula includes a correction factor C.

$$P = A - 2.5L - 0.9K + C$$

where $C = 3$ if $L < 20$

      $C = 2$ if $L \geq 20$ and < 21

      $C = 1$ if $L \geq 21$ and < 22

      $C = 0$ if $L \geq 22$ and < 24.5

      $C = -0.5$ if $L > 24.5$

Third Generation Formulas

With the advent of the third generation IOL power calculation formulas, prediction of post-operative ELP underwent further refinement. In the modern formulas ELP varies not only with axial length, but with corneal curvature as well. Hence, for two eyes having the same axial length but different average K values, the IOL would rest closer to the retina in the eye having the steeper cornea and closer to the cornea in the eye having the flatter cornea. The third generation theoretical formulas include the SRK/T formula, the Holladay formula and the Hoffer Q formula and give excellent results post-operatively.

The Lens Constants and Personalization

All IOL power calculations have constants, of which one is most familiar with the A-constant which is used in the SRK regression formulas and the SRK/T formula. The Holladay formula uses the Surgeon Factor or S factor which is distance from the anterior plane of the iris to the optical plane of the IOL. The Hoffer Q formula uses what is known as the personalized ACD-constant which is the average distance between the principle power plane of the cornea and that of the IOL. These constants are specific values depending upon the position of the principal plane of the lens to be implanted. Simple conversion equations are available to convert from one constant to another. For example, an A-constant of 118.5 corresponds to a Surgeon factor of 1.51 and an ACD-constant of 5.26.

These constants (A, S or ACD) need to be personalized based on the post-operative refractive results to take care of any consistent shift that might affect the IOL power calculations, namely the surgical technique, the measuring devices used, and the implant's style and manufacturer. When a new IOL is implanted, the surgeon should use the constant designated by the manufacturer. After having implanted 20 or more such implants, the A-constant is personalized by back-calculating the constant for each case using the formula of choice and taking the mean of these values. For this purpose one must ensure that all the cases being reviewed have the same parameters namely: the same surgeon, same technique, same A-scan biometry unit and technician taking the measurement, same keratometer and technician taking the measurement and the same IOL style from the same manufacturer. It is preferable to implant the new IOL in average eyes.

Fourth Generation Formulas

The development of fourth generation formulas has further refined prediction of the ELP so as to provide satisfactory results over the entire range of axial lengths and corneal powers. Hitherto ELP prediction was based on axial length and corneal radius of curvature. The newer formulas attempt more accurate ELP predictions based not only on axial length and K readings but on other pre-operatively determined parameters as well. The Holladay 2 formula takes into account the corneal white-to-white diameter, the pre-operative AC depth, the phakic lens thickness, and the patient's age and sex besides the axial length measurement and the K readings to accurately predict the post-operative AC depth (ELP).

Another fourth generation formula, the Haigis formula, takes a different approach. This is a hybrid formula utilizing both regression analysis and a theoretical component. Haigis realized that pre-operative AC depth and phakic lens thickness were the most important determinants of ELP prediction and double regression analysis of a large number of operated eyes for a given lens style gave the following relationship:

$$ELP = a_0 + a_1 AC + a_2 AL$$

where, AC is pre-operative AC depth (phakic AC depth), AL is axial length and a_0, a_1 and a_2 are three constants typical for a given IOL. Hence instead of a single constant, as in other formulas, each IOL style has a set of three numbers characterizing it. Initially, a_0, a_1 and a_2 are fixed values. Later after implanting a significant number of IOLs of a given style, these constants are modified based on post-operative analysis by a process known as optimization. The Haigis formula with no optimization performs as well as third generation theoretical formulas. With optimization of one constant (a_0) its performance is often better for short and long eyes. With triple optimization (a_0, a_1 and a_2) the formula works well for all axial lengths and all lens styles.

A *calibration* check should be performed regularly. It is accomplished by a model eye which is provided with the biometer. The instructions for calibration check are specific and provided with each instrument.

The Measurement of Axial Length

Axial length calculation must be very accurate as even a 1 mm error can lead to a miscalculation in the IOL power by 2.5 D. This error is more in very short eyes (3.75 D per 1 mm error in axial length measurement) and less in very long eyes (1.75 D per mm error in axial length).

Echography Principles

A-scan echography involves generation of sound waves in the ultrasonic range (well above 20 kHz) by a piezo-electric transducer probe. The probe emits multiple pulses of ultrasound wavefronts which are transmitted through different ocular media each of which has a specific velocity of sound. At the interface of two media, part of the sound is reflected back to the transducer and the rest is further transmitted to deeper tissues till another interface is encountered. The brief pauses in between pulses allow the transducer to receive returning echoes, which are then converted to electrical signals and recorded as an echograph, with each individual "echospike" plotted on a timeline. The times at which echo impulses are received can be used to compute distances between corresponding interfaces, knowing the velocity of sound in each medium by the following formula:

$$d = \frac{tv}{2}$$

where d is distance, t is the echospike time, and v is the time velocity. The denser the medium, the faster is the sound velocity. The generally accepted sound velocities in various media are:

Cornea and crystalline lens	1641 m/sec
Aqueous and vitreous	1532 m/sec
Dense cataract	1629 m/sec
Soft tissue (retina)	1550 m/sec
Silicone iil (1000 cSt)	980 m/sec
Silicone oil (5000 cSt)	1040 m/sec
PMMA IOL	2660 m/sec
Acrylic IOL	2200 m/sec
Silicone IOL	980 m/sec
Glass IOL	6040 m/sec

The *frequency* of the ultrasonic waves is determined by the rate at which piezoelectric element resonates. Higher the frequency the better the resolution, and lower the frequency the better the penetration i.e. the lesser is the absorption. All A-scan biometer transducers produce ultrasonic waves in the frequency range of 8 to12 MHz which penetrate the ocular media easily all the way to the back of the globe without getting absorbed significantly.

Due to the effect of absorption and scattering, the echoes received by the transducer from the posterior ocular structures are obviously weaker in intensity compared with those from the anterior structures. This is known as *attenuation*. If the echo is severely attenuated it would be barely distinguishable from background noise which is intrinsic to all sensitive electronic devices. On the other hand the initial signal from the transducer would be sufficiently strong to saturate the electronics and produce a high spike with a clipped or flat top. The difference between these two echo levels is known as the *usable dynamic range* of the biometer and is specified in decibels (dB). For performing meaningful biometry, the A-scan device should have usable dynamic range of at least 40 to 50 dB. Most modern biometers have a range of 60 to 80 dB.

The echograph in the A-scan display can be depicted with a *linear scale* or a *logarithmic scale*. Linear scaling produces well-defined echospikes but a large usable dynamic range cannot be achieved. The advantage of logarithmic scaling is that a larger usable dynamic range can be used and it allows better definition of weak echoes of posterior vitreous detachment, floaters and hemorrhage. A newer scale is the S-curve scale, which expands the mid-range portion of the display and compresses the upper and lower portions, thereby providing clear echospike tracings and increased dynamic range.

Another term used in echography is *sensitivity*, which is also measured in decibels. The device should be sensitive enough to detect weak echoes. Sensitivity can be improved by increasing the adjustable *gain* setting which electronically amplifies the echo signals. However, too much gain amplification would cause clipping of the echospikes and amplification of background noise.

Biometry Technique

The following points should be kept in mind while performing the scan for determining the axial length.

There are two techniques for performing ultrasonic biometry. In the *contact method* the probe is in direct contact with the cornea. In the *immersion method*, the patient is placed in a supine position and a scleral shell is fitted in the palpebral aperture filled with irrigating fluid or gonioscopic solution which acts as a coupling fluid between the cornea and the probe. The biometry probe is thus immersed in the solution 5 to 10 mm away from the cornea and causes no corneal compression.

The probe should be placed on the anaesthesized cornea in such a way that it points towards the macula. This is particularly important in myopes, who may have a staphyloma. There should be no fluid bridge between the probe and the cornea and the cornea should not be depressed. Corneal compression results in inadvertent shortening of axial length as a result of pressure from the probe in contact technique. It is maximum with solid and minimal with water-filled probes

The **mode** may be set to the operator's preference:

Manual mode

The advantage of a manual mode is that the examiner may dynamically scan the eye, looking for the best echo pattern that the eye is capable of producing . There may be delay in pressing the foot pedal and one may miss the right reading.

Automatic mode

In this, control of echo pattern interpretation is relinquished to the software algorithms inside the instrument. Though an instrument cannot make a better decision than the human brain, this mode is useful in uncooperative patients. It is the most commonly used mode by majority of the surgeons.

It is best to have an observer watch the echo patterns on the screen while the operator positions the probe in automatic mode.

The observer is looking and selecting in his mind what the right reading should be. If that coincides with the automatic mode, you can be sure of accuracy i.e. delay due to foot is avoided. Watching the screen ensures dynamic biometry as well as the static graph of automatic mode. The axial length of both eyes should be done for comparison.

ECHOGRAPH

The initial echospike in the A-scan display of the contact method (Fig. 5.1) is a combination of the pulse emitted by the probe itself as well as the reflection from the corneal surface, the second spike is from the anterior surface of the crystalline lens, the third spike represents the posterior lens surface, the fourth spike comes from the internal limiting membrane of the retina, and the last tall spike comes from the sclera. This spike is followed by a chain of reflective spikes from the orbit. In the immersion scan (Fig. 5.2), the initial spike comes from the probe itself which is followed by a double-peaked

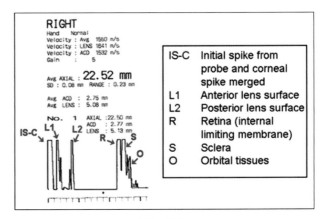

Fig. 5.1.

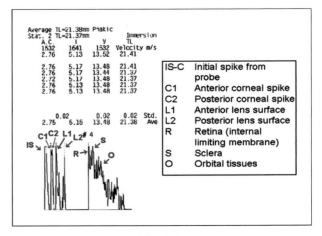

Fig. 5.2.

corneal spike representing the anterior and posterior surfaces of the cornea. Thereafter the spikes are similar to those seen in the echograph of the contact method.

A-scan biometry by immersion will display an axial length somewhat longer than that by the applanation technique, because there is no corneal compression and the displayed axial length is closer to the true axial length. The difference between applanation and immersion can be anywhere between 0.14 mm to 0.28 mm depending on the degree of corneal compression. Using a 10-MHz ultrasound transducer, by the immersion method, the typical accuracy for axial length measurements is within 0.12 mm, which translates to approximately 0.28 D of post-operative refractive error in an eye of average axial length. This error would be more for a shorter eye and less for a longer eye. A-scan biometry by immersion has better reproducibility, which leads to an overall increase in accuracy.

Characteristics of a good A-scan

1. Tall single peak from the cornea.
2. Tall echoes from anterior and posterior capsules.
3. Few to no echoes in the vitreous cavity.
4. Tall sharply rising echoes from retina with no staircase at the origin.
5. Medium to low echoes from the orbital fat.
6. There should be not much variation in the readings.
7. Deepest AC depth.
8. Largest reproducible axial length.

Selection of the scan

The scan with the maximum axial length, within the range obtained, should be selected. ***Repeat measurement should be done if***

1. Axial length is < 22 mm or > 25 mm.
2. Average corneal power is < 40 D or > 47 D.
3. If the difference between the two eyes is
   (a) Average corneal power > 1 D
   (b) Axial length > 0.5 mm
   (c) Emmetropic implant power > 1 D.

Avoiding errors in biometry

The most important source of error in axial length measurement by the contact method is corneal compression. This gives a falsely shorter axial length and leading to post-operative myopia. An error of 1 mm will give rise to approximately 3 diopters deviation from

the expected post-operative refraction. Care should be taken not to indent the cornea while taking the measurement by reviewing the anterior chamber depth recordings and identifying and deleting the shorter readings. Hand-held probes cause more compression than slit-lamp mounted probes. The immersion scan will cause no compression as mentioned previously.

Off-axis measurement occurs when the probe is not held perpendicular to the ocular surfaces. When the probe is held properly and aligned with the macula, the lens spikes rise sharply and are perpendicular to the baseline. A mildly misaligned probe is characterized by absence of the posterior lens spike or a very small one. A larger off-axis measurement in addition will show a jagged retinal pike ("stair-stepping") (Fig. 5.3). Absence of scleral spikes suggests alignment with the optic disc rather than the macula (Fig. 5.4).

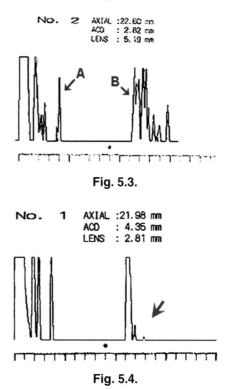

Fig. 5.3.

Fig. 5.4.

A-scan biometer features

A good biometer should have the following features:

1. A fixation light at the probe tip to aid in accurately measuring the length between the corneal apex and the macula.
2. Both contact and immersion scan capability.
3. A screen display which shows axial length, anterior chamber depth, lens thickness, vitreous cavity

length, and standard deviation. These are facilitated by the presence of electronic *gates* which are "electronic calipers" that measure the distance between two structures. It is desirable to have four or more gates representing the anterior corneal surface, the anterior lens surface, the posterior lens surface, and the anterior retinal surface.

4. Choice of measurement in automatic or manual mode. Most scans are performed in the automatic mode, in which the biometer automatically places a gate on what it believes to be the corneal spike, the anterior lens spike, the posterior lens spike, and the retinal spike, and is programmed to measure the distance between each pair of gates at a given velocity. Sometimes, when the quality of the scan is not satisfactory, one may need to measure in the manual mode, in which the operator presses a foot switch to capture the scan when it is seen to be of high quality.

5. Choice of setting different sound velocities. Measuring with individual velocity settings for the various media is more accurate than using an average velocity.

6. Storage of multiple scans, incorporation of various modern IOL power calculation formulas and option for reviewing data and allowing personalization of constants.

7. The printout should give the IOL power for emmetropia, the expected post-operative refractive error with any IOL power, and the IOL power with different formulas.

Partial Coherence Laser Interferometry

Routine ultrasonic biometry is an indispensable tool for axial length measurement, but has limitations of resolution since very high frequency sound waves are absorbed by ocular tissues. Partial Coherence Laser Interferometry also known as Optical Coherence Biometry is a relatively new technique for performing non-contact biometry using optical methods. Since it uses a partially coherent light wave with an extremely small wavelength (9.75×10^{-8} mm) to measure relatively large distances, its resolution is significantly higher than ultrasonic biometry. The commercial device developed by Zeiss Humphrey Systems in 1999, known as IOLMaster, performs extremely accurate axial length measurements. This technology has also been used in its tomographic variant as Optical Coherence Tomography (OCT) and has widespread clinical applications in ophthalmology.

The principle behind optical coherence biometry involves creating a dual beam using wavelets of infrared light of wavelength 780 nm. Two such coaxial beams I_m and I_f with short coherence length ($c \approx 130 \,\mu m$) are generated by the laser diode (LD) of a Michelson interferometer with the help of a beam splitter (BS1), a fixed mirror (M_f) and a movable measuring mirror (M_m) (Fig. 5.5).

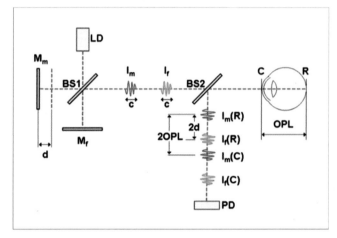

Fig. 5.5.

These two beams travel into the eye and are reflected from the cornea (C) and the retina (R). They then encounter a second beam splitter (BS2) which directs the partially reflected beams onto a photodetector (PD). The distance between the wavelets reflected from the cornea and the retina obviously equals twice the optical path length of the eye. In other words:

$$I_m(R) - I_m(C) \text{ or } I_f(R) - I_f(C) = 2\text{OPL}$$

If the displacement (*d*) of the movable mirror (M_m) is such that $I_f(R)$ and $I_m(C)$ are close enough, i.e. if $2\text{OPL} - 2d \leq c$, then these two wavelets will interfere and their intensity distribution will be sensed by the photodetector. In such a situation the distance *d* can be considered the optical length of the eye. Axial length (AL) is derived from optical path length (OPL) by knowing the average refractive index (*n*) of the eye using the formula: AL = OPL/*n*.

Longitudinal eye movements obviously do not affect the reading because of beam splitting. With this method the measurement is made up to the retinal pigment epithelium (RPE) unlike ultrasonic biometry where it is up to the internal limiting membrane. Since the patient fixates on the laser spot, the measurement is made along the visual axis at the centre of the macula. Moreover, the laser beam is very narrow and strikes the thinnest part of the fovea, which is not flat, but with thicker surrounding shoulders. Ultrasound biometry with its wider sound beam cannot make this distinction. All these features, along with its superior resolution, make optical coherence biometry extremely accurate, reproducible and user-independent. One can zoom in to the signal reflected from the back wall of the eye and distinguish between the internal limiting membrane, the retinal pigment epithelium and the choroid. This technique of optical biometry has been found to have a high resolution (12 μ) and precision (0.3–10 μ) in measuring intraocular distances as compared to conventional ultrasound (resolution of 200 μ and accuracy of 100–120 μ).

Besides being a non-contact device, there are other advantageous features of the IOLMaster such as measurement of anterior chamber depth, corneal radius of curvature, white-to-white diameter, measurement in aphakic mode, pseudophakic mode, and silicone-filled mode. This device includes all the modern day IOL power formulas including the Haigis formula, and can be used in conjunction with the Holladay 2 formula. It can also perform the calculation of IOL power in eyes having undergone myopic LASIK using the Haigis-L formula. However, due to the longer axial length measurement, it is necessary to calculate new lens constants for optical biometry. For this purpose, a User Group for Laser Interferometry Biometry (ULIB) was founded in 1999 with the intention to collect clinical data from all over the world and derive suitable constants for the IOLMaster.

Some of the situations where optical coherence biometry may not be possible are: nystagmus, severe tear film abnormalities, corneal scars, advanced cataracts, dense posterior subcapsular opacities, dense vitreous hemorrhage, membrane formation, maculopathy and retinal detachment.

Measurement of Corneal Power

The important factors to be considered while estimating corneal power are:

1. Instrumentation
2. Astigmatism
3. Corneal transplant
4. Previous refractive corneal surgery

Instrumentation

The corneal power is measured by a manual **keratometer** which measures the front surface of the eye and converts the radius of curvature obtained in diopters (K) using an index of refraction of 1.3375 ($K = 337.5/r$). This machine must be calibrated regularly to obtain accurate results. Contact lenses should be removed 1–2 weeks prior to estimation of K.

While doing keratometry, the patient should be instructed to look into the keratometer and care should be taken that the mires are focussed in the centre of the eye. To take care of the refractive error of the observer, the cross-hairs should be adjusted before starting the keratometry. Majority of patients with immature cataract can see the reflection of their own eye. If so, patient can be instructed into the centre of this reflection. In mature cataracts the patient is instructed to fixate the pin with the other eye. Keratometry may be difficult or impossible in conditions with irregular or distorted corneal surface. In such cases, keratometric readings of opposite eye may be used or topographic mapping may be employed. Both the minus signs and the vertical component of the plus signs should be superimposed completely. If there is any angle between them, rotate the keratometer till they can be completely superimposed.

Keratometry in Eyes with Corneal Transplant

A problem arises if a combined procedure is planned. Attempting to predict the post-operative keratometry is difficult so the corneal power of the other eye may be used or one can use an average of the surgeons' post-operative astigmatism, if available. Performing the IOL implantation after the corneal transplant has stabilized may be a better option.

Biometry and IOL Power Calculation in Special Situations

The Pseudophakic Eye

The pseudophakic A-scan pattern displays the initial spike followed by the double-peaked corneal spike in immersion biometry or a single initial spike which is merged with the corneal spike in the contact method. This is followed by a highly reflective spike from the anterior surface of the IOL following which there are usually multiple smaller echospikes which represent multiple reverberations between the anterior and posterior surfaces (Fig. 5.6). The display then shows the highly reflective retinal spike and the tapering scleral and orbital spikes. The operator must remember to lower the gain setting to differentiate between the main spikes and the artifacts.

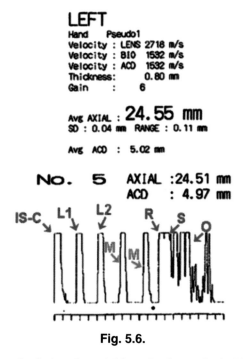

LEFT
Hand   Pseudo1
Velocity : LENS 2718 m/s
Velocity : 810   1532 m/s
Velocity : ACD 1532 m/s
Thickness: 0.80 mm
Gain   :   6

Avg AXIAL : **24.55** mm
SD : 0.04 mm RANGE : 0.11 mm

Avg ACD : 5.02 mm

NO. 5   AXIAL :24.51 mm
         ACD : 4.97 mm

Fig. 5.6.

For calculating the axial length of pseudophakic eyes the following average sound velocities are recommended:

An eye with a PMMA IOL   1555 m/sec
An eye with a silicone IOL   1476 m/sec
An eye with a glass IOL   1549 m/sec
An eye with an acrylic IOL   1554 m/sec

However, this method is prone to error especially in the case of silicone IOLs where the error may exceed 1.0 mm. For better results, Holladay has suggested biometry at a sound velocity of 1532 m/sec and then adding or subtracting a corrected axial length factor (CALF):

$$AL_{TRUE} = AL_{1532} + CALF$$
and $$CALF = T_L \times (1 - 1532/V_L)$$

where AL_{TRUE} is the true axial length, AL_{1532} is the length measured at a velocity of 1532 m/sec, T_L is the IOL thickness, and V_L is velocity of sound in various IOL materials as provided below:

PMMA (central thickness 0.6 to 0.8 mm)   2660 m/sec
Silicone (central thickness 1.2 to 1.5 mm) 980 m/sec
Glass (central thickness 0.3 to 0.4 mm)   6040 m/sec
Acrylic (central thickness 0.7 to 0.9 mm) 2200 m/sec

An alternate method which gives a close approximation of the true axial length has also been recommended by Holladay:

PMMA IOL	$AL_{1532} + 0.4$ mm
Acrylic IOL	$AL_{1532} + 0.2$ mm
Silicone IOL (new generation)	$AL_{1532} - 0.6$ mm
Silicone IOL (old generation)	$AL_{1532} - 0.8$ mm

The Aphakic Eye

The A-scan of the aphakic eye shows unique features (Fig. 5.7). The fovea may be difficult to localize due to the absence of the lens spikes. Sometimes, in aphakic eyes, one may encounter a strong echo signal after the corneal spike. This may be due to reflection from the iris, if the pupil is not fully dilated and the sound beam is wide, or it may due to reflection from posterior capsule remnants if an extracapsular surgery had been done, or it may occasionally be due to the anterior hyaloid face after an intracapsular cataract extraction. Axial length should be recorded using sound velocity of 1532 m/sec which is the velocity in aqueous and vitreous. Some biometers use an average velocity of 1534 m/sec to account for the cornea. However, if the biometer being used has a fixed velocity setting of 1550 m/sec one can use the following formula:

Aphakic AL = (1534/1550) × AL measured at 1550 m/sec

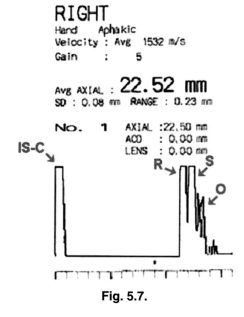

RIGHT
Hand   Aphakic
Velocity : Avg   1532 m/s
Gain   :   5

Avg AXIAL : **22.52** mm
SD : 0.08 mm RANGE : 0.23 mm

NO. 1   AXIAL :22.50 mm
         ACD : 0.00 mm
         LENS : 0.00 mm

Fig. 5.7.

Intumescent Cataract

Sound velocity in the clear crystalline lens is generally accepted to be 1641 m/sec. However, the sound velocity in the lens decreases with increase in age and the normal thickness of the lens increases from 4.01 mm at 1 year of age to 4.80 mm at 80 years of age. In the case of an intumescent cataract the water content of the lens increases with the result that the lens becomes thicker (more than 5.0 mm). Concomitantly sound velocity decreases to 1590 m/sec in an intumescent cataract. If an individual lens velocity of 1641 m/sec is used in this situation, the axial length will be falsely recorded approximately 0.15 mm longer, yielding a weaker IOL power leading to approximately +0.5 diopter post-operative hyperopia. Most biometry units use an average velocity setting of 1548 m/sec for estimating the axial length in such a situation.

Holladay has recommended a simple refinement to increase accuracy of axial length estimation for any type of cataract for any age. He advocates measuring axial length at a velocity of 1532 m/sec, which is the sound velocity in aqueous and vitreous, and correcting for the underestimation of the thicknesses of the cornea and the crystalline lens by simply adding a factor of 0.32 mm (Table 5.1).

The Highly Myopic Eye with Posterior Staphyloma

Posterior staphyloma is commonly found in pathological myopia, and one may encounter difficulties in measuring the axial length in such eyes. Suggestive findings during biometry are long axial length with inconsistent axial readings in both the measured eye as well as when compared with the fellow eye. Most staphylomata are located in the peripapillary region and are not centred around the macula with the result that the fovea is often present on the sloping wall of the staphyloma rather than in the bottom. Hence if the probe is directed towards the fovea, it is difficult to get a high quality sharply rising retinal spike since the sound beam will not strike perpendicular to the retinal surface and the display will show a saw-toothed appearance of the retinal spike. If the beam is then directed eccentric to the fovea towards the bottom of the pit so as to get a good retinal spike, an erroneously long axial length will be recorded. This can lead to significant errors because the anatomical axial length (distance from the corneal vertex to the posterior pole) may differ from the refractive axial length (distance from the corneal vertex to the fovea).

In this situation, using the immersion technique and with the patient fixating on the fixation light of the probe, it is preferable to select the most consistent readings even if the spikes are saw-toothed rather than the longest reading with a steeply rising retinal spike. If the cataract is not dense, performing partial coherence interferometry with the IOLMaster will give the refractive axial length accurately since the patient fixates on the target light.

Another method described in eyes with staphylomata is B-mode-guided biometry also known as Immersion Vector-A/B-scan. In this technique an immersion bath is used and with the help of a B-scan probe a horizontal axial section of the eye is recorded with a superimposed A-scan vector which displays corneal thickness, anterior chamber depth, lens thickness and vitreal length. The adequacy of the measurement is ascertained by visualizing the anterior and posterior corneal surfaces, the anterior and posterior lens surfaces, and simultaneously visualizing the vitreoretinal interface in a location temporal to the optic nerve (Fig. 5.8). The A-scan vector is then adjusted to pass through the centre of the corneal and the anterior and posterior lens echoes. Such an alignment will ensure that the vector intersects the retina in the region of the fovea wherever it may be situated.

Table 5.1. Calculation of True Axial Length (TAL)

Tissue	Velocity	Thickness	Underestimation
Cornea	1641 m/sec	0.55 mm (average)	$0.55 \times (1 - 1532/1641) = 0.04$ Adjustment required + 0.04 mm
Aqueous	1532 m/sec	No adjustment required	
Lens (e.g. for a 72-year-old patient)	$1659 - (72 - 10)/2 = 1628$ m/sec	$4.00 + 72/100 = 4.72$ mm	$4.72 \times (1 - 1532/1628) = 0.28$ Adjustment required + 0.28 mm
Aqueous	1532 m/sec	No adjustment required	

Therefore, True Axial Length (TAL) = Apparent Axial Length at 1532 m/sec (AAL_{1532}) + 0.04 + 0.28
or
$TAL = AAL_{1532} + 0.32$ mm

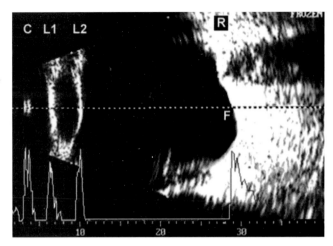

Fig. 5.8.

The Very Short Eye

In extremely short eyes (less than 20 mm) even a small axial length error can lead to a significant post-operative refractive error (3.75 diopters per millimeter). It is therefore imperative in this situation to perform accurate biometry by the immersion technique, or if the media permits, to perform optical coherence biometry with the IOLMaster. In such eyes with extremely short axial lengths, and often with a hyperopic spherical equivalent of +8.00 or greater, the calculated IOL power may exceed that available commercially, and placement of a single IOL would result in an unacceptable refractive outcome.

The solution would be to implant two IOLs in the eye at the same operative session (primary poly-pseudo-phakia). However, the original practice of stacking two acrylic lenses in the capsular bag has been abandoned due to interlenticular opacification and subsequent reduced visual acuity. It is now advocated to place two IOLs of different materials in different locations (e.g., a high power acrylic lens in the capsular bag and a biconvex silicone lens in the ciliary sulcus containing the residual power). After accurate biometry, the total power required is calculated for in-the-bag implantation using the Hoffer-Q formula or better still one of the fourth generation formulae such as Holladay-2 or Haigis. The highest commercially available power for the acrylic lens to be implanted in the capsular bag is deducted from this total, and the residual power is adjusted (reduced) for ciliary sulcus implantation of the second IOL (piggyback IOL).

With the recent manufacture of high IOL powers (up to 40 diopters) allowing single lenses to be implanted in eyes with extremely short axial length, the need for primary polypseudophakia would become less frequent.

Silicone-filled Eyes

Silicone oil is often placed temporarily in the vitreous cavity for various retinal conditions. When silicone oil removal is planned, the patient often has to undergo a concomitant cataract surgery requiring IOL power calculation. Measuring the axial length in an eye filled with silicone oil is a challenging exercise. The velocity of sound in silicone oil is reduced to 980 or 1040 m/sec depending upon the viscosity (1000 or 5000 centiStokes), and displays highly erroneous axial lengths (such as 35 mm) if a velocity of 1550 m/sec is used. Often the returning sound wave is so much attenuated that it is difficult to obtain good echoes.

One option is to measure the axial length at a velocity of 1532 m/sec and correct the velocity for the vitreous cavity depth by the following steps:

1. $VCD_{1532} = AL_{1532} - (ACD + LENS)$, where VCD_{1532} is the apparent vitreous cavity depth measured at 1532 m/sec, ACD is AC depth and LENS is lens thickness.

2. $VCD_{corrected} = VCD_{1532} \times 980*/1532$ (* or 1040 m/sec depending on the oil placed in the patient's eye)

3. $AL_{corrected} = VCD_{corrected} + ACD + LENS$

This method is not very reliable, as it often may not always be possible to know the viscosity of silicone oil used. Moreover the vitreous cavity may be partly filled with silicone oil making the measurement inaccurate. At times it may even be impossible to measure if the oil is emulsified. A better option is to perform silicone oil removal, and then perform biometry in the phakic mode with a sterile probe prior to cataract extraction. If the cataract is not advanced, measurement of the axial length by optical coherence biometry (IOLMaster) in the 'silicone filled eye' mode gives results superior to ultrasonic biometry.

IOL Power Calculation in Eyes after Previous Corneal Refractive Surgery

With the increasing popularity of procedures which aim to correct refractive errors and reduce dependence on glasses or contact lenses, it is vital to obtain a history in this regard from patients undergoing cataract surgery. This is especially relevant for cataract patients in their 40s and 50s. Performing routine keratometry for a patient, who has previously undergone Photo Refractive Keratectomy (PRK) or Laser in situ Keratomilieusis (LASIK) for the correction of myopia, will typically over-estimate the corneal power. Using these K-readings for

IOL power calculation will underestimate the power to be implanted and give rise to post-operative hypermetropia. This is because the assumptions used for routine keratometry no longer hold true.

In normal corneas the posterior radius of curvature is approximately 82% of the anterior radius of curvature. Excimer laser correction (PRK or LASIK) alters the anterior corneal radius of curvature without affecting the posterior radius of curvature and this percentage is reduced significantly due to selective flattening of the anterior surface. Using the keratometric index of 1.3375 will falsely estimate a higher corneal value in this situation. Moreover, as mentioned earlier, keratometry measures an area not in the central part of the cornea, but an annular area somewhat larger than 3 mm in diameter in the post-LASIK flattened cornea. This region would be close to the mid-peripheral steepened area at the edge of the ablated area and would further contribute to the overestimation of corneal power.

The vice versa is true for corneas having undergone hyperopic LASIK, which will give rise to post-operative myopic error. Various solutions have been advocated for determining corneal power after excimer laser surgery of which some are described below:

1. Clinical History Method

This method is used if the keratometry values prior to LASIK are known. Also one must know the amount of refractive correction achieved by the excimer laser procedure. For a given eye, the actual post-LASIK keratometry readings are disregarded, and instead the true corneal power (K_A) is calculated thus:

$$K_A = K_P + R_P - R_A$$

where K_P is the average corneal power prior to refractive surgery, R_P is the spherical equivalent of the refractive error prior to refractive surgery, and R_A is the stable refraction (spherical equivalent) achieved after refractive surgery but prior to the development of cataract. For example, consider an eye which has undergone LASIK in which the corneal power measured by keratometry is 40.50 D. According to the old records, the average K-reading and the refractive error prior to LASIK were 44.0 D and –5.0 D respectively. The records also show that after stabilization but before the development of cataract, the residual refractive error was –0.25 D. The post-LASIK true corneal power (K_A) to be used for IOL power estimation is therefore calculated as:

$$44.0 + (-5.0) - (-0.25) = 39.25 \text{ D}$$

If the K-reading of 40.50 D is used, instead of 39.25 D, for implant power estimation, it would lead to a post-operative hypermetropic error of over +1.0 D. Originally in this formula, all the spectacle plane powers were adjusted according to the vertex distance and calculated at the corneal plane. However this is not done so currently to avoid any overestimation of the true corneal power.

2. The Hard Contact Lens Method

Very often the pre-LASIK K-readings are not available. In this method the corneal power is re-measured instead of being recalculated. The patient's refraction is first determined, following which a plano hard contact lens of a known base curve is fitted on the cornea and an over-refraction is performed. If the refraction remains the same, the corneal curvature is equal to the base curve of the contact lens. If the over-refraction results in a higher myopic error, the difference between the over-refraction and the original refraction is algebraically added to the base curve of the contact lens. This would then yield a corneal power of value lesser than the base curve. Conversely, a more hyperopic change would increase this value. This method to derive the true corneal power (K_{TRUE}) can be represented as the following formula:

$$K_{TRUE} = C_{BASE} + C_{POWER} + R_{CL} - R_{BARE}$$

where C_{BASE} is the base curve of the hard contact lens in diopters, C_{POWER} is the power of the contact lens in diopters, R_{CL} is the over-refraction in diopters, and R_{BARE} is the refraction in diopters prior to insertion of the contact lens. For example, an eye with a refraction of –1.0 D and average K-reading of 32.0 D (by keratometry) is fitted with a plano contact lens of base curve 33.0 D. Over-refraction is performed which yields a refraction of –3.50 D. The true corneal power (K_{TRUE}) is calculated as:

$$K_{TRUE} = (33.0) + (0.0) + (-3.5) - (-1.0) = 30.5 \text{ D}$$

Using the average K-reading of 32.0 D instead of 30.5 D would give rise to 1.5 diopters of hypermetropia. One of the main drawbacks of this method, besides the non-availability of plano contact lenses in a clinical setting, is obtaining an accurate refraction in the presence of a cataract.

3. Modified Maloney Method

This is an excellent method when the pre-LASIK K-readings are not available and gives satisfactory results post-operatively. According to the original technique described, the central corneal power is estimated by placing the cursor at the exact centre of the Axial Map of the Zeiss Humphrey Atlas topographer to derive the true corneal power CP_{TRUE}:

$$CP_{TRUE} = CCP \times 1.114 - 6.1$$

This method can be applied to the central corneal power derived from the axial map of any corneal topography system for determining post refractive surgery corneal power. In the absence of topography, it could possibly be used on the K-readings obtained by routine keratometry, although the accuracy may suffer.

4. The Oculus Pentacam

The Oculus Pentacam is a rotational slit scanning device for evaluating the anterior segment. The 360° rotational camera works on the Scheimpflug principle to capture up to 50 slit images with excellent depth of focus, and includes information from the anterior corneal surface to the posterior crystalline lens capsule. Information provided by the Pentacam includes: anterior and posterior corneal topography with elevation maps, corneal pachymetry from limbus to limbus, 3D-chamber analysis (anterior chamber depth, chamber angle, chamber volume, etc.), lens densitometry, and tomography.

In addition to the traditional maps used in corneal topography, the Pentacam provides a unique "True Net Power" map which calculates point-to-point corneal powers by taking into account the anterior and posterior radii of curvature, and the refractive indices of air (1), cornea (1.376) and aqueous (1.336). This feature has been utilized in the Holladay Report programme of the Oculus Pentacam to provide accurate corneal power estimation in patients who have previously undergone corneal refractive surgery. For both myopic and even hyperopic LASIK, the 4.5 mm central zone has been shown to have a high correlation with the central corneal power calculated by the clinical history method. The reading generated from this zone is known as the "Equivalent K-reading" and is used for the purpose of IOL power calculation (Fig. 5.9).

5. The IOLMaster

The IOLMaster can be utilized for directly calculating the emmetropic IOL power in patients having undergone previous corneal refractive surgery for myopia. The axial length and anterior chamber depth as measured by partial coherence laser interferometry, and keratometry as measured by the auto-keratometer module of the IOLMaster are used by a special algorithm called the Haigis-L formula for this purpose. The advantage is that

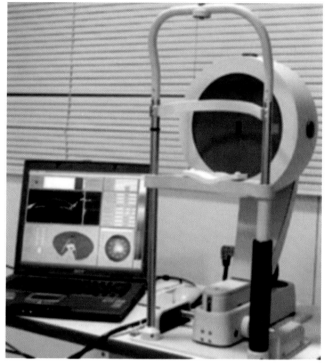

Fig. 5.9.

it utilizes the current K-reading values as measured by the IOLMaster, and no adjustment of the corneal power readings is necessary on the part of the operator.

After analyzing all the above methods, we have realized that if the following adjustments are made you will hit the target most of the time. Calculate the power as usual using the SRK-T formula. Additionally, 0.5–1.5 D may be added to this value as follows:

On biometry if you get a value of:

- Less than 13 D   Add 1.5 D
- 13-15   Add 1 D
- 16-20   Add 0.5 D
- 20 D or more   Don't add

These patients are usually happier if left myopic rather than hyperopic.

IOL Power Calculation after Radial Keratotomy (RK)

Unlike excimer laser ablation for myopia (LASIK and PRK), the ratio between the posterior and anterior corneal radii is not decreased for eyes that have previously undergone radial keratotomy (RK). Theoretically speaking, the K-readings therefore do not require any adjustment, especially if the optical zone is larger than 3.0 mm. However, studies have shown hypermetropic surprises after IOL implantation in eyes having undergone RK. If data previous to RK is available, the clinical history method should be applied as described for PRK or LASIK. If, however, this data is not forthcoming as is usually the case, it is preferable to perform corneal topography and directly estimate the central corneal power by averaging the data of the central 4.0 mm of the power map. Recently, an IOLMaster based formula, and an Oculus Pentacam method for calculating post-RK IOL power is available online (http://doctor-hill.com/iol-main/prior-keratorefractive.htm).

Scarred Corneas, Keratoconus

In such cases with irregular astigmatism, manual or auto-keratometry will be unreliable as the keratometry mires are likely to be severely distorted. Instead, corneal topography should be performed and the central corneal power estimated by averaging the data of the central 4.0 mm of the power map. If available the Oculus Pentacam may be a better alternative in this regard, since its "True Net Power" map gives central power based on anterior and posterior corneal topography. In the absence of topography and inability to get any meaningful K-readings by keratometry, one may be left with no choice but to use the K-readings of the fellow eye. An alternate approach that has been suggested is to do a hard contact lens trial and use the base curve of the best fitting contact lens as the K-readings for IOL power calculation.

Corneal Transplantation Combined with Cataract Surgery

The problem in this situation is that it is impossible to predict the central power of the donor graft prior to corneal transplantation combined with cataract surgery and IOL implantation (Triple Procedure). One approach is to use the surgeon's "average" post-keratoplasty central corneal power based on results of past keratoplasties performed by surgeon. However, this method is highly unreliable and can often lead to unpleasant post-operative refractive surprises after the Triple Procedure.

A better option is to perform corneal grafting and cataract extraction without IOL implantation (extra-capsular technique) in the first part of a planned two-stage procedure. Once cornea has stabilized after 6 to 8 months, secondary IOL implantation is performed and a posterior chamber IOL is placed in the ciliary sulcus over the intact posterior capsule. For the purpose of IOL power calculation the central corneal power is determined using corneal topography. Axial length is determined by ultrasonic biometry in the aphakic mode, or by partial coherence laser interferometry (IOLMaster).

Alternatively IOL power can be determined for secondary IOL implantation by performing accurate aphakic refraction and calculating the IOL power using the Refractive Vergence formula as given by Holladay:

$$IOL_e = \frac{1336}{\dfrac{1336}{\dfrac{1000}{\dfrac{1000}{PreRx} - V} + K_0} - ELP_0} - \frac{1336}{\dfrac{1336}{\dfrac{1000}{\dfrac{1000}{DPostRx} - V} + K_0} - ELP_0}$$

where, IOL_e is power of the secondary implant, ELP is effective lens position (anterior chamber, sulcus or bag), K is net corneal power, V is vertex distance whilst performing refraction, PreRx is the pre-operative refraction, and DPostRx is the desired post-op refraction.

The main advantage of this formula is that it is dependent mainly on refraction, and does not take axial length into consideration, which can be a potential source of error. Besides secondary IOL implantation for correction of aphakia, it is used for calculating the implant power of a phakic IOL which is placed in front of the crystalline lens to correct a refactive error, and to calculate the power of a piggyback IOL inserted in front of an existing IOL to correct a residual refractive error.

Selecting the Appropriate IOL Power

Choosing the correct power of the IOL involve not only using appropriate biometric calculations but patient's needs, expectation and profession should also be kept in mind. Most Indian patients are happy to be emmetropic. Professionals like doctors may like to be slightly myopic. Hypermetropia is usually not desirable. The refractive status and IOL power of the other eye need to be given due consideration. It is advisable to periodically analyze your own cases so that you can estimate the accuracy of your own biometry and make the necessary adjustments in future.

IOL Power Selection in Children

IOL power selection poses a special dilemma in children because of the problem of a rapidly growing eye. There is a steep axial length growth rate from birth (approximately 15 mm) to the age of 2 years (21 mm) of almost 6 mm which corresponds to almost 20 diopters of myopia. Concurrently corneal power drops from 54 D to 44 D, neutralizing 10 diopters of myopia. Between the ages of 2 to 5 years, axial growth slows to 0.4 mm per year and only increases another 1 mm from 5 to 10 years, while corneal power remains stable. As is evident this refractive instability makes it difficult to predict the final adult IOL power in a particular child, especially in the younger age group. If one were to implant a standard adult power for an average eye, it would lead to significant hypermetropia post-operatively and subsequent amblyopia. On the other hand, if one were to implant the emmetropic power, it would render the child highly myopic later in life

The solution to this dilemma is to partially undercorrect the emmetropic IOL power calculated and to correct the residual hyperopic refractive error with contact lenses or spectacles to prevent amblyopia. Close follow up is essential to monitor the ever changing refraction which undergoes a myopic shift. Ultimately, with this approach one expects a low to moderate myopia in later life. Based on this principle of undercorrection in children, IOL power selection guidelines have been recommended.

In children less than 2 years of age, axial length and corneal power is measured, and the emmetropic IOL power is undercorrected by 20%. Alternatively in this age group, only axial length measurement is considered for selecting the appropriate IOL power:

17 mm	+28 D
18 mm	+27 D
19 mm	+26 D
20 mm	+24 D
21 mm	+22 D

In the age group of 2 to 8 years, axial length and corneal power is measured, and the emmetropic IOL power is undercorrected by 10%.

Biometry: Important Considerations

- Do it yourself or have a reliable technician.
- Select the correct mode/velocity.
- Careful data input.
- Selection of the appropriate formula.
- Axial length comparable with other eye.
- IOL power compatible with history.
- Choose power suitable for patient (age, profession, needs).
- Estimate your own error (surgeon factor).

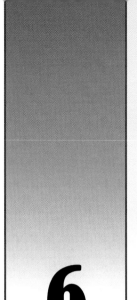

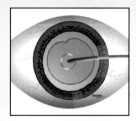

6

Incisions and Wound Construction

One of the main advantages of small incision cataract surgery is the reduction in post-operative astigmatism. Over the years, our experience with extra-capsular cataract extraction has shown that astigmatism is caused by wound gape/slippage and faulty suturing technique. Even a 1 mm of wound displacement can lead to astigmatism of upto 10 diopters. Also, the closer the incision to the centre of the cornea and the larger the incision, the more the astigmatism. Thus, now all attempts are directed at minimizing the surgically induced astigmatism by modifying the incision. **A small incision as far away from the centre of the cornea as possible, with no gape and no sutures is closest to the ideal incision.**

APPLIED ANATOMY (Figs. 6.1 & 6.2)

The surgical limbus is a zone of 1–2 mm marking the transition between the sclera and the cornea. The anterior limbus is bluish and the posterior limbus is whitish in colour, the junction overlies the Schwalbe's line anteriorly. The conjunctival insertion is variable and tends to regress posteriorly temporally. The attachment of Tenon's fascia is approximately 1 mm further posterior to the conjunctiva. Disturbance of the Tenon's leads to chemosis during surgery.

It is important to keep in mind the curvature of the corneal dome, **both** in the vertical direction (from limbus to the centre of the cornea) **and** in the horizontal direction (from side-to-side) while advancing the knives, to maintain the correct planes.

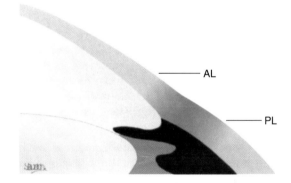

Fig. 6.1. Limbus—side view. AL = Anterior limbus; PL = Posterior limbus.

Astigmatic neutral funnel (Figs. 6.3, 6.4 & 6.5)

It has been seen that an incision of 3–3.5 mm at the limbus results in minimal astigmatism of 0.25–0.50 D and for all practical purposes can be considered astigmatically neutral. The concept of an astigmatic neutral funnel was derived from 2 mathematical equations:

- Corneal surgically-induced astigmatism is directly proportional to the cube of the length of the incision.
- Corneal surgically-induced astigmatism is inversely proportional to the distance of the incision from the centre of the cornea.

Keeping this in mind, the concept of an ***astigmatic neutral funnel*** has evolved. The mouth of the funnel is along the limbus and it flares out as we move posteriorly. Making the incision within this funnel will result in least

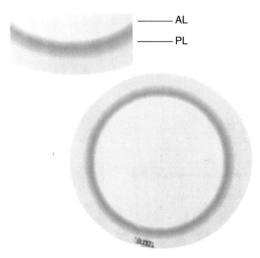

Fig. 6.2. Surgical limbus—top view. AL = Anterior limbus; PL = Posterior limbus.

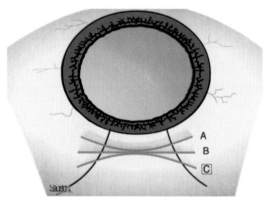

Fig. 6.3. Astigmatic neutral funnel. Note that for the same chord length and at the same distance from the limbus amount of incision falling out of astigmatic neutral funnel is least in frown and most in concave. A = Concave towards limbus; B = Straight line incision; C = 'Frown' incision convex towards limbus.

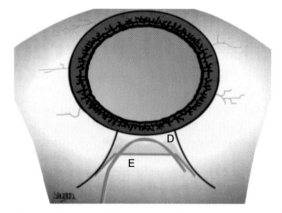

Fig. 6.4. Other modifications of incisions within the astigmatic neutral funnel. D = Trapezoid incision; E = J-shaped incision.

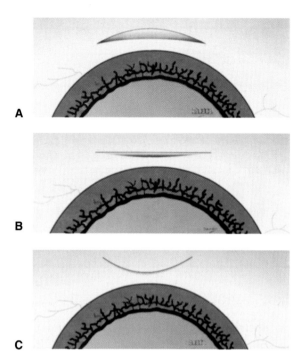

Fig. 6.5. Wound gape in different types of incision. (A) Concave incision: has maximum wound gape. (B) Straight incision: moderate gape. (C) Convex (frown) incision: minimum gape.

astigmatism. The shape of the incision may be *'Frown'* (convex towards the limbus), *'Smile'* (concave towards the limbus) or *'Straight'*. For the same chord length of incision and at the same distance from the limbus, a convex incision would extend slightly outside the funnel followed in decreasing order by straight and concave. **Wound gape due to sagging** of the wound is also in the same order. Various other incisions have been designed namely trapezoid and J-incision to decrease the wound gape, and keep the incision totally in the funnel.

Self-sealing incision (Fig. 6.6A & B)

The advantage of a self-sealing incision, not requiring sutures, is obvious. The features of an incision that make it self-sealing are:

• Creation of a corneal valve
• Square incisions are self-sealing

It is the inner corneal lip of the wound that functions as a valve. With the normal IOP of the eye, this lip gets pushed up against the dome of the cornea thus sealing the wound. Usually, 1.75 mm is adequate for the formation of a good corneal valve, with an incision of upto 4 mm. The corneal lip needs to be of adequate length *all along*; a ragged or irregular corneal lip will not

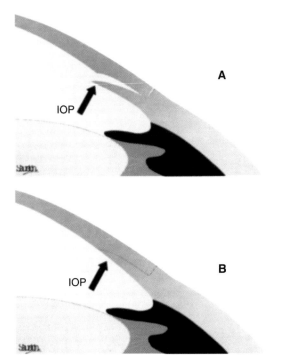

Fig. 6.6. Corneal valve. (A) Valve open. (B) Soft corneal lip acts as a valve and is closed by the IOP. More the IOP the better is the valve action.

function as a good valve. The larger the corneal lip, the better the sealing action. However, you must keep in mind that enlarging the lip more than 2 mm results in encroachment onto the centre of the cornea which can decrease the visibility for the rest of the surgery. When planning for a 5.5 mm optic IOL, a slightly larger corneal valve is required. In these cases, one should start the incision a little more posteriorly.

INSTRUMENTS

15° blade/MVR blade, keratome (2.8–3.2 mm) and crescent knife are needed. Keratomes and crescent knives are available as bevel up and bevel down, with the bevel up being more commonly used. These instruments are available in steel, diamond and crystal. Diamond blade is available with a cutting side and without a cutting side, the former being better. Diamond, being the hardest material, provides a smoother cut. However, it is expensive and there is recurring cost of cleaning it. If not maintained well it may lose its sharpness after 50 to 100 cases because of adherence of microscopic cotton fibres. Also since the tactile feedback is absent, the chances of a premature entry are high. It can also easily cut through in case of any accidental movement by the patient. Steel blades are as good as diamond if used for

limited number of cases. I prefer using Alcon knives which last for 5 to 7 cases if handled properly. ETO is ideal for sterilization. Autoclaving blunts these instruments and use of formalin gas chamber and chemicals (Cidex) is questionable.

PRE-REQUISITES (Photos 6.1 to 6.4)

Sharp instruments and a tense eyeball are the prerequisites for good incision. Exchange aqueous with VES from the side port to obtain adequate IOP before starting the incision.

SIDE PORT INCISION (SPI) (Photos 6.5 to 6.8)

SPI is made on the left hand side of the main port for a right handed surgeon. Location of SPI can be varied according to the nucleotomy technique used. For divide and conquer and central chop, the SPI is made 3 clock hours away from the main port. This makes removal of sub-incisional cortex easier. A position of 2 clock hours is good for peripheral chop, however, removal of sub-incisional cortex is tougher. Therefore, practically, a location between 2 to 3 clock hours is ideal for all purposes.

The size of the side port should be 1 to 1.5 mm. A clear corneal square tunnel is preferable. A scleral tunnel would not only bleed more, but also increase the incidence of iris prolapse, being closer to the iris root. The sclera also does not swell, rather it retracts increasing the incidence of wound leak.

A 15° blade/MVR blade may be used. Enter with the knife pointed towards the ciliary body 150–180° away creating a uniplanar 1.5 mm × 1.5 mm square tunnel. After entry, rotate the knife so that the cutting edge of the knife is turned away from the capsule, towards the corneal apex, preventing accidental capsular injury. This size of tunnel allows free instrument movement with minimum leak. A larger tunnel would lead to iris prolapse and unstable chamber. A tight tunnel leads to localized corneal whitening or edema. One should take care that the knife is sharp to allow for smooth movement. Counter-pressure by a toothed forceps/chopper can be applied on the other side to assist this. If the knife is blunt one tends to use more force for entering and the knife may go in with a jerk damaging the capsule.

SCLERAL TUNNEL / SCLERAL POCKET

An ideal tunnel would be square, self-sealing, lying within the astigmatic neutral funnel and extending 1.75

mm into cornea. However, a square configuration would result in too long a tunnel if PMMA lens was to be inserted (5.5 mm × 5.5 mm). This would make manipulation of the phaco probe difficult. Practically, an ideal tunnel is that which has a minimum width of 3 mm in the centre and flares out at the periphery. A 1.75 mm corneal lip is maintained all along the incision, parallel to the limbus. A depth of 1/3 to 1/2 thickness of sclera is ideal (300 μ to 500 μ).

Technique (Photos 6.9 to 6.32)

After placing superior rectus and inferior rectus bridle sutures close to the muscle insertion, a fornix based conjunctival flap is made. The sclera is bared of Tenon's. The length of the incision is marked and light cautery is applied along the area to be dissected.

Initial groove

The initial groove is made with a 15° blade or 11 No. blade. This groove is 1.5 mm away from the limbus at the centre and at about 1/2 scleral thickness depth (500 to 600 microns). As described previously, the initial groove may be frown-shaped or straight. Practically, the latter is as good as the former and easier to make. Usually the starting point of the groove is not deep enough and a reverse sweep with the knife should be made to ensure uniform depth. Beginners tend to make a shallow cut and may be required to repeat at the same site. One must endeavour to make the groove in one single motion.

Making the tunnel (Fig. 6.7A & B)

The tunnel is constructed with a sharp crescent knife. Engage the tip of the crescent knife in the centre of the groove at adequate depth (300–400 microns) and advance the knife from outside-in with slight sideward movements. Once initial central tunnel is made, the knife is moved from inside out to extend the tunnel to 1 mm to the periphery. For the corneal lip, the tunnel is extended further with outside-in sweeping motion. Corneal dissection is much easier than scleral dissection. The corneal valve must be 1.75 mm long and circumferential to the limbus. Because of the curvature of the crescent knife, the inner lip tends to be shorter at the extremes. The corneal pocket should be enlarged by rounding off the edges to ensure an adequate inner lip.

Internal incision is made with the help of 2.75 mm keratome. Put VES into the tunnel to assist in visualizing the extent and shape of the internal end of the tunnel. VES also lubricates the passage and prevents the knife

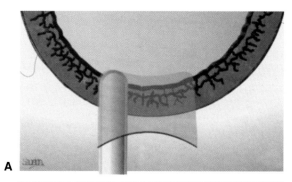

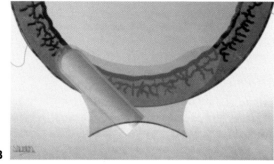

Fig. 6.7. (A) Note that outer incision is larger but the curvilinear part of the inner end is smaller. Inner curvilinear lip should be larger or equal to the outer incision for effective corneal valve action. (B) Enlarging the inner pocket on both sides.

from getting caught in the bed. Lift the scleral lip with the help of a rounded repositor or forceps, and gently introduce the keratome with side to side movement. Change the direction of the keratome by lifting the handle so that the tip now points towards the opposite ciliary body. This will create a dimple in the cornea before perforating. (Note: Eyeball *must* be well pressurized otherwise perforation won't occur.) Once the tip perforates the cornea, turn the handle downwards to make the blade parallel to iris plane or even tilt a little upwards and advance further. If the direction of the keratome isn't changed immediately after perforation, the corneal valve assumes a triangular configuration with 1.75 mm length in the centre and much less on the sides. I prefer to advance the knife only upto the shoulder of the knife. If the knife is advanced fully, it may enter the AC with a jerk and the tunnel may get cut on the sides while withdrawing the knife. One must remove the knife gently to avoid unplanned extension of the tunnel.

The section has to be enlarged during the insertion of IOL depending on the size of the IOL. Inflate the bag and the eye with VES. For a PMMA IOL, a 5.2 mm keratome is ideal for this purpose as it has a blunt tip and does not get entangled in the tissue. Also, this ensures that the section is of adequate size. If a crescent knife or 3.2 mm keratome is used, the strokes should be from outside in. Do not cut while withdrawing as this decreases the width of the corneal lip, thereby decreasing the self-sealing capacity. Avoid cutting in multiple planes.

PROBLEMS

1. Scleral disinsertion (Fig. 6.8)

If the initial cut is more than 80% to 90% deep, it results in wound gape leading to astigmatism. If it occurs, it should be sutured at the end of phacoemulsification.

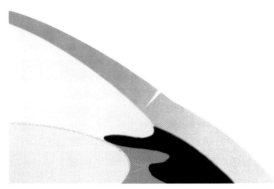

Fig. 6.8. Scleral disinsertion. See the gape at the external wound because of the deep initial cut.

2. Torn edges (Fig. 6.9A & B)

This occurs because the surgeon moves his knife parallel to the floor rather than along the curvature of the eyeball especially on side-to-side movement. The knife has to be tilted a little towards the side of motion of the blade.

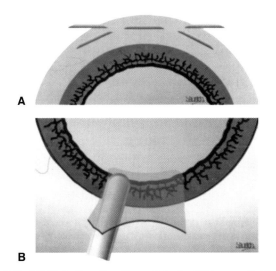

Fig. 6.9. (A) Note the direction of blade. If it is parallel to the floor, it will cut the edges. The blade must dip on the side to avoid cutting the edges. (B) Torn edges due to not following the curvature of the globe.

The problem is increased when the initial groove is small. During enlargement of the incision with a 5.2 mm keratome, the surgeon tends to lift the section and cuts the edges in the process. This can be avoided by pressing the keratome against the globe (to flatten the curvature) and pointing the tip upwards. Concentrate on the external wound while enlarging the incision till the shoulder has entered the section. *Now* concentrate on the internal lip. Holding the flap with the toothed forceps may cause a tear.

3. Premature entry (Fig. 6.10)

Early perforation of the cornea results in a premature entry into the AC. The smaller corneal lip thus produced will not have an efficient valvular function. Premature entry results in unstable AC and repeated iris prolapse, which leads to miosis, making the surgery difficult.

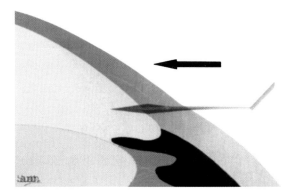

Fig. 6.10. Premature entry. Advancing the knife parallel to the floor (not following the curvature of the cornea) leads to premature entry.

Premature entry can be due to a number of reasons. The initial groove may have been too deep thus leading to a deeper plane of dissection. Too sharp a knife may also result in an uncontrolled entry. One of the common causes of premature entry is the failure to move the knife in accordance with the curvature of the corneal dome.

If the initial groove is too deep and you have recognized this in time, you can try to come to a more superficial plane. This may be facilitated with the use of a bevel-up knife. Alternatively, one can make another groove 1 mm in front of the initial incision and repeat dissection in a more superficial plane. To prevent premature entry due to incorrect advancement of the knife, the tip should be pointed slightly towards the ceiling rather than the floor while advancing.

If the premature corneal entry has *already* been made, the further course taken depends upon the type of cataract and degree of mydriasis. In case of soft cataract, with fully dilated pupil and no iris prolapse, one may proceed with the surgery as planned. If the pupil is **not** well dilated or there is repeated iris prolapse or the cataract is **hard** then the surgery will have to be modified. There are a couple of options available: you can either make another tunnel at a different site or convert to ECCE. If the initial tunnel is made at 12 O'clock, one can suture the initial incision and complete the nucleotomy from a clear corneal temporal incision. The original 12 O'clock tunnel can be used for lens insertion. After IOL insertion inflate the globe with air, constrict the pupil and if required suture the wound.

4. Thin flap

Shallow initial groove is the commonest cause of thin flap. Once the scleral dissection is started in one plane, it is difficult to change the plane. Too sharp or too blunt a knife may also cause the same problem.

5. Thin and shredded flap

If a blunt knife is used, one ends up tearing the flap instead of cutting it. This results in a thin and shredded flap and at times even button-holing.

If thin flap is detected early, i.e. before the tunnel has reached the cornea, stop. Deepen the initial groove and dissect again in a deeper plane. Change the knife if it is blunt. Another alternative is to leave this incision and make another groove 1 mm in front of the initial incision or make a fresh groove at a new site. If the whole tunnel has been constructed, and the cataract is soft, surgery may be attempted from the same incision.

6. Too long corneal valve

This happens when a sharp crescent knife is used in a pressurized eye. If the pocket is too long, perforate the globe 1/2 mm behind.

CLEAR CORNEAL INCISION

With the advent of foldable IOLs, the size of the incision has further decreased making it possible to make self-sealing corneal incisions. Clear corneal incisions have the advantage of not requiring cautery. The temporal approach is specially suited for a clear corneal incision since the horizontal diameter of the cornea is usually 1 mm more than the vertical and the tunnel interferes less with the visibility. The other advantage of the temporal incision is ease of surgery, especially in deep-set eyes, where the eyebrow and supraorbital margin can

interfere with the movement of the probe. There is less pooling of fluid in fornices, better red reflex and less chance of oar-locking of instruments in the temporal approach. However, temporal scleral incision is not recommended since it is cosmetically unacceptable.

Phacoemulsification under topical anaesthesia is more convenient with a corneal incision since cautery, which is quite painful, is not required. Also, lack of bleeding with the corneal incision means improved visibility during surgery.

Types of Corneal Incision (Figs. 6.11 to 6.14)

- Triplanar
- Biplanar
- Uniplanar
- Hinged

Sharp instruments and pressurized eye are two essential requirements for any incision, corneal or scleral.

Triplanar incision

The initial vertical cut is made with a No. 11 blade or a 15° knife, far away from the centre of the cornea, without cutting the conjunctiva. The cut should be 300–500 μ deep and 2.75 mm in width. The dissection is done with a crescent knife (squarish dissection, 1.75 mm × 2.75 mm). Inner lip is straight and parallel to the initial incision. Then, viscoelastic is injected into the tunnel and AC entered with 2.75 keratome. Advantage of this incision is that it is a well-controlled incision with an excellent valve. The only disadvantage is that it takes slightly longer time and additional instruments (crescent knife) are required.

Hinged incision

Initial groove is 600 μ or more and the tunnel is made at 300 μ as in the triplanar incision. The valve action is supposed to be better.

Biplanar corneal incision (Photos 6.33 to 6.36) (Figs. 6.15 to 6.18)

A well made **biplanar** corneal incision is as effective as the triplanar incision. However, the chances of premature entry and torn edges are more. After the initial groove, the keratome is used directly to make 1.75 mm corneal valve and then the direction is changed to enter the AC (no crescent knife is used). It virtually becomes a triplanar incision. Note the direction of knife in each step as shown in the diagrams.

TYPES OF CORNEAL INCISION

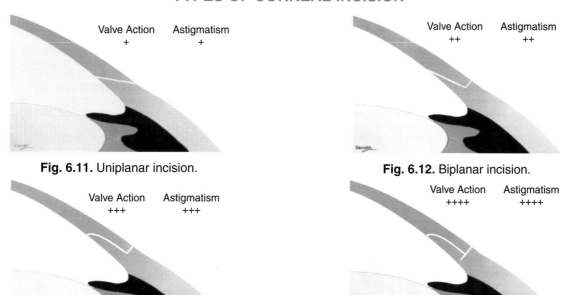

Valve Action
+

Astigmatism
+

Fig. 6.11. Uniplanar incision.

Valve Action
++

Astigmatism
++

Fig. 6.12. Biplanar incision.

Valve Action
+++

Astigmatism
+++

Fig. 6.13. Triplanar incision.

Valve Action
++++

Astigmatism
++++

Fig. 6.14. Hinged incision.

Note the relationship of valve action and astigmatism in different types of incisions.

BIPLANAR CORNEAL INCISION

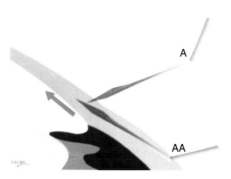

Fig. 6.15. Movement of knife. Knife 'A' represents initial direction. After engaging the knife 'AA' is moved along the curvature of the cornea. Note the base dips down and the tip points forward. The red arrow indicates the direction of advancement of the knife.

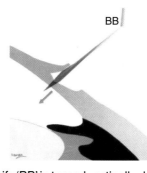

Fig. 6.16. Knife 'BB' is turned vertically down for perforating the cornea.

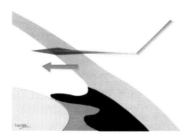

Fig. 6.17. Knife is made horizontal again, parallel to the iris and advancing upto the shoulder.

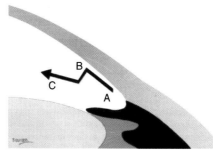

Fig. 6.18. Direction of keratomes for wound construction. Creation of: A = Tunnel; B = Perforation; C = Enlargement of initial wound.

Uniplanar clear corneal incision
(Photos 6.37 to 6.40)

Biplanar and *triplanar* incisions sometimes result in persistent post-operative irritation to the patient due to slight wound gape. With the advent of diamond knife/very sharp knives it is now possible to make the incision without the initial groove. The post-operative irritation is reduced. However, the outer flap is very thin and tends to roll into the tunnel while entering the phaco tip into the AC (this may result in corneal burn). It is also very difficult to control the course of the incision. The cut may be irregular and the valve action is not as good as in the previous two incisions. Practically, these complications are seen very rarely because the valve seals due to corneal oedema. Even if the wound leaks and the AC collapses, pseudophako-corneal touch does not occur due to backward angulation of the IOL placed in the bag. Iris prolapse is also fortunately rare.

I personally feel that the beginners should initially start with *triplanar* incision. Once the surgeon is comfortable with the feel of tissue, he can shift to *biplanar* incision. *Uniplanar* incision is not recommended except in expert hands.

LIMBAL INCISION (Fig. 6.19)

The clear corneal incision tends to come closer to centre and this may cause glare to the patient particularly during pupillary mydriasis. There is no protection by the conjunctiva and wound healing is slow. Chances of corneal burn are high, especially in hard cataract. Therefore, some surgeons advocate *posterior limbal incision*.

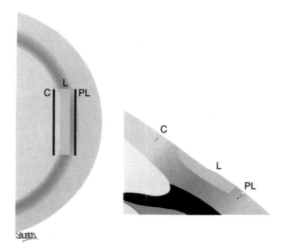

Fig. 6.19. Recommended site of limbal incision is represented by green area. C = clear cornea, L = limbal incision, PL = posterior limbus.

This can be done with or without conjunctival detachment and cautery. Problems include bleeding and chemosis in the latter incision due to the disturbance of the Tenon's and conjunctiva. Bleeding usually stops by the end of surgery. However, during surgery chemosis may hamper the smooth progress, and disinsertion of the conjunctiva and Tenon's may be required. We feel that a limbal incision, as far away from the centre of the cornea as possible without disturbing the conjunctiva, is a good compromise between a clear corneal and a posterior limbal incision.

Modified temporal incision (corneolimbal / limboscleral) (Photos 6.41 to 6.52) (Fig. 6.20)

This incision is a modification of *temporal clear corneal triplanar* incision for a PMMA lens. This incorporates the advantages of temporal clear corneal incision and is better than the superior scleral incisions.

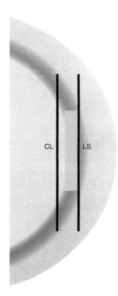

Fig. 6.20. Modified temporal incision for 5.5 mm IOL. CL = Corneolimbal—central 3 mm in cornea; LS = Limboscleral—central 3 mm in limbus.

The site of the initial groove is the same as for *clear corneal* and is extended 1 mm on either side. Slight bleeding may be present but usually does not obscure the view. Incision should not cut the conjunctiva in the central 3 mm, to avoid the chemosis. Aim for a tunnel approximately 2 mm long. If the same incision is shifted 1/2 mm to 1 mm behind, a *limboscleral* incision can be constructed. Enlargement of incision is done in the same way as for scleral tunnel. This incision may be biplanar or triplanar. Uniplanar incision is a poor choice.

PROBLEMS OF CORNEAL AND LIMBAL INCISIONS

1. Torn edges

They are very common with a corneal tunnel, particularly during the enlargement. This is due to failure to understand the curvature of cornea. While advancing the knife, beginners tend to lift up the flap and concentrate on the tip of the keratome. In such a situation the shoulder of the knife may cut the edges of the external wound. During entry one should press the shoulder of the knife *downwards* against the floor of tunnel (to flatten the curvature) and point the knife slightly upwards. Once the shoulder has passed the external wound concentrate on the internal wound enlargement.

2. Premature entry

Much more common in clear corneal incision because of the use of sharper knife. It is most frequently seen in uniplanar incision.

3. Long tunnel

Commoner in soft eyeball like myopes/inadequate VSD. This is because it is difficult to penetrate the cornea in a soft eye.

4. Leaky wound

If AC is not too unstable, cataract is not too hard and pupil not too small; one can proceed to phaco from the same port. In the event of difficulty, one can tighten the wound by placing one interrupted suture at one end of the tunnel or still better to make a fresh incision after closing this incision with 10-0 suture. In case of a leaky wound with iris prolapse it is best to close this incision and make a fresh one to continue with the surgery.

PRESSURISING THE EYE

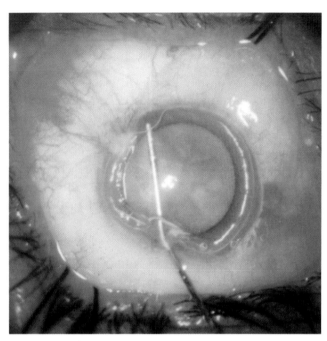

Photo 6.1. Note the position of the cannula going to the opposite angle from the side port.

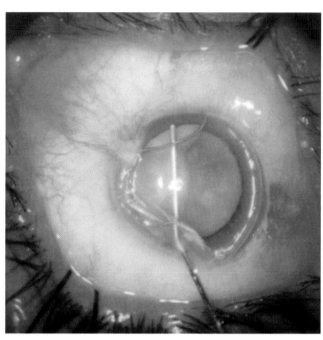

Photo 6.2. Creation of bolus of viscoelastic and simultaneous pressing the lip of the wound for the removal of BSS/air or both.

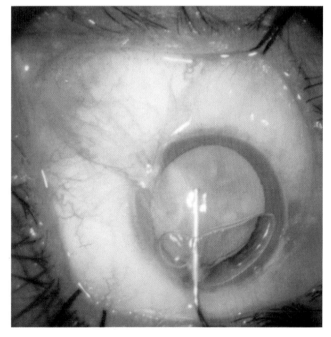

Photo 6.3. Enlarging the bolus by keeping the cannula inside the bolus.

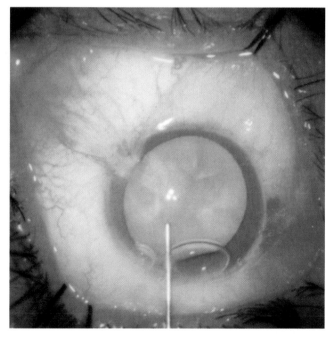

Photo 6.4. Complete replacement of air and BSS being done.

SIDE PORT

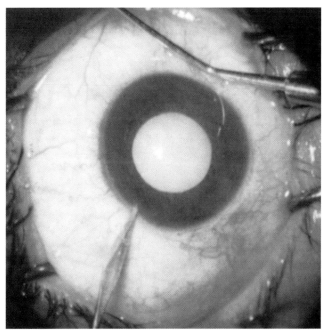

Photo 6.5. See the position of 15° blade between 2 & 3 O'clock into the clean cornea from the main incision. Cut edge is pointing away from the main incision. Counter pressure at the opposite limbus.

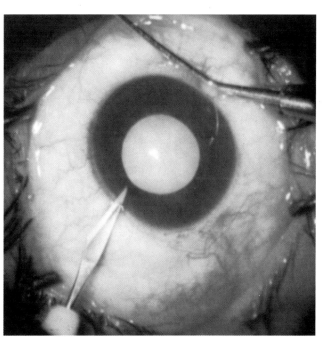

Photo 6.6. Knife advanced into corneal lamellae.

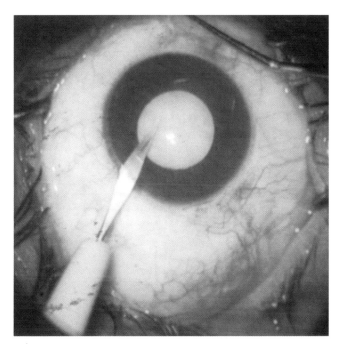

Photo 6.7. After perforation advance till the required width of the incision is achieved.

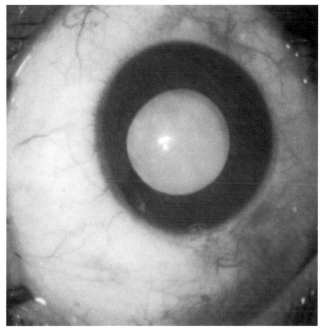

Photo 6.8. Creation of square side port.

SCLERAL POCKET

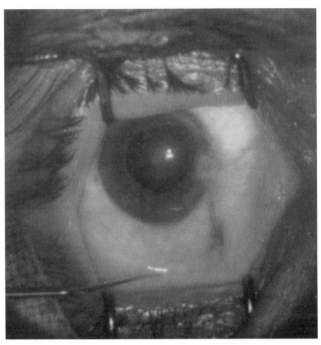

Photo 6.9. Inadequate exposure of the eyeball.

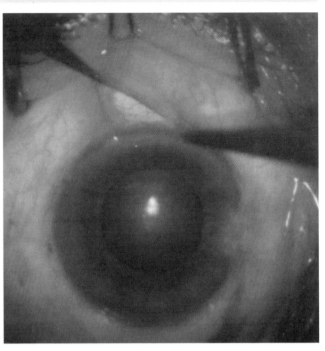

Photo 6.10. Adequate exposure of the eyeball after I.R. and S.R. bridle sutures. Note the Tenon's attachment and exposure.

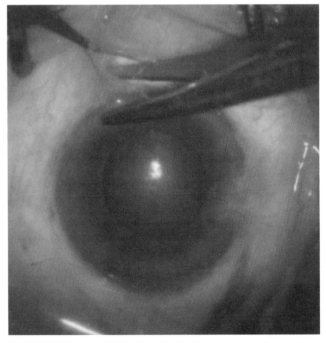

Photo 6.11. Detach the Tenon's to bare the sclera completely.

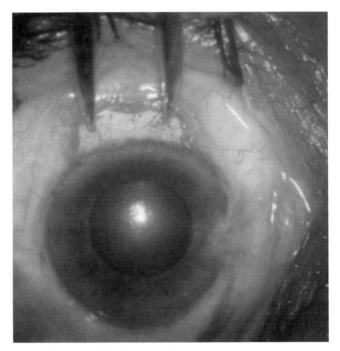

Photo 6.12. Measure the size of the incision.

SCLERAL POCKET (Contd.)

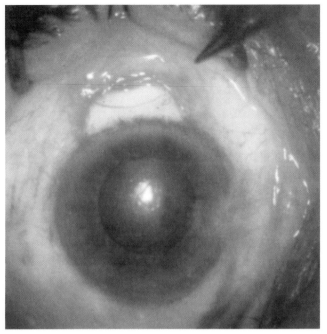

Photo 6.13. (After a light cautery) Make a frown incision 1.5 mm away from the limbus centrally 5.5 mm in length.

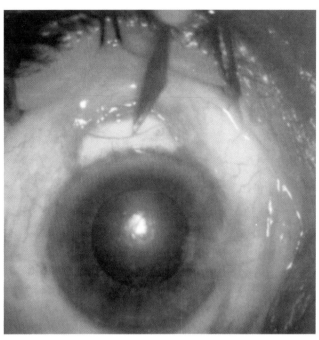

Photo 6.14. Reverse sweep of the knife to attain equal depth.

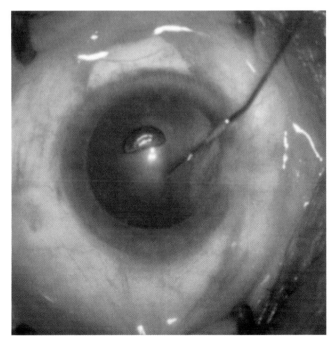

Photo 6.15. Replace the aqueous with VES from the side port to pressurize the eye.

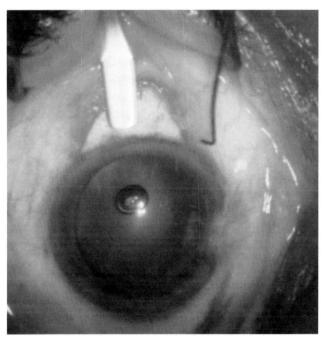

Photo 6.16. Lifting the flap in the centre with crescent knife.

SCLERAL POCKET (Contd.)

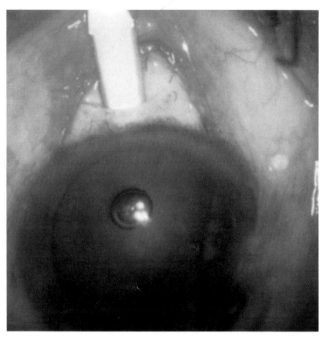

Photo 6.17. Going 1 mm into sclera with an outside-in motion centrally.

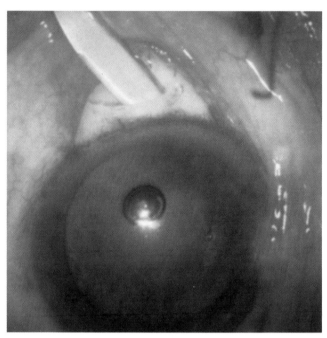

Photo 6.18. Extending onto one side by inside-out motion.

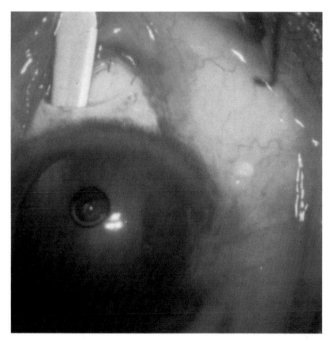

Photo 6.19. Inside-out motion on the other side.

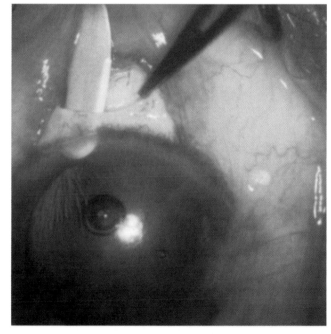

Photo 6.20. Outside-in motion used to extend the tunnel into the clear cornea. Note the site of forceps used to grip.

SCLERAL POCKET (Contd.)

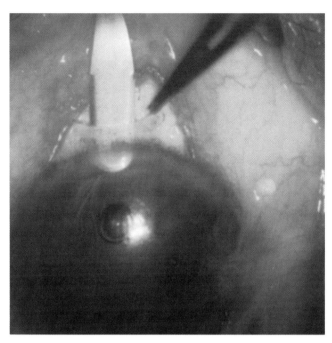

Photo 6.21. Enlarging the pockets laterally by inside-out motion.

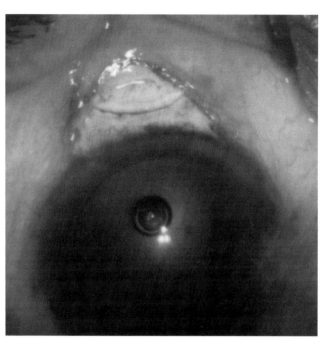

Photo 6.22. Stained tunnel. Note that outer incision is larger but the curvilinear part of the inner end is smaller. Inner curvilinear lip should be larger or equal to the outer incision for effective corneal valve action.

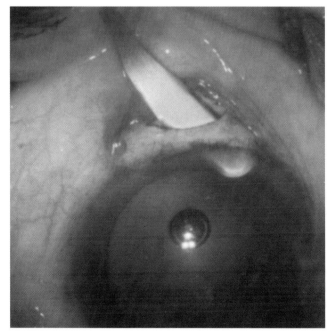

Photos 6.23 & 6.24. Enlarging the inner pocket on both sides.

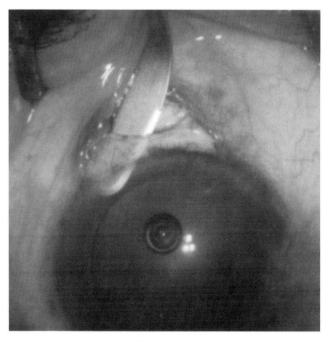

Photo 6.24.

SCLERAL POCKET (Contd.)

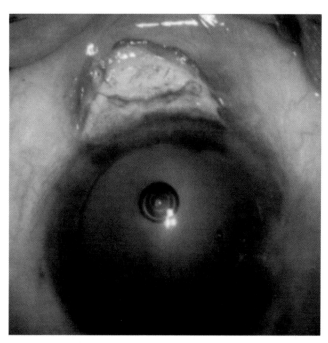

Photo 6.25. Stained tunnel showing adequately sized inner curvilinear pocket.

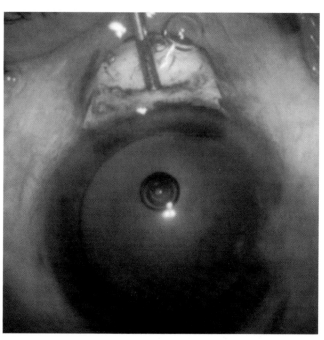

Photo 6.26. Injecting VES into the tunnel to lubricate and facilitate entry of keratome and to identify the internal limit of scleral pocket.

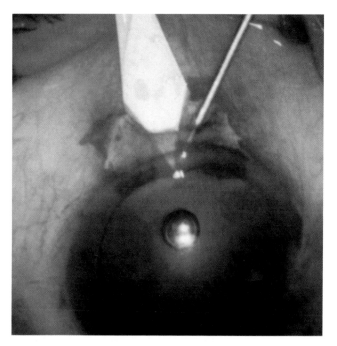

Photo 6.27. Rounded repositor used to help insert the keratome.

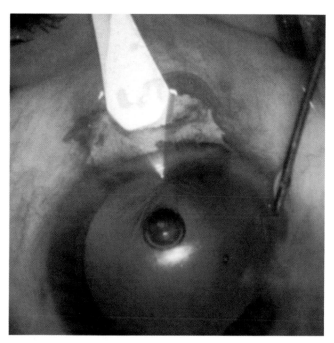

Photo 6.28. Creation of corneal dimple first and perforation by pointing the tip downwards.

SCLERAL POCKET (Contd.)

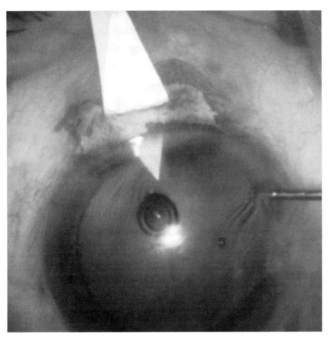

Photo 6.29. Once the tip is in, knife is turned to make the blade parallel to iris to enlarge the incision.

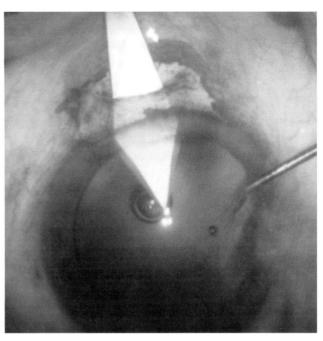

Photo 6.30. Advance the knife upto the shoulder only and then withdraw.

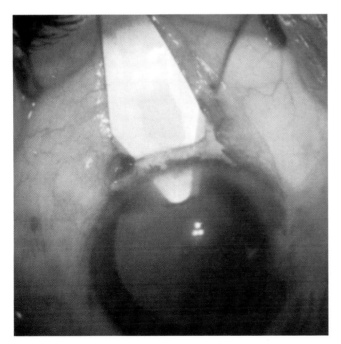

Photo 6.31. Advancing the section before PMMA IOL insertion with 5.2 keratome inside in a pressurized eye.

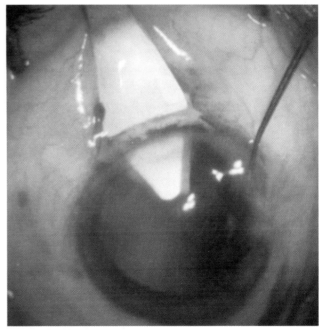

Photo 6.32. Point the tip slightly forwards, press the blade down to flatten the globe and advance further while concentrating on the shoulder to avoid cutting the outer edge. Once the shoulder is in then concentrate on the internal incision.

BIPLANAR INCISION

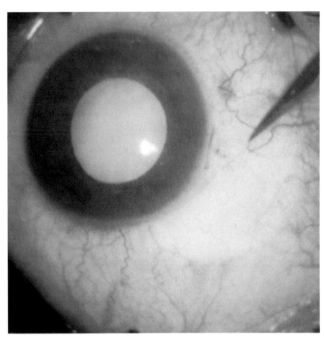

Photo 6.33. Creation of a straight cut 300 μ to 500 μ deep.

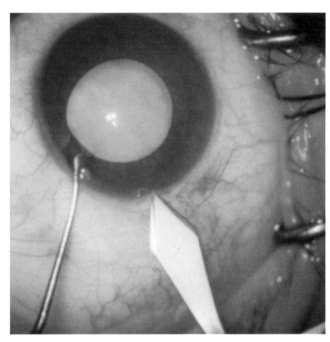

Photo 6.34. Engaging the keratome at the depth of the section. Note the stabilization of globe with second instrument.

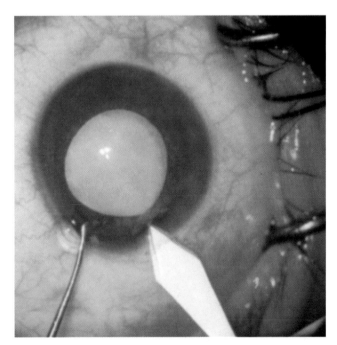

Photo 6.35. After advancing keratome forwards along the corneal curvature the tip is pointed backwards to create corneal dimpling before perforation.

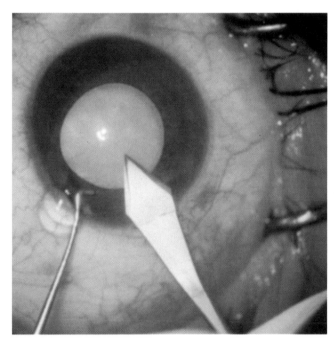

Photo 6.36. After perforation advancing the keratome parallel to the iris upto the shoulder.

UNIPLANAR INCISION

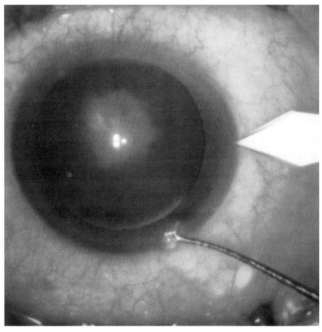

Photo 6.37. Stabilization of globe with chopper at side port. Keratome positioned at the limbus without any straight cut.

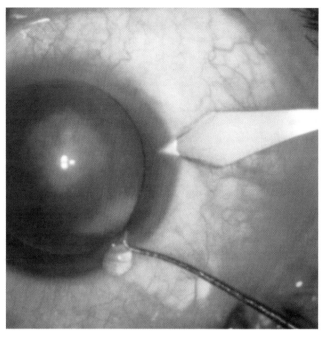

Photo 6.38. Initial entry made keeping the knife horizontal or slightly downwards.

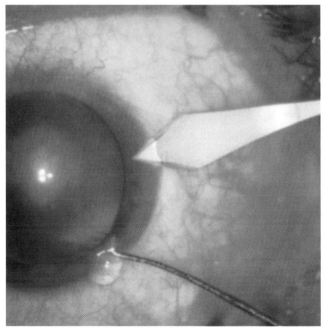

Photo 6.39. Advance further along the corneal curvature upto the required length (tip pointing forwards).

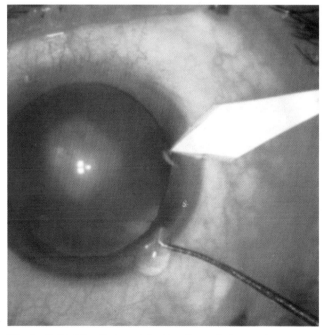

Photo 6.40. The tip is pointed backwards to create corneal dimpling before perforation.

MODIFIED TEMPORAL LIMBOSCLERAL TRIPLANAR INCISION

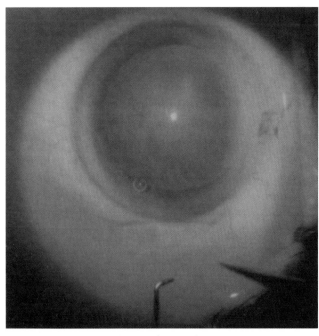

Photo 6.41. Initial sclerolimbal 5–5.5 mm groove—300 µ to 500 µ deep (central 3 mm at the limbus and rest 1 mm on either side onto sclera).

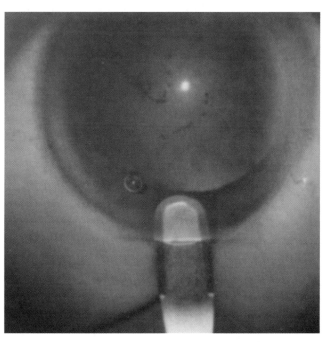

Photo 6.42. Creation of central tunnel with crescent knife using outside-in motion.

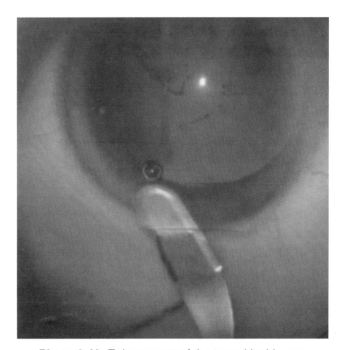

Photo 6.43. Enlargement of the tunnel inside-out.

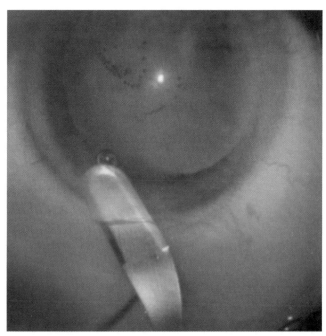

Photo 6.44. Making the inner pocket larger than the outer pocket (rounding off).

MODIFIED TEMPORAL LIMBOSCLERAL TRIPLANAR INCISION (Contd.)

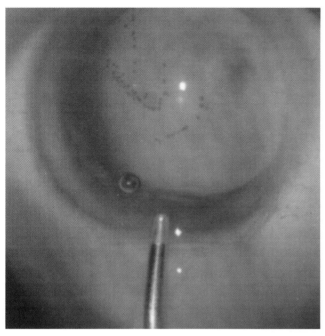

Photo 6.45. Injection of VES in the tunnel to define the tunnel, identify the internal limit and facilitate the keratome entry.

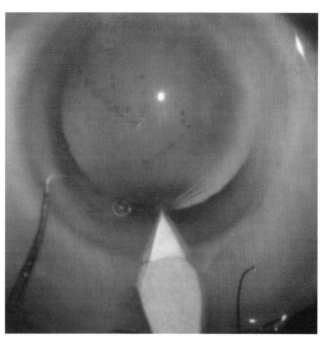

Photo 6.46. Creation of dimple.

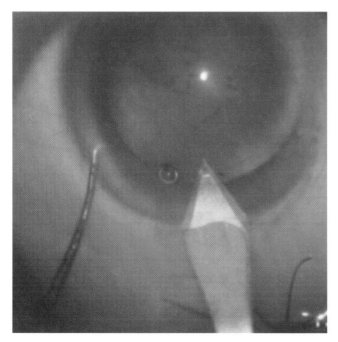

Photo 6.47. Perforation.

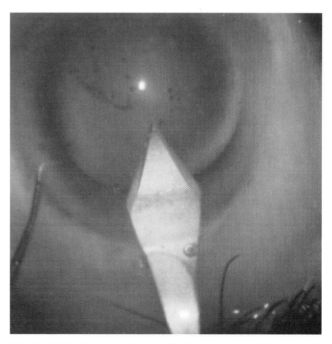

Photo 6.48. Advance the knife further parallel to the iris plane upto the shoulder of keratome.

MODIFIED TEMPORAL LIMBOSCLERAL TRIPLANAR INCISION (Contd.)

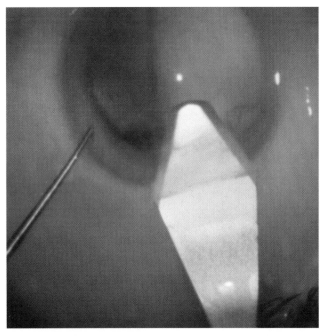

Photo 6.49. Enlarging the incision for IOL insertion. Concentrate at the external wound.

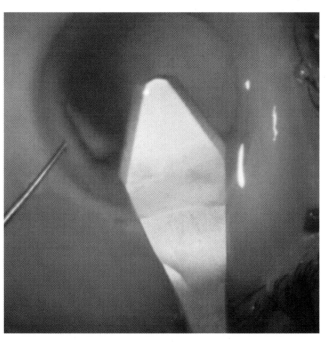

Photo 6.50. Advance the shoulder beyond the internal wound parallel to the iris plane.

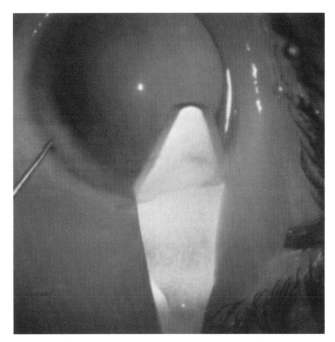

Photo 6.51. Enlarging the incision outside-in.

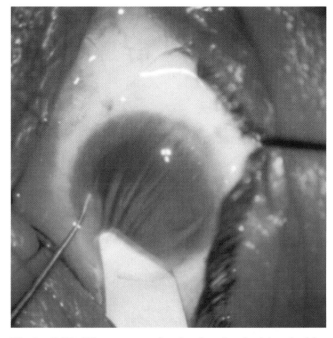

Photo 6.52. Wrong way of enlarging the incision inside-out.

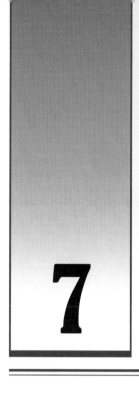

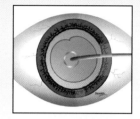

7

Continuous Curvilinear Capsulorrhexis

The single most important development that has made phaco and Small Incision Cataract Surgery popular is Continuous Curvilinear Capsulorrhexis (CCC). The continuity of CCC gives strength to the capsule to withstand wide fluctuations in IOP as well as bombardment with the phaco probe and nuclear fragments. The CCC not only maintains the integrity of the capsular bag but also keeps the nuclear fragments in the posterior chamber. This facilitates posterior chamber phaco, which helps to safeguard the cornea. With the advent of CCC, the problems of optic decentralization and pupillary capture have become almost non-existent. This has permitted evolution of the small optic lens, thereby reducing the incision size. It has also effectively reduced the posterior capsular opacification rate by ensuring that the IOL remains in the bag, in close contact with the posterior capsule, thus preventing migration of the epithelial cells.

APPLIED ANATOMY (Figs. 7.1 & 7.2)

The capsular bag is 10–11 mm in diameter. The thickness of the capsule varies in the different parts. Zonular fibres are attached to the lens capsule in a criss-cross pattern at the equator, anterior and posterior surfaces of the lens, and leave about 6–7 mm of central capsule clear. The anterior capsule is a basement membrane with a lining of proliferating epithelium. The young anterior capsule is very elastic, i.e. it stretches a lot before tearing. With advancing age the capsule becomes firmer. Between the age of 40 to 60 years it is usually easiest to handle. On further maturation, it may become atrophic or fibrotic,

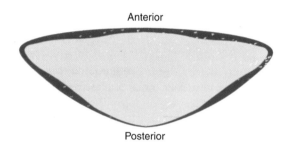

Fig. 7.1. Thickness of the capsule. Note that it is thinnest at the posterior pole and thickest at the insertion of zonular fibres.

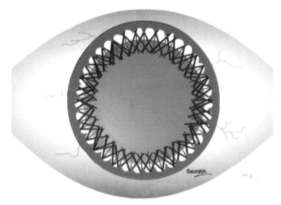

Fig. 7.2. Zonular attachment to the capsule. Note that the CCC should be kept within the central 6–7 mm to avoid the areas of zonular attachment. (The iris is not shown in the diagram.)

with or without calcification. Calcification is very common with hypermature, morgagnian absorbed cataract. In the hard nuclear cataract the capsule tends to be atrophic.

65

As soon as the capsule is opened, there is a tendency for the lens to be propelled out. This happens because of multiple factors, one of the most important factors is intralenticular pressure (ILP). ILP depends upon the fluid content of the bag and is therefore high in childhood and intumescent cataracts, whereas it is low in nuclear cataracts. Other factors which tend to push the nucleus out of CCC include vitreous upthrust, scleral rigidity, orbital fat in obese patients, tone of the rectus muscles, micro-retrobulbar haemorrhages, pressure by the lid, wire speculum and bridle sutures. These factors may also cause extension of CCC to the periphery.

PHYSICS OF CAPSULORRHEXIS
(Figs. 7.3 to 7.9)

Understanding the direction and the type of forces is essential to create a continuous curvilinear capsulo-rrhexis.

Types of force

1. **Ripping:** Using a ripping motion, the tear obtained will be uncontrolled. Since many fibres are pulled, all at different angles and with differing force, the break-point will not be simultaneous and thus the tear will be uncontrolled.

2. **Shearing:** In this, one fibre is broken at a time. Thus, the tear is more controlled and requires much less force.

Tangential force (Figs. 7.5 to 7.9)

A line perpendicular to the radius at any point on a circle is the tangent at that point. Any force applied in this direction is **Tangential Force**. The direction of tangential force is continuously changing. Movement of the needle should be curvilinear along the proposed margin of CCC (nearly superimposing). If the angle of the force is not changed as the flap advances, the angle will be more than 90° and the cut will extend to periphery. If the angle of the force is less than 90° then cut end will move in resulting in a CCC smaller than planned. The above two principles can be utilized in increasing or decreasing the size of CCC.

SIZE OF CCC

The optic size of the phaco-profile IOLs varies between 5.5 mm ± 0.5 mm. The CCC should cover the optic of the IOL by 0.25 mm circumferentially. Thus the ideal CCC is 5 mm ± 0.5 mm and well centred. This presses

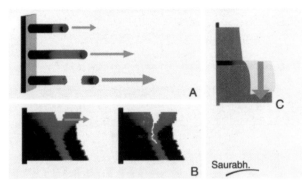

Fig. 7.3. (A) With the application of force (red arrow), the fibre stretches and then breaks. The blue zone denotes the stretch of the fibre. (B) **Ripping force:** When the same force (red arrow) is applied to a sheet of fibres, there is varying force on the different fibres which stretch and break at different sites resulting in an uncontrolled uneven tear. (C) **Shearing force** causes stretch of one fibre at a time, a controlled tear is obtained.

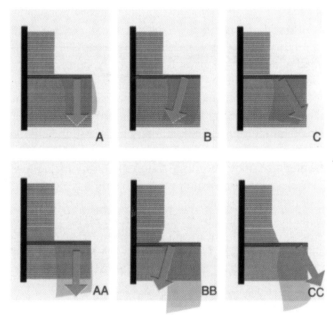

Fig. 7.4. Direction of shearing force—By varying the direction of force (red arrow) the direction of the tear can be controlled.

the IOL optic against the posterior capsule, preventing opaci-fication, keeps the IOL centred and does not interfere with the visualization of posterior segment. This size of CCC is good enough for easy removal of majority of the cataracts and is also easiest to control. A larger CCC (> 5.5 mm) has a high tendency to go to the area of zonular fibres. The zonular fibres do not only interfere with the smooth movement of CCC, but also tend to pull it outwards.

TANGENTIAL FORCE

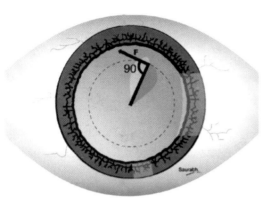

Fig. 7.5. Arrow shows the direction of tangential force 'F' to be applied.

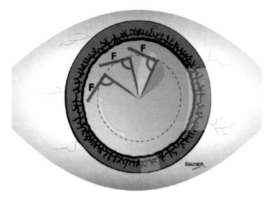

Fig. 7.6. Note that direction of force 'F' is continuously changing as the CCC proceeds.

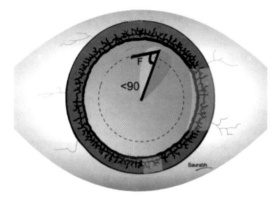

Fig. 7.7. The size of CCC can be reduced by decreasing the angle of the force applied to less than 90 degree.

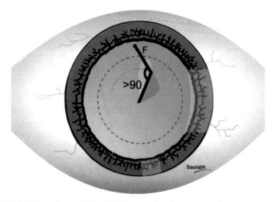

Fig. 7.8. The size of the CCC can be increased by increasing the angle of the force applied to more than 90 degree.

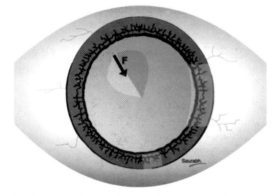

Fig. 7.9A. Applying a ripping force towards the centre instead of a tangential shearing force will result in a tear (dotted line).

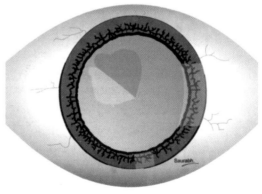

Fig. 7.9B. "Flower petal" CCC due to application of uncontrolled ripping force.

INSTRUMENTS (Fig. 7.10)

Cystitome

The cystitome is usually made out of 26 G needle by turning the tip twice. The first turn is at the bevel which may be turned out (more common) or in. For this, the tip of the needle is held at the hub with a CV needle holder (at the fulcrum of the needle holder for a better grip, if needle is held closer to the tip of the needle holder then grip will not be good) and turned by 1/3rd of the bevel

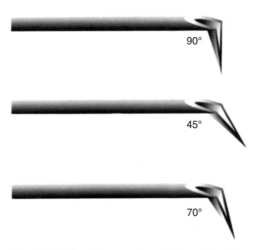

Fig. 7.10. Cystitome—Angulation of the tip.

length. For a shallow chamber, a smaller tip is made. Normally recommended angle is 90° but we personally prefer 70° to provide better visualization of the tip during CCC while maintaining a reasonably good grip. With a 90° turn, the grip is excellent but visualization of the tip is hampered. Visualisation is better with 45° turn but the hold is poor.

The second turn of the needle is at the junction of the hub and the needle. This may be by 60° or according to the convenience of the surgeon. Too large a turn at the hub may bring the surgeon's fingers in the field of view. The needle is then mounted on a Leur-locked syringe.

Forceps

In certain situations, forceps are useful. Utratta's is ideal but McPherson's can also be used. Many modifications of Utratta forceps have been introduced. The forceps should have reasonably good tensile strength so that one can feel when one is holding the capsule. On release, the forceps should open easily. With repeated autoclaving they tend to lose this elasticity. A good Utratta forceps is an essential instrument for all phaco surgeons. Co-axial capsular rhexis forceps are very useful particularly while doing microphaco. Additionally, they can be used from the side port, whenever rhexis has gone out or has a tendency to do so.

PRE-REQUISITES

The pre-requisites for a good CCC are:

1. Good akinesia
2. Moderate hypotony: For phacoemulsification, moderate hypotony is required. The eye should not

be very soft (as required for ECCE) since nucleotomy becomes difficult.

3. Good red reflex: Following measures should be taken for a good red reflex:
   - The lipid layer of the tear film is removed by scrubbing with a betadine-soaked swabstick and washing with BSS simultaneously. Clean thoroughly till there are no oily/shiny reflexes.
   - Position the eyeball and head in such a way so as to obtain a good red reflex.
   - Remove all the annoying reflexes which are usually caused by the eye drapes, steridrape and pooled fluids. This can be achieved by decreasing the diameter of the light beam so that there is less light on the drapes and by avoiding the use of steridrape.
   - Microscope settings: Use high magnification. Focus on the capsule or the iridocapsular junction. Bedewing appearance of the capsule may be seen when focussed exactly.
   - The pupil should be well dilated with mydriatic. We routinely use intracameral adrenaline, 0.05–0.1 ml of 1 : 10 dilution. 0.3 to 0.5 ml adrenaline in 1 : 1000 dilution may be added to 500 ml of irrigation fluid for sustained dilatation.
   - The aqueous in AC should be totally replaced with viscoelastic. The addition of VES on the cornea removes the lipid layer, increases clarity and prevents drying. It also acts as a positive lens and enhances visibility.
   - Before entering the AC, pressurize the eyeball with viscoelastic till the lens-iris diaphragm moves backwards and the chamber is flat/concave in centre. Approximate IOP should be 30–35 mmHg. In soft eye conditions, there is no need to make the eye too concave. Too high IOP is not required. In a cramped chamber, IOP rise occurs early; do not make it too concave. ***Under no circumstances should rhexis be done in a shallow AC with a convex lens-iris diaphragm.***
   - Rhexis can be done from the main port or side port. Advantage of side port rhexis is that there is no leakage of viscoelastic, but there is less manoeuvrability. Rhexis from main port obviously means better manoeuvrability, but there is more leakage and one needs to keep reforming the chamber.

TECHNIQUES OF CCC

CCC can be done either with cystitome or forceps or a combination of the two.

NEEDLE CCC

Initiation

The AC should be well formed with VES. Before injecting into the AC, depress the plunger outside to remove air and then enter with the plunger depressed or else air will be drawn into the cannula. The cystitome is mounted on a viscoelastic-filled syringe, taking care that it is tightly fixed. With gentle pressure on the plunger (to prevent an air bubble from entering) enter the tunnel with knee of the turned bevel. Keeping the direction of the tunnel in mind, advance the cystitome forward with a gentle sideways motion till you reach the inner lip. Once you reach the inner lip of the wound, turn the needle such that the tip enters first (knee first can cause Descemet's tear). If you find it difficult to enter the tunnel with the cystitome, the tunnel can be opened by lifting the roof with a rounded iris repositor.

Linear cut (Fig. 7.11)

The needle is kept vertical at the exact centre or slightly left of the centre of the pupil. Press it gently downwards to perforate the capsule. Now tilt the needle slightly towards the right and move in a linear fashion towards the right creating a cut of approximately 1.5 mm in length. Linear extension can also be done by multiple punctures as in 'can opener technique' from uncut to cut area.

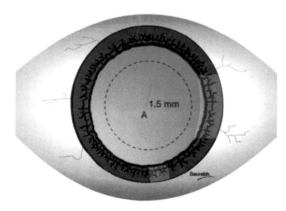

Fig. 7.11. Initiation of CCC—horizontal cut of 1.5 mm is made, starting from the centre 'A'.

Raising the flap (Fig. 7.12)

The needle is then brought to the junction of medial 2/3rd and lateral 1/3rd of the cut. Put the needle under

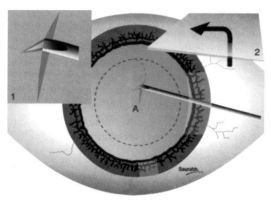

Fig. 7.12. Lift the flap by placing the cystitome at the junction of the central 2/3rd and the outer 1/3rd of the initial cut (inset 1) and lifting up and then pushing the flap down (inset 2 showing direction of force). Correct application of forces will result in a curvilinear extension of 1–1.5 mm as shown by the dotted line.

the cut edge and try to lift the cut edge *up towards* the ceiling. After stress is created, snap open the flap. The initial force will be directed towards the ceiling and as soon as you get the feeling of give-way then turn it down, giving a curvilinear extension of approximately 1 mm and 1 to 1½ hours in radial fashion. Now the cut end is approximately 2.5 mm from the centre and if the rhexis is continued parallel to the pupillary border, it will be 5 mm in diameter.

Problems in Initiation (Figs. 7.13 to 7.15)

1. The initial puncture may be slightly to the right of the centre. If the CCC is continued, it will end up eccentric. To correct this, extend the initial cut towards centre by cutting from uncut to cut area. If the initial puncture is towards the left, you may continue with CCC. The only problem faced in this situation is that the flap is large in size.
2. While trying to make the initial cut, the needle must not be pushed too deep into the cataract as this disturbs the cortical fibres, which then interfere with the visibility of the cut edge. While attempting to lift the flap also one has to take care not to disturb the cortex.
3. At times the needle edges are not sharp and instead of a single linear cut, a triangular tear is obtained. The guiding principle is – turn triangular flap if possible. A triangular flap will have an upper and lower edge. If both these tears are equal and not very large, then the tear close to the incision may be extended towards the periphery and turned downwards to create a flap for CCC, so that the other tear

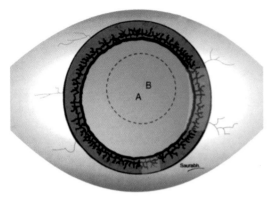

Fig. 7.13. Problems in initiation. Initiation off axis—Starting away from the centre 'A' will result in an off centre CCC.

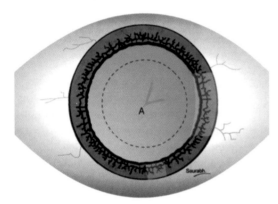

Fig. 7.14A. Triangular flap at initiation.

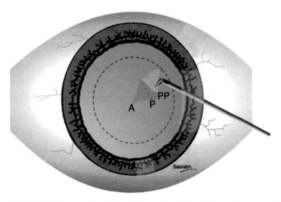

Fig. 7.14B. Proceed with raising the flap from the proximal cut edge 'P' to 'PP'.

will get incorporated into the flap. Some surgeons plan the initiation of CCC with creation of triangular flap. To deliberately create a triangular flap, place the tilted needle on the centre and pull the capsule towards the right without perforating the capsule. The advantage of this technique is that snap opening is avoided and since the capsule is not perforated, the cortical fibres are not disturbed.

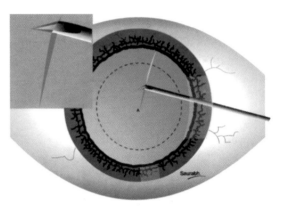

Fig. 7.15. Problems in initiation—If the flap is lifted from the periphery of the initial cut (inset), the tear will go to the periphery instead of making a curvilinear extension.

4. If the needle is kept at the peripheral edge of the cut to snap open, instead of at the junction of 2/3rd and 1/3rd, the cut end, instead of extending curvilinearly, gets extended further towards the periphery. Another mistake is trying to push the flap downwards instead of upwards. The needle keeps slipping and a good grip is not obtained. This may disturb the cortical matter or cause the cut to extend peripherally.

Continuation of CCC (Figs. 7.16 to 7.20)

There should be sufficient amount of flap so that it can be turned over such that the anterior surface of the flap is touching the intact capsule. This can be achieved by either pushing it over with the cystitome or using VES, or a combination of both. Once it starts lifting, push it down with cystitome and keep it pressed for a couple of seconds. If it is large enough and the chamber is stable, it will stay down. However, if it is small (i.e. small curvilinear extension) or the AC is shallow (not enough VES) then the flap will keep turning back. In that case you will have to increase the curvilinear extension if you want to complete the CCC with cystitome. In order to achieve this position, you either push the flap at the peripheral end or release at the centre if required. At this point, it is to be emphasized that you need to have a mental picture of your proposed CCC with relation to the pupillary border before progressing.

The needle is kept on the line of proposed CCC approximately 1 mm away from the cut end, for good control. To initiate the movement, the flap is gradually stretched such that there is a tactile feedback before it gives way and tears. If the needle is too close to the cut end, it tears too soon and you are not able to maintain

CONTINUATION OF CCC

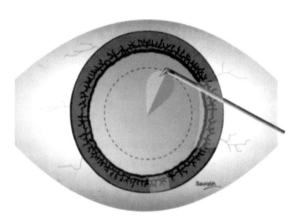

Fig. 7.16. Turning the flap—The flap is turned over so that it lies on the uncut surface of the capsule.

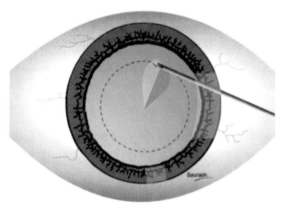

Fig. 7.17. The flap is moved so that the cut edge lies beyond the proposed line of CCC.

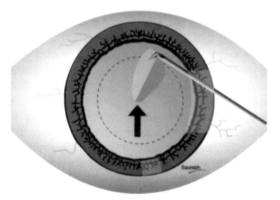

Fig. 7.18. If it is not moving, release at the centre so that it can move.

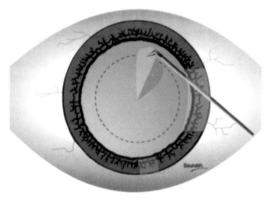

Fig. 7.19. Shearing force is applied such that the flap moves on or parallel to proposed line of CCC.

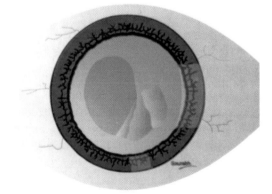

Fig. 7.20A. As the CCC progresses, the flap will enlarge and get crumpled.

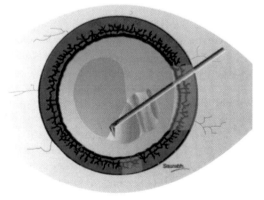

Fig. 7.20B. The flap must be smoothened out before advancing. Note that the corner of the incision is used for correct placement of the cystitome.

control. If you keep too far away, applying a tangential force is difficult and you lose control of the direction. Normally, in one push, you can achieve 1–3 clock hours of CCC. The flap should be flat without any wrinkles.

Beginners may need to repeatedly flatten the flap and try to move it. It may need over 6–12 strokes for completion. The needle should be kept lightly on the flap so that it can push the flap. The cystitome should be slid along the flap, gradually increasing the pressure till the resistance is overcome and the flap starts moving. Pushing it down causes dimpling of the capsule and then the CCC will not proceed smoothly.

As in driving, you watch the road and not the steering wheel, similarly, after positioning the needle, concentrate on the movement of the advancing end of the CCC and do not look at the needle. There should be no fold between the cut end and the needle—if it appears you will definitely lose control of CCC. You must immediately stop and reposition the flap before proceeding.

Completion of CCC (Figs. 7.21 & 7.22)

Usually it is possible to comfortably come up to the left of the incision, i.e. 8 clock hours. When the CCC reaches sub-incisional area there are some problems. Visibility is poor due to the corneal tunnel. The flap is now large and tends to flow out of the section. There is less space

Completion of CCC

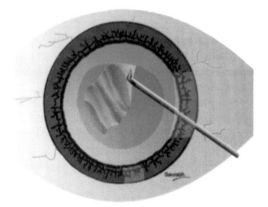

Fig. 7.21. As the CCC nears completion, the large flap tends to flow out of the section obscuring visibility. Reposit the flap towards the centre so that the endpoint is clearly seen. Also note the use of left corner of the incision.

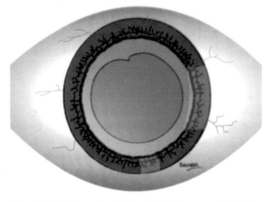

Fig. 7.22. Complete the CCC from outside-in.

to manoeuvre the instruments. Take the flap well away from the incision and spread it so that it lies towards the centre with the edge lying flat over the uncut capsule. Using the full length of the incision, the needle is angulated from the corner of the incision so that the flap is pulled towards the centre of incision or beyond, if possible. Reposition the flap and now use the other corner of the incision to push the flap. Once you have crossed the incision, the flap should be positioned so that you can visualise the point of finish. CCC is completed from outside-in to have a perfect round CCC.

If one finds it difficult to complete the CCC, then one can make the rhexis a little smaller at 12 O'clock/sub-incisional area. Once you reach the sub-incisional area, presume that the rhexis is going out and start making it smaller. Though you will get a pear-shaped rhexis, it will not pose any problem during surgery. Also, one can finish the rhexis with forceps or use the side port for completion of CCC with the cystitome.

FORCEPS CCC

Though CCC can be done comfortably in most situations with the cystitome, there are some circumstances in which the forceps is invaluable. Thus, knowledge of this technique is important.

The biggest disadvantage of the forceps is that it is bulky and because of the flat grip, initially seems difficult to manoeuvre. Also, it causes more wound leak and distortion of the cornea. It is particularly difficult to use if you are using low viscosity viscoelastic, e.g. methyl cellulose. Thus, it is better used with high viscosity visco-elastic, e.g. Healon GV/Healon. It cannot be used from the side port or under air/BSS. Also, when initiating the CCC, the puncture may not be as comfortable with the forceps; so it is better to initiate with the needle and then continue with forceps. The biggest advantage of the forceps is that the grip on the flap is very good and no counter-pressure is required. Also, it is easier to change the direction of the flap. Forceps is particularly useful in fibrotic, atrophic and elastic (i.e. paediatric) capsules and in soft cataract with high intralenticular pressure (morgagnian and intumescent) where one is not able to get a good counter-pressure. Posterior CCC and paediatric cataracts are not possible with cystitome and require use of forceps. Co-axial forceps are very good for the purpose as they can be easily passed from the side port causing minimal viscoelastic leak.

Technique (Photos 7.1 to 7.18)

All other pre-requisites are the same. It is advisable to use high viscosity VES and perform it through the main port. Forceps are introduced horizontally and then made vertical. With the closed tip, perforate the capsule in the centre to raise the flap. Alternatively, one can open the tip, pinch the capsule and then tear.

This flap created should be well within the desired CCC size. Once the grip on the flap has been obtained the CCC is initiated. The flap is brought to the desired line of CCC. The ideal grip is close to the leading edge with one tooth on the undersurface and one tooth on the anterior surface of the flap. However, if the flap is lying flat one can hold with the undersurface as well. Usually, it is possible to complete more clock hours of CCC at one go than with the cystitome.

After making the initial quadrant one should release the flap in a way that it is in a suitable position for holding again (i.e. in a vertical position). This repositioning should be done before releasing the flap. Therefore in the cross-incisional area the flap should be radial to the incision. For sub-incisional area the periphery of the torn flap should point towards the incision (thus the torn edge should always be pointing to the incision site).

COMBINATION CCC (Photos 7.19 to 7.28)

It is easier to initiate the CCC with a needle. After raising the flap and completing the initial quadrant, the flap can now be comfortably advanced with the forceps up to the sub-incisional area. Completion is more convenient with the needle. For anticlockwise CCC, right half of the CCC is easier with the needle and left half is easier with the forceps.

Loss of control of CCC (Photos 7.29 to 7.35)

Why we lose control

In some rare situations the tear runs out as soon as the capsule is opened. This is because of high intralenticular pressure (ILP). However, usually the cause of losing control is not paying due attention to the pre-requisites. The surgeon may have to pay heavily for his reluctance to do canthotomy or for proceeding in a hurry in the presence of inadequate hypotony. In high risk cases, high viscosity viscoelastic is a good investment to prevent the CCC from extending. **Application of wrong forces (cutting, ripping) or the right force in wrong manner, are major causes of extension of CCC in the hands of beginners.**

Some beginners use the edge of needle to cut the capsule like a paper knife. This results in an uncontrolled tear. Application of a ripping force leads to uncontrolled CCC. Inability to position the flap beyond the presumed line of CCC, or not holding the flap on the undersurface result in failure in applying tangential force. Force applied in such situations is usually ripping in nature. Some beginners, in their enthusiasm to obtain a good grip on the flap, press the needle too hard. Thus, the force is transmitted to the anterior surface of the capsule lying below, resulting in tear by ripping as if no flap has been turned. Beginners may inadvertently apply ripping force by trying to pull the flap radially, fearing that the CCC may go out and thus a flower petal shaped CCC is obtained. Also, if the needle is kept too close to the cut edge, application of shearing force is difficult. Sometimes, even experts may use ripping force when they are in a hurry.

In a properly applied shearing force, the initial CCC comes out perfectly. After a point, one needs to regrasp the flap. This may be indicated by the appearance of a fold between the cut edge and the cystitome. If CCC is continued with the flap in this position, then it will rip open.

It is important to recognize early that the CCC is going out and stop immediately and manage appropriately. Early recognition is possible if one concentrates on keeping the CCC parallel to the pupillary border.

How to regain control (Photos 7.36 to 7.49)

Correct any missing pre-requisite, i.e. red reflex, deep chamber, etc. *Identification of the exact location of the cut edge is absolutely essential.* For this, increase the magnification, improve visibility by putting VE on cornea and smoothen out the disturbed capsule and cortical fibres with a rounded repositor. **DO NOT PANIC.** After identifying the cut edge, with the cystitome, turn the flap such that it now lies along the proposed new margin of CCC. Now apply a tangential force with the cystitome on the line of proposed CCC. Once the flap starts moving *then* change the direction to bring the CCC into the original proposed line (i.e. smaller). This change of direction may be slow if you are in the cross-incisional area or rapidly if you are in sub-incisional area. The same thing can be done with the forceps if the flap is in a position that is more comfortable to hold with the forceps. The grip may be better with forceps especially when you are in the periphery where the zonular attachments may prevent the smooth movement of the flap with the cystitome.

If this fails you can try a planned ripping. Keeping the flap radial try to pull it towards the centre with some force. At times this may work.

Since cross-incisional control of CCC is easier, depending on the site of extension, one can use a cystitome from the side port or, another valvular tunnel (2–2.8 mm) can be made 90° to the site and you can try to control the CCC from there. Enlarging the existing side port will result in a leaking wound that will hamper the rest of the surgery. The surgeon can even change his sitting position (i.e. from temporal to superior) for further convenience.

If you cannot complete the CCC from the point of loss, you can try to make a flap from the other side. There are various techniques:

1. Raise a flap from the starting point. Proceed clockwise.
2. **Create a T**—Either create a horizontal flap and cut with Vannas in the middle. Or give a radial cut with cystitome, pull the flap towards the incision. Then give a cut with Vannas at the radial cut to complete the CCC on the other side.

The attempt is to complete the CCC by taking the flap from outside in so that there are no cones. If you are not able to do so, then integrity of CCC is doubtful and you should probably convert.

DYES IN CCC (Photos 7.50 to 7.60)

Dyes are indicated in cases where the visibility of anterior capsule is poor like in hypermature and morgagnian cataract. There is no red reflex and no contrast. Therefore, identification of cut end is difficult in such situations. Some beginners find it easy to perform CCC under dye even in immature cataract. This could be of use in immature cataract if the operating microscope does not have co-axial light. Dyes are not a substitute to learning to do good CCC. Additional advantage of the dye is that the CCC margin can be identified during nucleotomy, but I/A is difficult as subcapsular fibres are not clearly visible.

Trypan blue and indocyanine green (ICG) are the commonly used dyes. Both the dyes are effective and without any side effects. ICG is expensive. Therefore, trypan blue is more popular. It is commercially manufactured in India. Trypan blue in a vial can be autoclaved and re-used but repeated autoclaving may increase the concentration. For one time use autoclaving is not needed.

Technique

To prevent corneal staining, inject air into AC through the side port. Air bubble should be of moderate size reaching up to or beyond pupillary border (6–7 mm diameter). Do not try to inflate the eye completely from limbus to limbus, since the air starts leaking as soon as trypan blue is injected and chamber may collapse. If the cornea gets stained in the periphery, do not worry, as it does not interfere with the surgery.

Trypan blue is taken in a syringe with 27 G cannula. Go beneath the air bubble to centre of the capsule and inject. Keep spreading the dye on the capsule. Make sure that whole of capsule is adequately covered with the dye. Now quickly replace the dye, air and aqueous with VE by starting the injection from the cross-incisional area. This will push both the dye and air out of the side port incision. In this manner corneal staining is prevented and if slight staining is present, it is washed off as soon as phaco is started. Now CCC is done as usual or one can attempt to do sinusoidal CCC. The amount of dye and duration of leaving it in AC is immaterial as long as the capsule is adequately stained and cornea is not.

If you have injected the viscoelastics already such as in small pupil for placement of iris retractors, or after starting the CCC you find visibility is not good, then one can simply stain and place the dye between anterior capsule and the viscoelastic substance. It will serve the purpose.

ENLARGEMENT OF CCC (Fig. 7.23)

Since chances of a small CCC extending to the periphery are less, so beginners tend to make small CCC. In a soft/moderately hard cataract it is usually possible to complete phaco and CCC may be enlarged after putting the IOL. In grade IV cataract or above it is difficult to perform phaco from CCC less than 4 mm. Therefore, in these cases one should enlarge the CCC before attempting phaco.

Right side of CCC is cut obliquely with Vannas for a millimetre. The triangular flap is grasped with Utrata forceps and the desired rim of CCC is removed, ideally all around for 360° by repeatedly regrasping the flap. However, even removal of 180° or so facilitates the surgery to a large extent. If the CCC is good enough for the type of cataract present, then it is best to enlarge it after IOL insertion. The optic size gives a good idea about size of CCC required, the visibility improves and even if it goes out, there is no danger of nucleus drop. It is

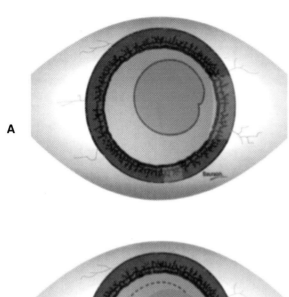

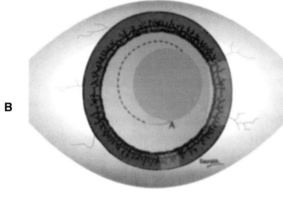

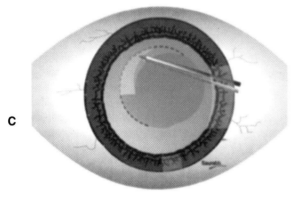

Fig. 7.23. Enlarging the CCC. (A) A small eccentric CCC created. (B) Make a nick with the Vannas at 'A'. (C) Enlarge the CCC by starting from the cut end removing a strip with the Utrata forceps.

necessary to enlarge a small CCC, since there are higher chances of capsular contracture syndrome, PCO and management of posterior segment disease will be difficult

if you don't. Therefore, enlargement in myopes and diabetics is desirable. Enlargement after capsular contracture syndrome may be difficult. It is not easy to laser the CCC and patient is subjected to an additional intraocular surgery.

CCC IN YOUNG PATIENTS (Photos 7.61 to 7.67)

The direction of force should be centripetal. No attempt should be made to spread the flap along the proposed line of CCC. Proceed slowly as the CCC has a tendency to extend peripherally.

POSTERIOR CAPSULORRHEXIS

There are a few indications for primary PCC. This is required in cases where there is a thick posterior capsular plaque. Also in cases where there is a small PC rent, this can be converted into a PCC to avoid inadvertent extension. Pediatric cataracts remain the most common indication.

Technique

Inflate the bag with Healon. Just above the centre, perforate the PC with a 26 G needle attached to Healon GV. Inject a few drops into the space between PC and anterior hyaloid face to separate them. While withdrawing the needle make a radial cut (1–2 mm long). Now using the Vannas make a small perpendicular cut to create a triangular flap. This flap can now be easily grasped with the Utrata forceps. Tear it along the proposed line of PCC; usually 4 mm is adequate.

One needs to continuously regrasp the flap close to the cut edge since the posterior capsule is very stretchable. The stretchability means that the whole of the capsule gets pulled and at times so distorted that one cannot visualize where the rhexis is going, i.e., along the proposed margin or into the periphery. Trying to initiate CCC with needle is difficult because of the stretchability of the capsule. The capsule tends to go out of focus and there is no counter-pressure for the cystitome.

If the PCR is in or around the central area and there is only cortex/epinucleus remaining then this can be converted into a smooth round opening which will not get extended. This is particularly useful if a foldable implant is planned, more so the silicon lenses.

FORCEPS CCC

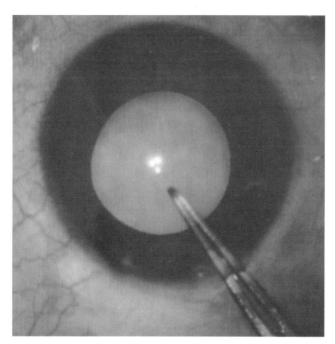

Photo 7.1. Enter with the closed forceps.

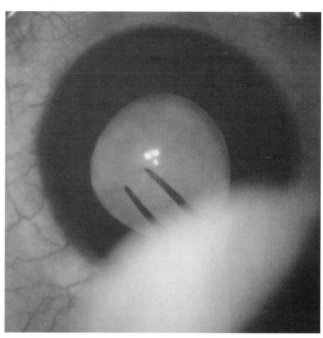

Photo 7.2. Open the forceps and pinch the capsule to create flap.

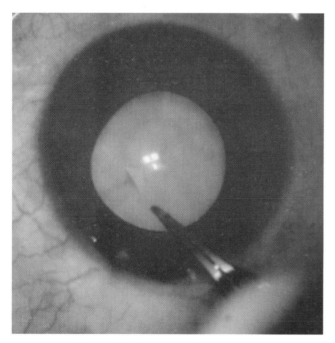

Photo 7.3. Triangular flap created.

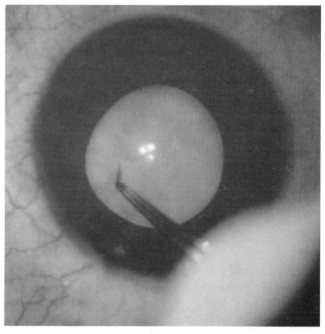

Photo 7.4. Hold the edge of flap towards the incision to incorporate the other cut end into the CCC.

FORCEPS CCC (Contd.)

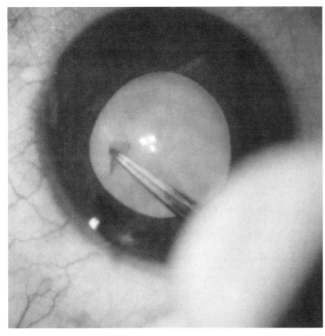

Photo 7.5. Hold the flap and start rotating in a clockwise direction. Note the incorporation of both cut ends of triangular flap.

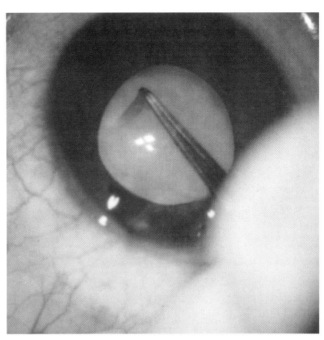

Photo 7.6. 2–3 clock hours of CCC completed in one stroke.

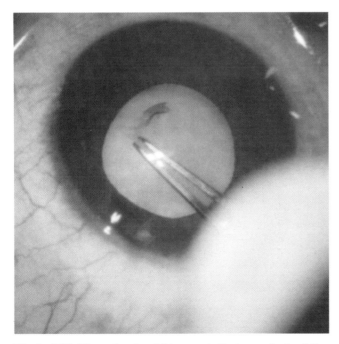

Photo 7.7. The grip should be such that one limb of the forceps is on the undersurface and the other on the anterior surface of the flap.

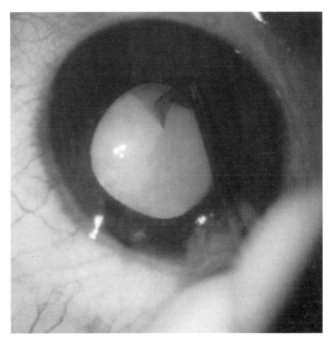

Photo 7.8. Another 2 clock hours of CCC completed. Note the cut end of CCC parallel to pupil.

FORCEPS CCC (Contd.)

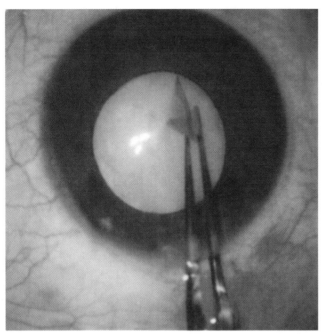

Photo 7.9. Before leaving the flap, it needs to be positioned for the next grip such that it is lying radial to the pupillary border.

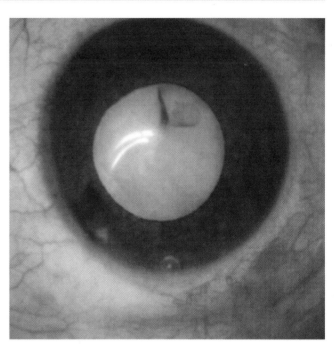

Photo 7.10. Flap radial to pupillary border.

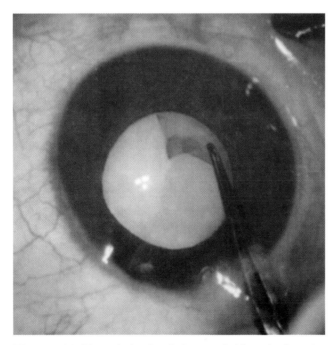

Photo 7.11. Though the flap is kept radial for gripping, the force remains tangenital and thus the flap is pulled along the pupillary margin.

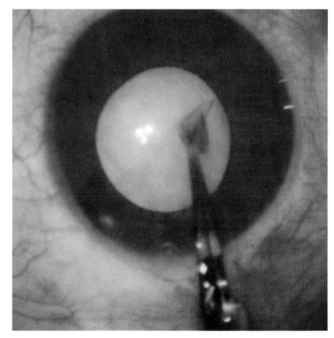

Photo 7.12. Two more clock hours completed. Note the cut end is left pointing towards the incision for a comfortable grip.

FORCEPS CCC (Contd.)

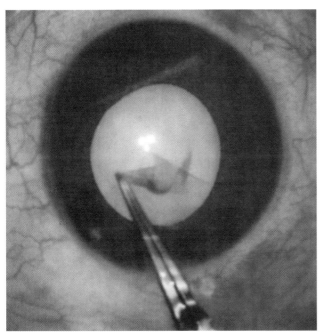

Photo 7.13. Two more clock hours to reach sub-incisional area.

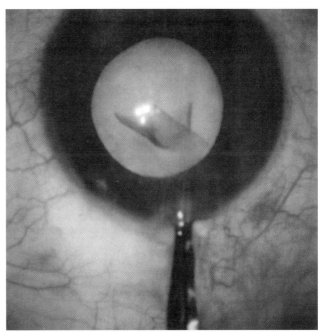

Photo 7.14. Note that the cut end of the flap is lying flat and parallel to the pupillary border. At this position, however, the CCC can be easily held from below and above. This is not possible in the cross-incisional area where one needs to leave the flap standing and vertical.

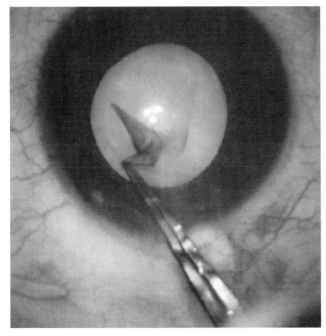

Photo 7.15. The flap is advanced past the sub-incisional area and regrasped.

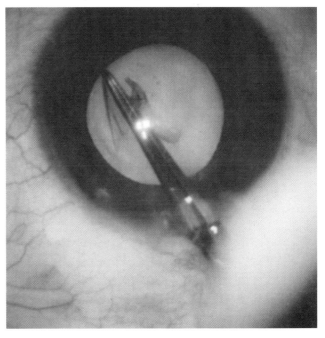

Photo 7.16. Under direct vision, the rhexis is completed from outside-in.

FORCEPS CCC (Contd.)

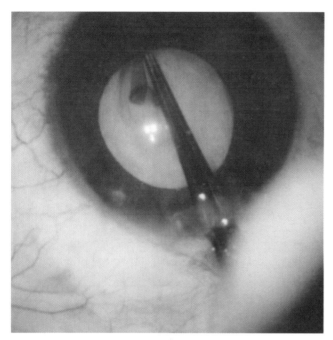

Photo 7.17. Keep holding the flap.

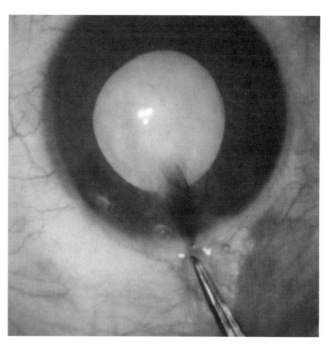

Photo 7.18. Pull the flap out of chamber.

COMBINATION CCC

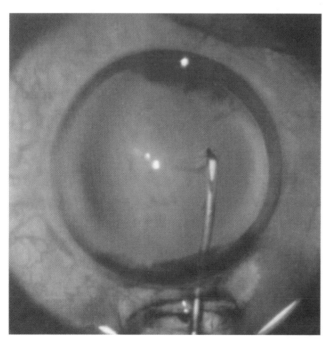

Photo 7.19. Initiation – Note the position of the needle. The flap is being lifted to create a curvilinear extension.

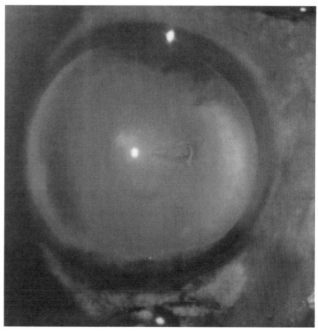

Photo 7.20. Curvilinear extension created and the flap is turned down. Antero-under grip with forceps is difficult.

COMBINATION CCC (Contd.)

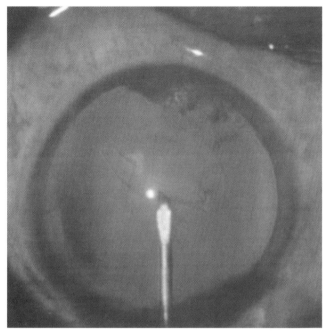

Photo 7.21. First quadrant is completed with needle.

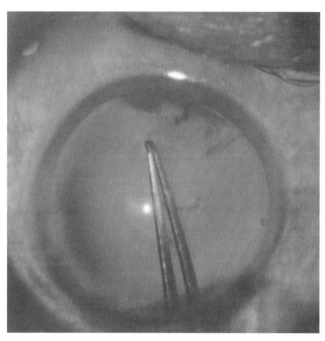

Photo 7.22. Ideal position for antero-under grip of the flap.

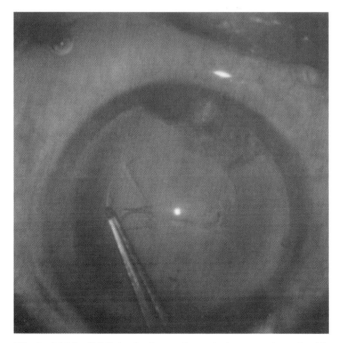

Photo 7.23. CCC in 2nd quadrant being continued with forceps.

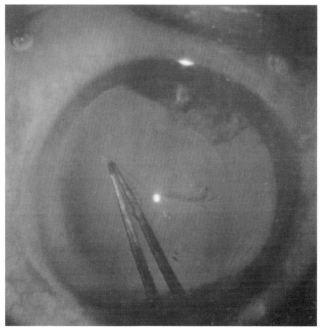

Photo 7.24. Flap left radially to regrasp with antero-under grip.

COMBINATION CCC (Contd.)

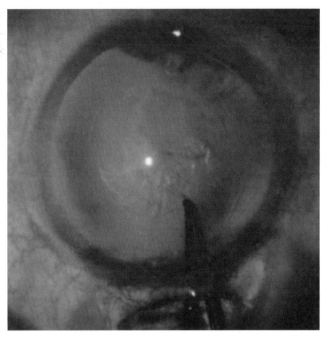

Photo 7.25. CCC advanced with forceps upto the sub-incisional area.

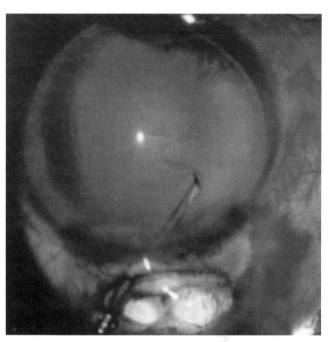

Photo 7.26. In sub-incisional area the antero-under forceps grip is difficult. It is easier to advance from this position with the needle.

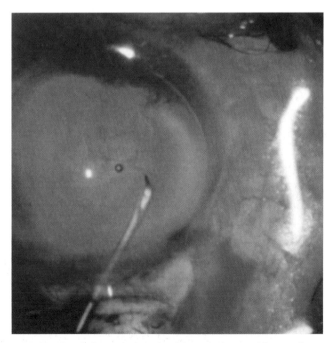

Photo 7.27. Completing the last quadrant with needle.

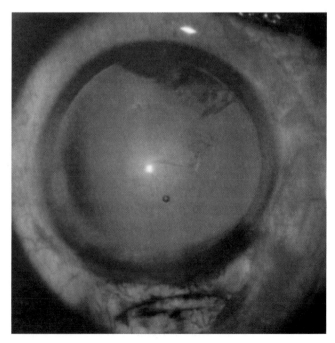

Photo 7.28. Completion of CCC from outside-in.

LOSS OF CONTROL

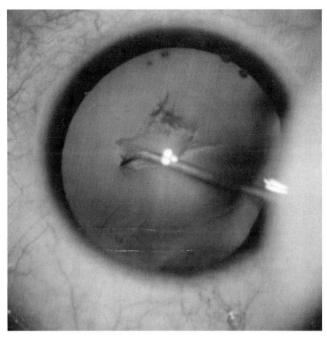

Photo 7.29. Tearing the cut edge like a paper knife instead of turning over and using the undersurface. Note the placement of the needle at the margin of inadequately turned flap. Needle being used to cut the flap.

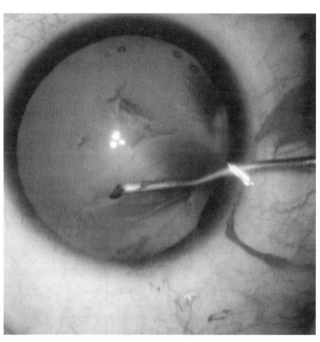

Photo 7.30. Needle kept at the edge of turned flap and attempt is being made to pull the flap by ripping force.

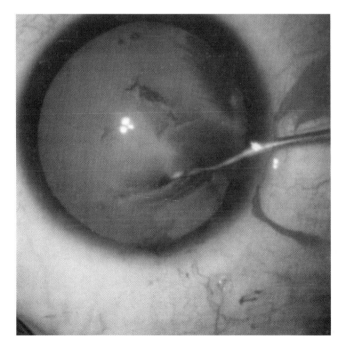

Photo 7.31. CCC being attempted on a crumpled flap, i.e. inadequately spread flap.

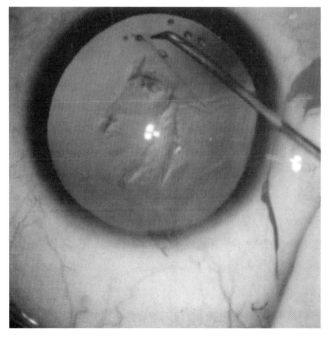

Photo 7.32. Attempt being made to continue CCC while stretch line has appeared. Now the tangenital force application is not possible.

LOSS OF CONTROL (Contd.)

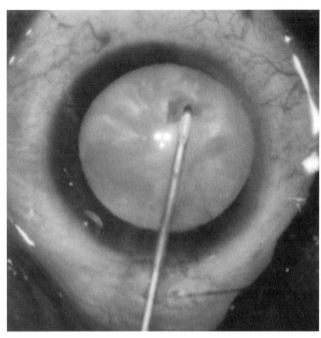

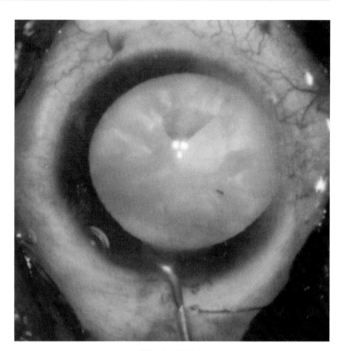

Photos 7.33, 7.34 & 7.35. High intralenticular pressure leading to loss of control of CCC. Note the tendency for the CCC to run out.

Photo 7.34.

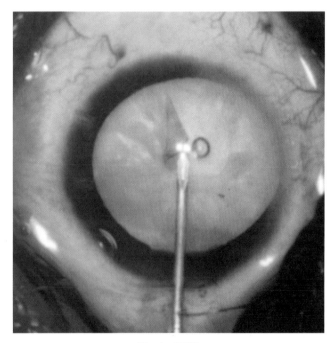

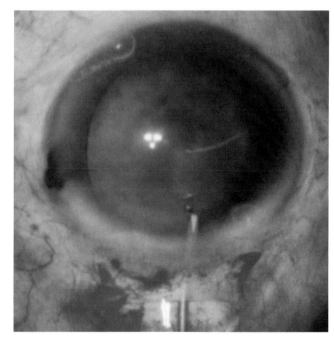

Photo 7.35.

Photo 7.36. Initial cut is large. Any attempt to make a curvilinear extension will go to periphery.

REGAINING CONTROL 1

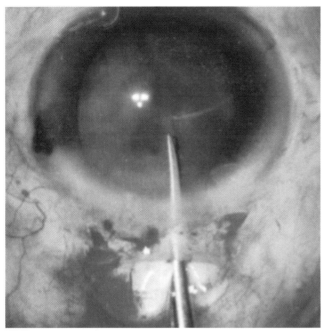

Photo 7.37. Radial cut perpendicular to the horizontal cut is made with Vannas.

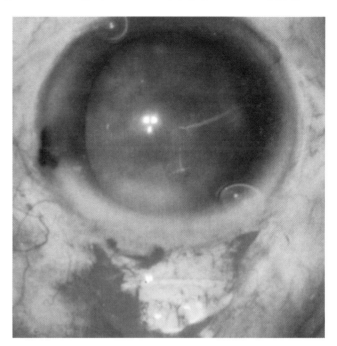

Photo 7.38. Creation of 'T' making two flaps.

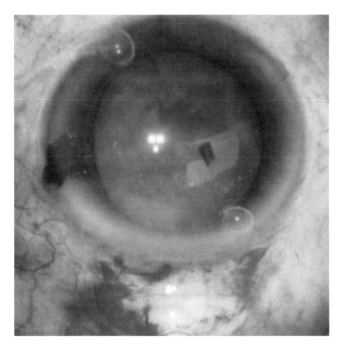

Photo 7.39. Lifting and completing CCC on one side. Attempt should have been made to complete from outside-in to avoid the creation of cone.

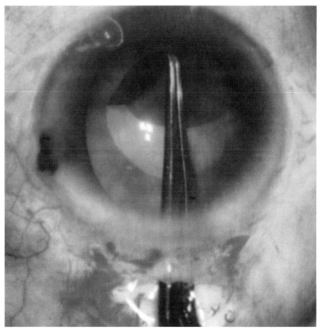

Photo 7.40. Lifting the other flap to make a controlled CCC.

REGAINING CONTROL 1 (Contd.)

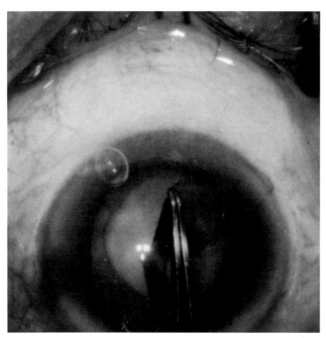

Photo 7.41. Attempt made to enlarge the CCC to complete from outside-in to eliminate the cone. Attachment of zonular fibres preventing the CCC from proceeding. Stretch line can be seen at the site of zonular attachment.

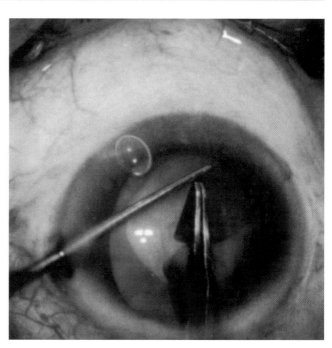

Photo 7.42. Breaking the zonules with rounded repositor.

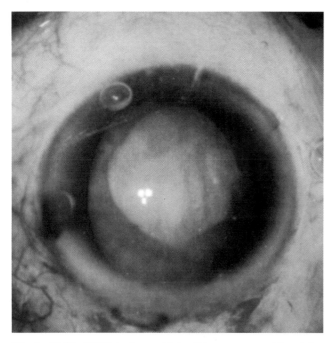

Photo 7.43. CCC is brought in. The cone could not be incorporated.

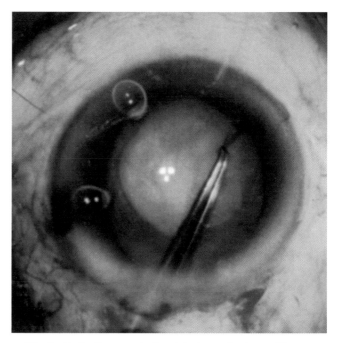

Photo 7.44. Removal of a strip to make it curvilinear.

REGAINING CONTROL 2

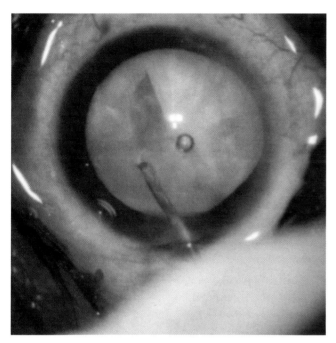

Photo 7.45. Make a radial cut.

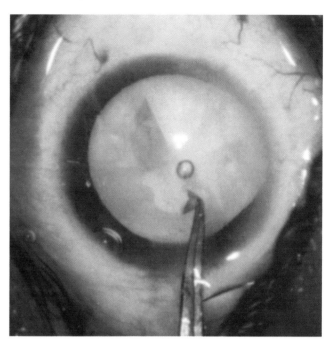

Photo 7.46. Pull the flap on one side to complete the CCC on that side.

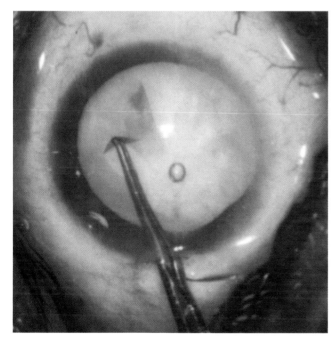

Photo 7.47. Push the other flap.

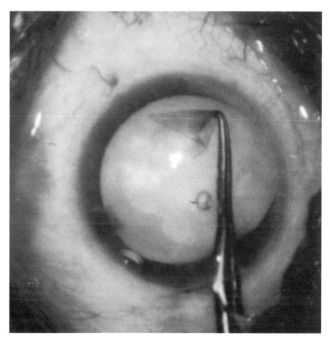

Photo 7.48. Complete the CCC on the other side.

DYES IN CCC (CONTROLLED METHOD)

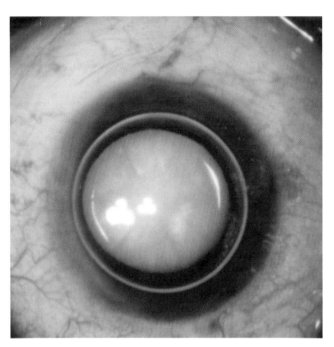

Photo 7.49. AC filled with air.

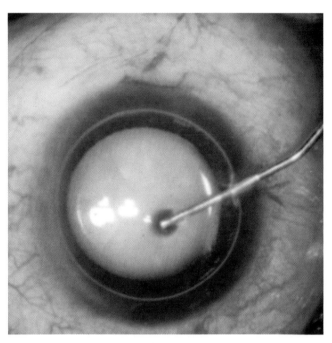

Photo 7.50. 27 G cannula attached to trypan blue dye filled syringe. Release of small amount of dye.

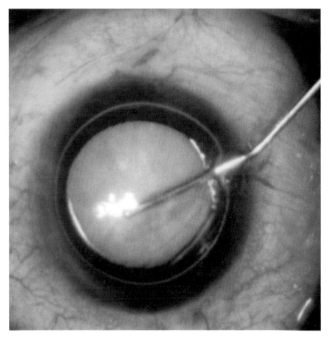

Photo 7.51. Sweep the cannula sideways to spread the dye.

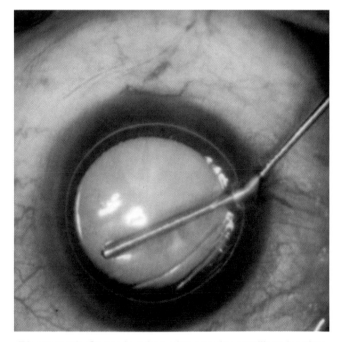

Photo 7.52. Cannula taken close to the pupillary border.

DYES IN CCC (CONTROLLED METHOD) (Contd.)

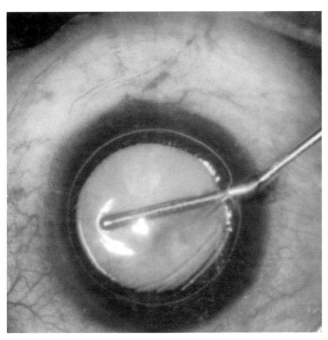

Photo 7.53. Go to another site and repeat the procedure.

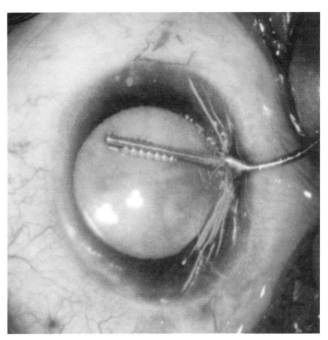

Photo 7.54. Repeat the procedure close to incision.

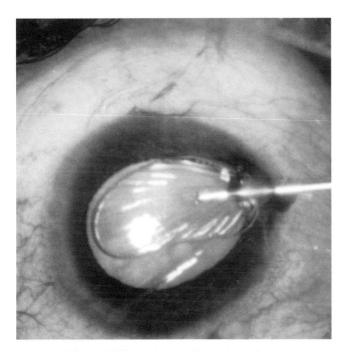

Photo 7.55. Leakage of air takes place.

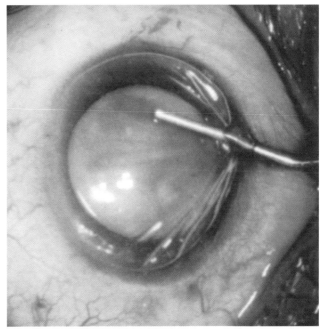

Photo 7.56. Inflate the AC and proceed to the new area.

DYES IN CCC (USUAL METHOD)

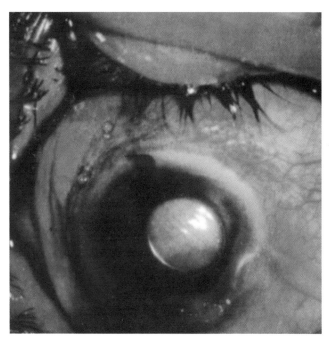

Photo 7.57. Inject dye under air.

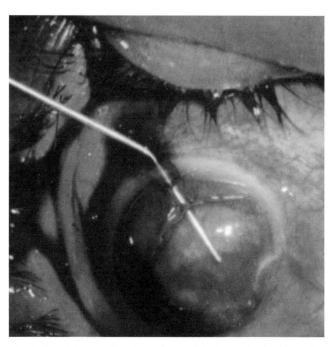

Photo 7.58. Immediately replace with viscoelastic. Note the dark staining.

NEEDLE CCC IN YOUNG PATIENT

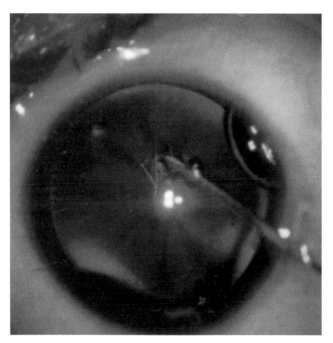

Photo 7.59. Raising the flap.

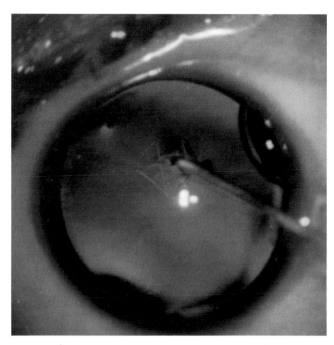

Photo 7.60. Flap turned down. Note that no attempt is made to spread it along the proposed line of CCC.

NEEDLE CCC IN YOUNG PATIENT (Contd.)

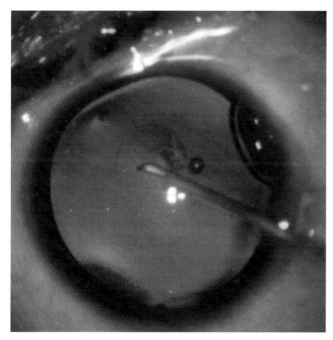

Photo 7.61. Note the position of the needle, closer to the centre, so that a radial force can be applied.

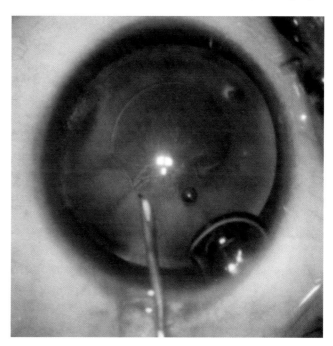

Photo 7.62. Flap flattened out to grip from the undersurface. No attempt is made to spread it along the proposed line of CCC.

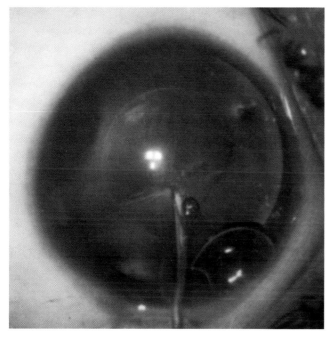

Photo 7.63. Note the centripetal direction of pull. Stretch line is visible.

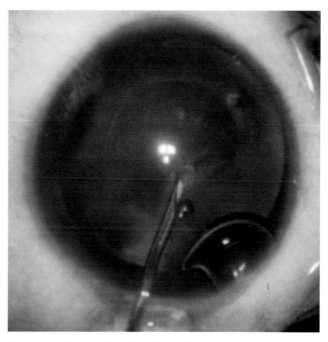

Photo 7.64. Note the direction of force towards the centre of anterior capsule.

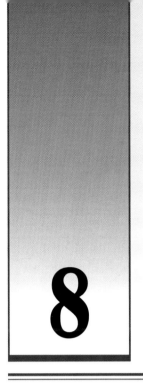

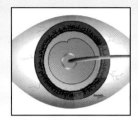

8 Hydroprocedures

The aim of hydroprocedures is to divide the cataractous lens into 3 distinct zones. Each zone requires to be removed in a specific way and separation facilitates this removal. The three parts of the lens are:

(a) Capsule with or without cortex
(b) Epinucleus
(c) Nucleus

Separation also *facilitates rotation*, so that the nucleus and epinucleus can be rotated and brought into the direct line of attack. The epinuclear plate created acts as a *cushion, protecting* the PC during phacoemulsification. Hydrodelineation also decreases the size (horizontal diameter) of the nucleus, thus enabling *prolapse of nuclear fragments* out of the rhexis margin, into the CSZ for phacoaspiration. At the outset we would like to mention that hydroprocedures are not to be taken lightly as this is the step which can lead to nucleus drop even in the hands of experts.

APPLIED ANATOMY (Fig. 8.1)

The peripheral cortical fibres are adherent along the capsule of the lens. The central fibres are the densest and cannot be separated easily. The mid zone, however, is compressible and can be separated easily. This mid zone is what decreases with advancing age and increasing sclerosis of the cataract. Therefore, in a soft cataract, one can easily go deeper into the lens. The mid zone can be decided by the plane of delineation selected by the

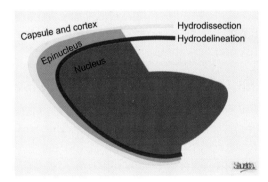

Fig. 8.1. Anatomy of the lens demonstrating planes for hydrodissection and hydrodelineation.

surgeon. The thicker the mid zone, the more is the cushion and the safer is the phacoemulsification.

INSTRUMENTS

The instruments required for this step consist of a syringe and cannula. The syringe may be glass or plastic and of 1–2 ml capacity. A 2 ml syringe gives a good grip and adequate amount of fluid for injection. Glass syringes are usually smoother and easier to use, though, if it is an ill-fitting piston, there may be fluid leak. It is good practice to use the same type of syringe and capacity every time, to get accustomed to the feel while injecting. This tactile feedback of the movement of the plunger is particularly important when you cannot see the wave as in cases with poor glow or small pupils. The cannula may vary from 26–30 G. A 27 G cannula (the one with Healon packing) is ideal; it may be straight or bent.

HYDRODISSECTION

Hydrodissection is the separation of the cataractous lens from the capsule by a mechanical fluid wave.

PRE-REQUISITES

The first step is to **partially remove the viscoelastic** from the chamber, especially if one has used higher viscosity agents like Healon GV and Healon. This is important since the fluid injected during hydrodissection will put undue pressure on the posterior capsule if the viscoelastic is already pressing on the CCC from the front. The fluid injected tends to move the lens forward and if there is too much of viscoelastic in the AC, the force will be transmitted to the posterior capsule increasing the chance of rupture. The method of removal is by depressing the posterior lip of the section. Before hydrodissection, one should **check the syringe and cannula** that is to be used. The piston should move smoothly and the cannula should not be loose.

TECHNIQUE (Figs. 8.2 to 8.8) (Photos 8.1 to 8.4)

Hydroprocedures are performed through the main entry. **The side port should never be used** as this may result in increased pressure on the PC if too much fluid is injected since there will be no other way for the fluid to come out of the chamber. If at all the side port is used (as is commonly done by beginners especially for the sub-incisional area), the chamber should be partly collapsed and a small amount of fluid should be gently injected to separate the anterior and equatorial fibres only.

The cannula is introduced just under (2–3 mm) the CCC as close to the undersurface of capsule as possible.

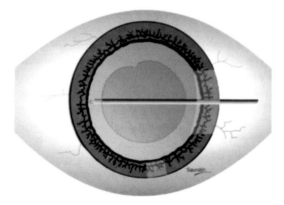

Fig. 8.2. Correct position of cannula for hydrodissection. Note that the tip of the cannula must be at least 1.5 mm under the CCC margin.

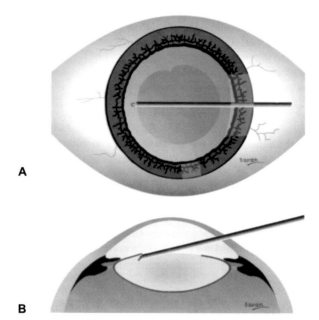

Fig. 8.3. Improper position of cannula. (A) top view, (B) side view.

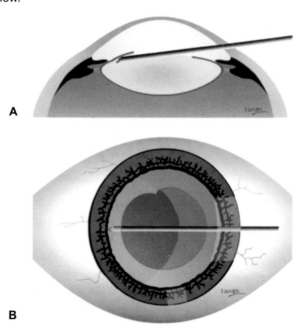

Fig. 8.4. (A) Tenting of the CCC margin before injecting with a jerk. (B) Injected fluid travels as a wave around the lens.

After tenting the CCC upward, the fluid is injected with a jerk. If it is not injected with a jerk, the fluid tends to come back into the AC and does not form a wave. Therefore, being 2–3 mm inside the CCC ensures that there is sufficient resistance to prevent regurgitation and the jerk results in a jet formation that travels as a wave beyond the equator of the lens. As the wave becomes

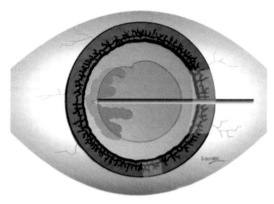

Fig. 8.5. Regurgitation of the injected fluid with no hydrodissection either due to improper placement or gentle injection.

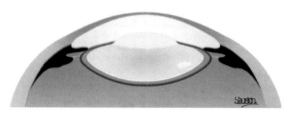

Fig. 8.6. Injection of sufficient fluid. CCC becomes taut, nucleus bulges forward and AC becomes shallow.

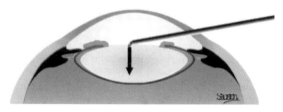

Fig. 8.7. Compression hydro. Gentle pressure in the centre allows the fluid to come anteriorly and the wave to be completed on all sides.

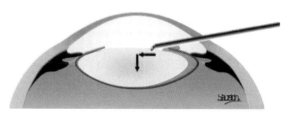

Fig. 8.8. Controlled compression hydro. Nucleus is first pushed to one side and then down to allow the fluid to safely come anterior in that quadrant. The procedure can be repeated at different sites.

visible along the PC, the speed of injection may be slowed down and when the wave is visible posteriorly, at the end opposite to where injection was initiated, the injection is stopped. If you are watchful you will see that when sufficient fluid has been injected, the lens comes anteriorly, the CCC gets stretched and the AC becomes

shallow. This is the ideal amount and more than this can lead to PCT.

A gentle pressure on the centre of the nucleus will release the fluid forward and one can actually see the separation taking place from the equator to the CCC margin; this is called **compression hydrodissection**. If this is seen all round then it is fine otherwise one can press on the nucleus on the side where the separation is not seen. Pressing on the centre may increase the risk of PCT particularly in a small CCC and in cases with a fragile posterior capsule. Our preferred method of releasing this trapped fluid is to place the Sinskey hook/chopper close to the CCC margin on one side, move the nucleus to the opposite side and then press slightly downwards for release of the fluid. This sideways movement on one side increases the resistance of outflow of fluid on that side and decreases the resistance on the same side, thus facilitating regurgitation without any pressure on the posterior capsule. This can be called modified compression hydrodissection.

If the hydrodissection does not appear to be complete or one has not been able to visualize the wave, hydro can be repeated at a different site. Alternatively, **mini-hydrodissection**, that is injection of fluid upto the anterior and equatorial fibres, can be performed at multiple sites.

Site for hydrodissection

If using the bent cannula, one can start 90° away from the main port. If using the straight cannula one should start 180° away from the main wound.

Cortical cleaving hydrodissection

In this, an attempt is made to separate the whole of the cortex from the capsule so that there is less cortical material to be aspirated later. The fluid is injected as close to the undersurface of the CCC as possible. Here we are attempting to separate the most adherent fibres and the movement of the fluid wave is not smooth. This wave moves very slowly and stops as soon as you stop injecting. In fact you may see a greyish reflex in the centre of the red reflex which can be confused with a PCT. You have to keep injecting till the lens comes forward. The disadvantage is that this is more difficult to perform and if some of the fibres are adherent, there is a possibility of a PCT. Also the few fibres that remain are more difficult to aspirate as it is not possible to create a vacuum seal and get a good grip on them. We see no real advantage in attempting this type of hydrodissection.

Special Situations

1. Small CCC (Fig. 8.9)

In a small CCC the chance of fluid entrapment under the CCC is high. It may be prudent to avoid a complete wave and instead perform mini-hydros at multiple sites.

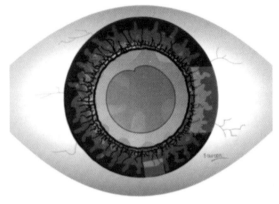

Fig. 8.9. Note small pupil and small CCC. Mini hydro performed by multiple injections. Note multiple small waves meeting posteriorly.

2. Large CCC (Fig. 8.10)

In case of a large CCC, there is a tendency for the nucleus to prolapse into the AC. You will have to reposit the nucleus back into the bag unless supracapsular phaco is planned. It is better to inject where rim of the capsule is less to prevent this happening. If a cortical sheet prolapses along with the nucleus, remove it with visco-expression as this can decrease the visibility.

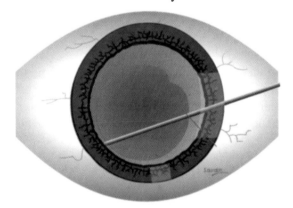

Fig. 8.10. Large eccentric CCC. Inject the fluid from the side of the CCC with the small rim to avoid the nucleus prolapsing into the AC.

3. Eccentric CCC (Fig. 8.11)

In case of an eccentric CCC it is better to inject such that fluid can come out of the normal side without entrapment or prolapse.

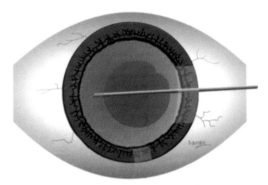

Fig. 8.11. Eccentric CCC. Inject from the side with the larger rim to prevent fluid entrapment which may cause PCT.

4. Hypermature Morgagnian cataract

These cases usually require minimal or no hydro-dissection. The nucleus is quite mobile; too much mobility can hamper the trenching. In these cases, the wave will not be seen; instead one must look for movement of the nucleus.

HYDRODELINEATION

The aim of this manoeuvre is to create the smallest possible nucleus with the thickest possible epinuclear plate. This would result in minimal use of phaco power with the maximal cushioning effect.

PRE-REQUISITES

The pre-requisites are the same as for hydrodissection. However, some amount of viscoelastic may be reinjected in the chamber if it has completely come out.

TECHNIQUE (Fig. 8.12) (Photo 8.5)

For hydrodelineation, the cannula is embedded into the centre of the nucleus (without pushing it backwards) and simultaneously advancing towards the CCC margin. Once well under the CCC margin, the cannula is directed slightly obliquely vitreousward and towards the periphery and fluid is injected with a jerk. The cannula should make an angle of 45° from the surface of the lens (floor) (cf. hydrodissection where cannula is tilted up). No wave will be seen, and instead a golden ring reflex or a gray reflex is seen. The posterior separation is usually quicker while the anterior fibres may remain adherent which may get separated by pushing the nucleus down—**compression delineation**.

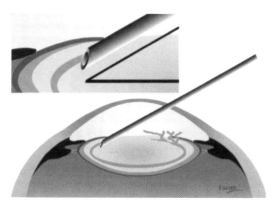

Fig. 8.12. Hydrodelineation. Injection of fluid into the substance of nucleus. Note angulation in inset. Also note that the tip is well under the CCC margin to prevent regurgitation.

Note: The fluid must be injected *beneath* the CCC margin, otherwise the fluid injected will just regurgitate into the AC without accomplishing anything. Also, some amount of viscoelastic over the CCC may help in directing the fluid wave into the substance of the lens and delineating the nucleus.

In case the ring reflex is not seen or is incomplete, one can repeat the injection at another site trying to go a little deeper and with a little more force. One can shift the nucleus from side-to-side to determine if the ring is complete. Beginners may find it difficult if they try to go too deep to delineate a very small nucleus. It is easier to create a ring superficially and one can then try to create *another* ring by going a little deeper.

Mini-delineation/mechanical delineation

In hard cataracts there may be almost no epinuclear plate. One can then scratch the anterior layers of the lens to create a plane of entry for delineation. Introduce the cannula as deep as possible and then inject; you should be able to achieve some delineation posteriorly. One can mechanically lift up the fibres already scratched to complete the delineation anteriorly. In these cases you get a thin epinuclear plate, though it doesn't provide much of a cushion, still dampens the bright red reflex, which reassures the beginner that the capsule is intact.

Soft cataracts

In softer cataracts one may see a bright golden reflex even if the anterior fibres are still adherent. You can perform mini-hydro to complete it anteriorly. Two or more delineation rings can also help you to remove the nucleus in layers.

Partial delineation ring

Sometimes one only succeeds in a partial delineation ring. To complete it, inject the fluid from close to the visible margin trying to be in the same plane. However, no damage is done if rings of differing diameters are created.

ROTATION OF THE NUCLEUS

Single-handed rotation (Fig. 8.13)

After completing the hydroprocedures, one should see if the nucleus is rotating easily. For this, the eye should be well pressurised i.e. fill the chamber with viscoelastic. The nucleus is then rotated with a Sinskey hook or with a chopper. The instrument should be placed close to the CCC, even inside the CCC if possible, and the nucleus is pushed towards the periphery of the lens and then rotated. The common mistake is to rotate trying to bring the instrument to the centre whereas the aim should be to take the counter-pressure from the periphery. Let the whole of the nucleus and the epinuclear plate rotate. Rotation of 2–3 clock hours is usually sufficient to confirm the mobility. Once you see that it is moving you can rotate it back to decrease the stress on the zonules. Unnecessary rotation can cause zonular dehiscence particularly in susceptible cases such as high myopes, pseudoexfoliative syndrome and traumatic cases.

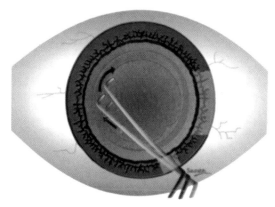

Fig. 8.13. Rotation of the nucleus: Single-handed technique. The nucleus is pushed from the central position 'S' towards the periphery 'P' and then rotated 'R'. Note the decrease in the delineation ring on the side that is being pushed.

Bimanual rotation (Fig. 8.14)

Bimanual rotation may be done with 2 Sinskey hooks or with one Sinskey hook and a chopper. Once again the eye must be fully pressurized. The 2 instruments are positioned 180° apart and should be pushed towards each other to get a grip on the nucleus. They are then moved

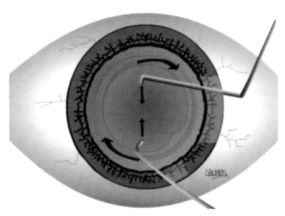

Fig. 8.14. Rotation of the nucleus: Bimanual technique—Both instruments are pushed towards each other for counter-pressure 'CP' and then rotated 'R'.

in opposite directions to rotate the nucleus, taking counter-pressure from each other.

Non-rotation of nucleus

The nucleus will not rotate if the hydrodissection is incomplete. If after successfully completing the hydro-dissection the nucleus still does not rotate, especially in a hard cataract; there may be fibrous adhesions and it will be prudent not to do phaco in these cases as there is a high chance of PCT. The nucleus will not rotate easily if there is a dialysis so the surgeon should be cautious. In a soft cataract it is difficult to get a grip on the nucleus and rotation is difficult. However, in soft cataracts rotation is not always essential.

In cases with hard cataract, pseudoexfoliation syndrome or those in which rotation has been difficult, one should reverse the rotation to decrease the torsional stretch on the zonules.

POSTERIOR CAPSULAR TEAR DURING HYDRODISSECTION (Fig. 8.15)

There are three reasons for posterior capsular tear during the hydroprocedures:

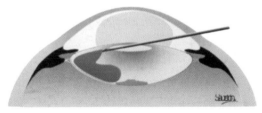

Fig. 8.15. Causes of PCT during hydroprocedures. Note the bolus of VE in AC, small CCC, large quantity of injected fluid and inherent weakness of PC in posterior polar cataract.

1. *Block to outflow:* The outflow may be blocked due to increased resistance offered by viscoelastic in the chamber or a small CCC/small pupil. Also, injecting from the side port, when the main wound is well sealed, can lead to a PCT.

2. *Injection of too much fluid:* Injection of too much fluid with too much force or using a faulty technique/wrong syringe and cannula can lead to PCT.

3. *Inherent weakness:* Weak capsule may be seen in case of posterior polar cataract, high myopes, post-vitrectomy, traumatic cataracts, pseudoexfoliative syndromes and some cases of posterior subcapsular cataract. In these cases one can avoid hydro-dissection (since this step can lead to a nuclear drop) and perform a careful hydrodelineation.

Dos and Don'ts of Hydroprocedures

Do

1. Remove some viscoelastic before starting hydro-dissection.
2. Inject from the main port only.
3. Focus below the CCC (between the CCC and PC) so that the wave is visible.
4. Use the same type of syringe and cannula (same brand) in each case.
5. Tent up the CCC margin before injecting.
6. Make sure the cannula is radial to the CCC and well inside the CCC (2–3 mm).
7. Start injecting with a jerk and slow down once you see the wave.
8. Inject an adequate amount of fluid.

Don't

1. Use the side port for hydroprocedures.
2. Use a very large syringe/sticky syringe.

HYDRODISSECTION

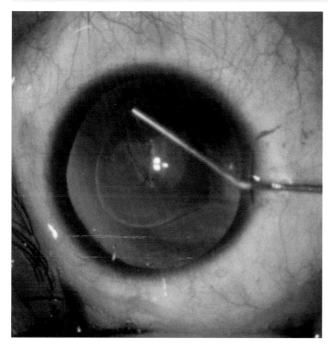

Photo 8.1. Cannula tenting up the anterior capsule.

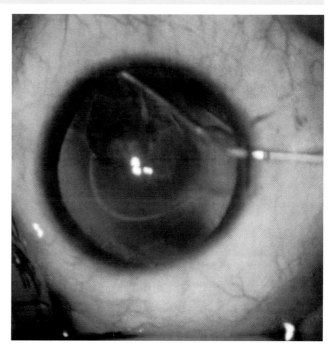

Photo 8.2. Fluid is injected with a jerk to create a wave.

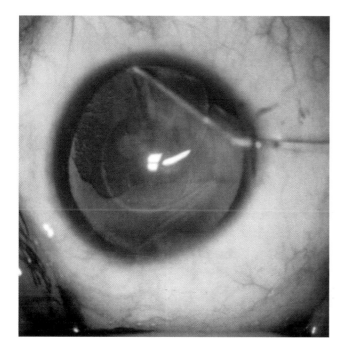

Photo 8.3. The wave has progressed slowly along the posterior capsule, as cortical cleaving hydrodissection was performed.

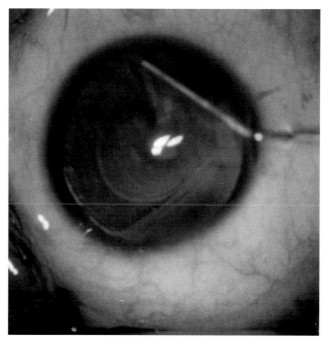

Photo 8.4. Stop injecting once the wave crosses the midline and allow it to proceed with its own momentum.

HYDRODELINEATION

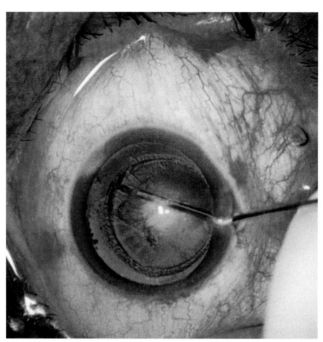

Photo 8.5. Posterior polar cataract. Hydrodissection should not be done, only hydrodelineation to be done. Note the appearance of golden ring reflex.

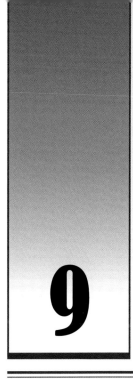

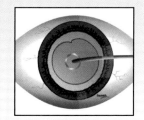

9 Nucleotomy

For the success of small incision surgery, we need to use ultrasonic energy for the disintegration of the nucleus as the rest of the lens can be removed by aspiration alone. The purpose of this step is to remove the central core of the nucleus, piece by piece, using minimum phaco energy and without damaging the surrounding structures especially the cornea and the posterior capsule. A good knowledge of the anatomy of the nucleus, the instruments and basic hand motions inside the eye can make this complicated procedure rather easy.

APPLIED ANATOMY (Figs. 9.1 & 9.2)

From the surgical viewpoint, the lens is divided into four parts: a central hard nucleus surrounded by an epinuclear (EN) plate of varying thickness and the outermost thin layer of the cortex and capsule. The central hard nucleus is densest in the centre while the outer nucleus is softer. As the age advances, the water content of the lens decreases and the density of the nucleus increases. There is accompanying sclerosis of the epinuclear material which results in a sclerosed EN plate of decreased thickness and leathery fibres. The sclerosis of the nucleus and posterior leathery fibres of the nucleus assume greater importance when attempting nucleotomy, as these fibres will not separate easily if the trench is not deep enough. The increasing density of the nucleus in old age also results in a downward (more posterior) placement of the densest part of nucleus. Thus, the trench has to be almost 90% of the thickness of the lens if a complete crack is to

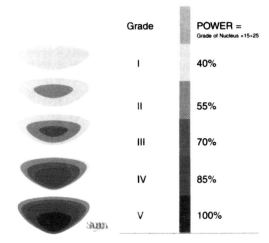

Fig. 9.1. Grades and density of the nucleus. With increasing grade and density, more phaco power is required.

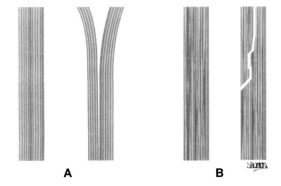

Fig. 9.2. (A) The less sclerosed fibres can be easily separated. (B) With increasing sclerosis, the cleavage planes are lost.

be obtained. Otherwise the central core of nucleus will remain unbroken with a crack in the surrounding softer outer nucleus. With further sclerosis, the fibres get so compressed that the cleavage planes are virtually lost making separation very difficult.

The greater curvature of the lens posteriorly as compared to the anterior surface is of special relevance to the phaco surgeon. It is important to note that this curvature varies, achieving almost a conical shape, as the age of the patients increases and the lens gets harder. The movement of the phaco probe while trenching *must* follow this curvature if adequate depth is to be achieved and capsular injury is to be avoided. The red reflex may be visible from the periphery even in a shallow trench so one should change the direction of the probe accordingly.

INSTRUMENTS

1. Phaco tip

The phaco tip is a vital instrument for nucleotomy. Various types of tip are available. Most tips are made of titanium. All the tips must have a tapered hub. This reduces air bubble formation in the anterior chamber. Teflon-coated tips have an advantage of preventing corneal burn.

The **Standard** or regular tip is most commonly used. It has a 0.9 mm inner diameter and 1.1 mm outer diameter.

The **Microflow** tip is useful in soft cataracts especially those less than grade 3. The internal diameter ranges from 0.45 to 0.6 mm, depending upon the manufacturer. As the fluid drawn out by the small bore is less, the amount of surge is decreased allowing one to work safely at higher vacuum levels. The smaller surface area, however, results in a decreased holding power for the same vacuum as compared to a regular tip. This tip is, therefore, not recommended for hard and hypermature cataract.

The **Kelman** tip has a downward angulation. This is ideal for sculpting in hard cataracts and eyes with deep AC. In a shallow AC this downward angulation increases the chances of PC damage. Beginners are advised to avoid this tip or else switch to a regular tip after the trench has been made. A modification of Kelman tip is the bell-shaped **Kelman flared** tip. The wider area of this tip allows more power transmission and is, therefore, ideal for hard cataract.

The **Cobra** tip has the base of microflow tip proximally and that of regular tip distally. This configuration enables it to aspirate a big piece and emulsify it within its walls.

2. Choppers (Fig. 9.3)

The chopper is an invaluable aid to phacoemulsification. Apart from actually chopping or splitting the nucleus, it can be used for stabilizing the globe, rotating the nucleus, feeding the tip and even protecting the PC. The chopper has a handle, a horizontal part and a vertical part. The length of the horizontal portion of an ideal chopper should be 12 mm. This allows easy access to all the capsular fornices. The vertical portion should be 1.25 ± 0.25 in length. This part is similar in all choppers whether blunt tipped or sharp tipped and is triangular in cross-section i.e. an inner cutting edge and an outer rounded smooth edge. The lower part of the vertical portion differs depending on whether it is blunt or sharp. The thickness of the chopper should be uniform ranging from 0.75–1 mm, so as to facilitate its entry and manoeuvrability through the side port.

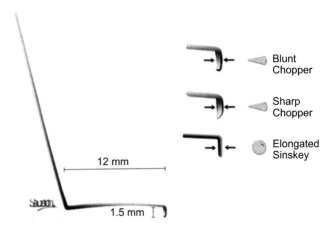

Fig. 9.3. Various tips of the choppers available.

There are a variety of choppers available. ***Blunt chopper*** with a ball is one of the earlier models. The ball-shaped end, however, was not found to have any advantage over the blunt chopper without the ball in preventing posterior capsular damage. In fact, the ball increases the length of the vertical part without adding to the cutting ability. The ***Sharp tipped chopper*** was introduced with the advent of Karate chop technique of nucleotomy. Nowadays the trend is towards smaller choppers which are used for splitting rather than chopping. An ***elongated Sinskey*** is thinner than the traditional chopper and has a good splitting action. The cross-section of the vertical portion is rounded. This instrument perhaps serves all the purposes of the chopper and is easier to manoeuvre in the anterior chamber.

NUCLEOTOMY

The most popular methods of nucleotomy are "*Divide and Conquer*", "*Chopping*" or a combination of the two i.e. "*Stop and Chop*" and "*Flip and Chip*". In *Stop and Chop* we start with a trench as in *Divide and Conquer*, stop after the first trench and then proceed with chopping techniques. Irrespective of the type of procedure certain steps are common to all, which are discussed as follows:

Entering the eye

Always enter a formed chamber, by partially filling the chamber with viscoelastic, to avoid touching the iris or cornea. Touching the iris can lead to meiosis and entering in a shallow chamber can lead to a corneal touch or Descemet's detachment. One can enter with the infusion on though this is not essential. It is to be noted that if you switch the infusion on after entering the AC then there are chances of a small air bubble coming in the AC.

Depress the lower lip of the wound and then introduce the metallic part of the tip. Now lift the upper lip of the wound and guide the sleeve in. Once the sleeve is in, lift the probe and direct the tip downwards to prevent Descemet's detachment. The motions here are similar to those while making the corneal tunnel.

Though the earlier teaching was to enter with the bevel down, it is now thought to be irrelevant. In fact it is more cumbersome to rotate the probe 180 degrees after entering with the bevel down.

Removal of the anterior epinuclear plate (Fig. 9.4)

Removal of the anterior epinuclear plate helps in baring the nucleus for trenching. This can be done mechanically by scraping with a Sinskey hook or chopper. For this, you have to first inflate the chamber. Then insert the chopper close to the CCC and pull towards the centre in a scratching motion. This manoeuvre should be repeated 20 times radially. The loose tissue can be then expressed

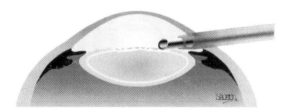

Fig. 9.4. Removal of the anterior epinuclear plate.

by depressing the lower lip of the wound. Alternatively, one may use minimum phaco and a vacuum setting of 60–70 mmHg to remove the epinucleus and cortex from the central area within the CCC margins. Here, first only vacuum is tried. Any area not getting aspirated is then given a short burst of phaco energy by bringing the probe close but still keeping a safe distance from the CCC margins (0.5 mm).

TRENCHING

Trenching involves making a groove into the nucleus. All nucleotomy techniques require some form of a trench to facilitate the breaking of the nucleus into smaller pieces and easy removal. This step is of vital importance for the *Stop & Chop* and *Divide & Conquer* techniques.

Settings for Trenching

Trenching should be performed at low vacuum settings (i.e. 20 ± 10 mmHg) since we are trying to sculpt the nucleus and don't want to hold it. The power setting will depend on the hardness of the nucleus. **A practical formula that may be applied is power = grade of nucleus × 15 + 25.** It is better to keep the setting at the highest required and control the actual energy delivered by the foot pedal. The phaco is kept in linear mode for better control. The ideal power is that at which there is no wasting of energy and no movement of the nucleus. Bubbles in the AC are indicative of wasted energy i.e. giving phaco energy when there is no tissue in front to emulsify. Too little power or moving the probe too fast results in pushing the nucleus without cutting it leading to zonular stress. The speed of the probe should match the rate of emulsification such that no power is wasted and the nucleus is not pushed. The sleeve may be withdrawn to expose the tip more (1–2 mm) to allow deeper access without obstruction by the sleeve.

Dimensions of the Trench

Before starting the trench, the surgeon should decide the size of the trench required. This is dependent on the hardness of the cataract – the harder cataracts usually have a large nucleus and require a deep trench. The estimation of the trench dimensions starts pre-operatively with the assessment of the hardness of the cataract by slit lamp examination and keeping the age of the patient in mind. The intraoperative factors to be considered start with the thickness of the anterior epinuclear plate – thinner the plate, larger the nucleus. The size and reflex of the delineation ring are also important indicators – larger delineation ring indicates a larger nucleus meaning thereby that a larger trench will be required. A grey ring, barely visible or not becoming wider on side-to-side movement of the nucleus is suggestive of a hard nucleus. The presence of a bright golden ring reflex usually indicates a soft cataract and a smaller nucleus. The other clue to the hardness of the cataract is the ease at which the probe is moving through the cataract.

Length of the trench (Figs. 9.5 & 9.6)

The surgeon should maintain a mental picture of the size of the CCC throughout trenching. The length of the trench should be just short of the CCC, i.e. approximately 4–5 mm. Once the superficial trench has been made, at least a tip deep, one can go under the CCC and increase the length. If you reach the delineation margin it is called a **relaxing nucleotomy**. However, while lengthening the trench, one should always be able to visualize the tip. There is no need to go under the CCC except in hard cataracts, very soft cataracts and in small CCC.

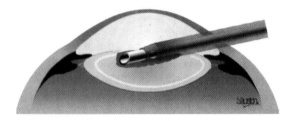

Fig. 9.5. Length of the trench: The trench should be just short of the CCC.

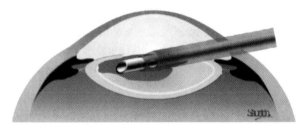

Fig. 9.6. Relaxing nucleotomy.

Width (Fig. 9.7)

The trench should be '2 tip diameters' wide in order to comfortably accommodate the sleeve. One may make a central groove and then widen both the sides by tilting the probe with the bevel facing the centre. It is better to widen the trench layer by layer before deepening it otherwise the sleeve may get stuck in a narrow trench.

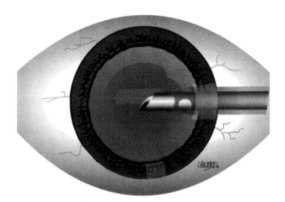

Fig. 9.7. Increasing the width of the trench. Note the bevel facing the centre.

Starting the trench (Figs. 9.8 & 9.9)

It is best to start at the centre of the nucleus or just proximal to the centre and move towards the CCC in the cross-incisional axis. The larger exposure of the tip, the downward angulation required for trenching and the higher chances of incisional corneal edema (due to the infusion ports being inside the wound) make it difficult especially for a beginner to start the trench in the sub-incisional area. It is, therefore, better to start at the centre, make a trench in the cross-incisional axis, rotate the nucleus and then complete the trench.

The movement of the probe and the foot control are vital during trenching. The nucleus needs to be sculpted using a **shaving action** which requires a minimal downward angulation without causing occlusion. ***In fact, there***

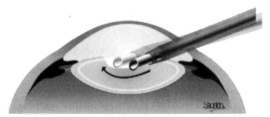

Fig. 9.8. Shaving action while trenching. To maintain the shaving action, the angulation of the tip is such that the tip is lifted up and the handle depressed using the incision as the fulcrum while moving forward.

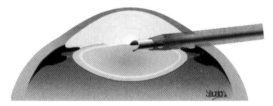

Fig. 9.9. Movement of tip such that less than half tip diameter is occluded.

should be no occlusion of the tip at any stage during trenching. The forward stroke consists of a shaving action with an attempt to move into the nucleus by a depth less than half the diameter of the tip. If one goes in too deep there may be occlusion of the tip. Another indication of having gone too deep is milking of the nucleus and clouding of the AC. On the return stroke, care should be taken that no phaco or aspiration is used. In systems with CIM (continuous irrigation mode), one can take the foot off the pedal as the AC is maintained by the CIM. In other systems one has to train oneself to come to position 1 or else remove the infusion tube from the pinch valve so that infusion remains on all the time.

The phaco power is used on the forward stroke and the speed of movement is adjusted according to the hardness of the cataract. The movement of probe is faster in softer cataract. In harder cataracts a well-demarcated edge will be visible and the movement is slower. Also, there may be the formation of tongue-shaped nuclear projections. However, these can be broken from the attached end easily with a chopper.

The trench is widened and deepened uniformly with multiple strokes. The nucleus needs to be rotated to bring the sub-incisional nucleus into the cross-incisional area for better access. The eye must first be pressurized by filling the chamber with viscoelastic. The instrument (chopper or dialer) is introduced into the periphery of the trench and rotated clockwise. One can use a single-handed or a double-handed technique. Pressurizing the eye before attempting rotation not only decreases the corneal striae and improves visibility but also facilitates smooth movement of the nucleus. Trying to rotate the nucleus in a soft eye can lead to posterior capsule damage. After gaining proficiency, the phaco probe need not be removed and the second instrument in the left hand can be used for rotating.

Completing the trench

After 180 degrees nucleus rotation, trenching is performed in the opposite half. For completing the trench, one should start superficially similar to the first half. There is a tendency to go too deep so one must be careful to continue the shaving action till the trench is of uniform depth.

Assessment of depth (Fig. 9.10A & B)

The most important aspect of trenching is achieving adequate depth. In a moderate grade nucleus, the red

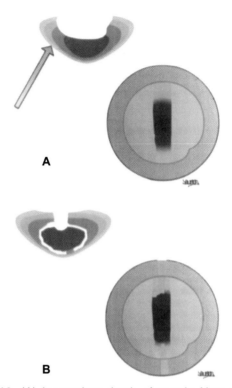

Fig. 9.10. (A) Incomplete depth of trench: Note that the peripheral glow is visible but the central hard nucleus is still intact. (B) Attempted crack in exonucleus only. Endonucleus left intact.

reflex is usually visible in the periphery first. In order to get the same reflex in the centre one may need to rotate the nucleus once or twice. Hardest part of the nucleus is at the centre or just below the centre of the nucleus; posterior to this, nucleus is comparatively softer. After emulsifying the central hard nucleus, the probe will suddenly move easily through the posterior softer nucleus if the power isn't decreased proportionately by foot control. Once you are deep enough there may be a sudden *'give way'* feeling as the emulsification of the last bit of the harder nucleus gives way to the relatively softer outer nucleus. Thus, one must proceed carefully as one is going deeper, and should reduce both the motion of the probe and the power to avoid suddenly going right through the epinucleus and posterior capsule.

While trenching, it is prudent to keep the magnification low-moderate as higher magnification decreases the operative field and reduces the range of depth perception. The eyeball should be placed such that the red reflex is visible, either by manipulating the bridle sutures or by rotating the head or by intraoperative positioning of the globe with the second instrument. Though most authors describe that one should be 2–3 tips deep, the visibility of the red reflex is a better guide in moderate cataracts. If you are unsure of the depth, it is better to withdraw the probe, fill the eye with viscoelastic and then assess. If the depth seems adequate, try to crack the nucleus. If it doesn't break easily then don't try to crack it as you may end up cracking the outer nucleus (exonucleus) with an intact inner hard nucleus (endonucleus). You should carefully try to deepen the trench by continuing the shaving action before attempting the splitting again. The endonucleus, though small, may be difficult to handle, as it is usually closely adherent to the rest of the nucleus.

Difficulties in trenching

Too wide a trench

Sometimes the trench becomes too wide especially in softer cataracts. Decrease the power and try to decrease the width as one goes deeper.

Too narrow a trench (Fig. 9.7)

After the initial groove is made on the surface it is sometimes difficult to widen as the probe tends to slip into the same groove. To widen this one should turn the bevel of the probe towards the centre and then apply power. Or else the initial groove should not be vertical but slightly radial so as to make a 'V' shaped trench.

Bumps in the depth (Figs. 9.11, 9.12A & B)

Sometimes due to lack of smooth actions the trench has an uneven surface or even a large bump in the centre. This is more likely if a "Spud" (Khurpi) like action is used rather than a shaving action. If the red reflex is visible anywhere between the bumps, then crack the nucleus. Otherwise the bumps need to be shaved off carefully to achieve a level surface.

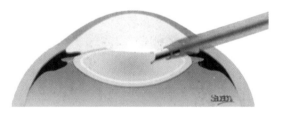

Fig. 9.11. Complete occlusion of the tip.

V-SHAPED OR VICTORY TRENCH
(Photos 9.21 to 9.36) (Fig. 9.13A, B, C & D)

A useful modification of the trench is a 'V' trench. In this, the initial stroke is made slightly radially instead of in the straight axis. The second stroke is also made

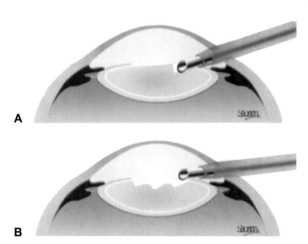

Fig. 9.12. (A) 'Khurpi' action instead of 'shaving' action. (B) Repeated 'Khurpi' action leads to uneven bumps.

radially to complete a 'V'. The trench is gradually deepened in the same shape. The nucleus is rotated and then similar strokes are made on the other side to make an 'X' pattern. The trench is then deepened as normal, keeping the peripheral curvature in mind.

The advantage of this 'V' trench is that there is a wider space to work in. Also the tendency to get stuck in the same groove is avoided. After making and rotating the first V the wider part of the V becomes sub-incisional which accommodates the sleeve of the phaco tip very easily. This is our preferred mode of trenching particularly in hard and mature cataracts.

SPLITTING (Figs. 9.14 to 9.17)

If the trench is good it makes splitting of the nucleus easier. Before attempting the crack one should keep in mind the direction of forces to be applied. For example, before breaking, any object stretches till break-point and then breaks. How much the tissue will stretch depends not only on the quality and type of the tissue but also on the distance between the forces or length of the tissue between the forces. If the forces are far away from each other, because of excessive stress, more space will be needed. While splitting the nucleus, we need opposing forces to be closer to each other, *vertically as well as horizontally*. If we try to break the nucleus by keeping both instruments (the forces) far away, we won't be able to reach the break-point and the two halves will keep on springing back.

One should put two instruments (either the phaco probe and chopper or two choppers) as deep as possible in the trench. The instruments must be **close** together both vertically *and* horizontally. The force is applied in

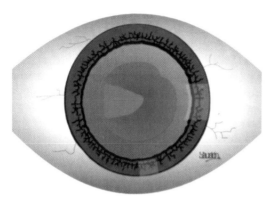

A. Make the first 'V'.

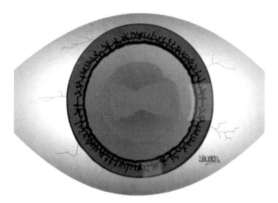

B. Deepen the centre.

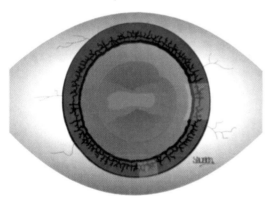

C. Rotate and complete to make an 'X' shape.

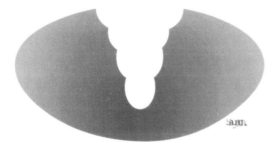

D. Depth of 'V' trench.

Fig. 9.13. V-trench or victory trench.

SPLITTING THE NUCLEUS

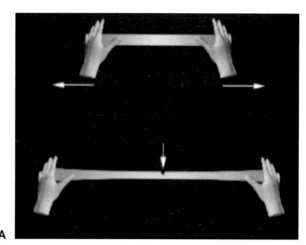

A

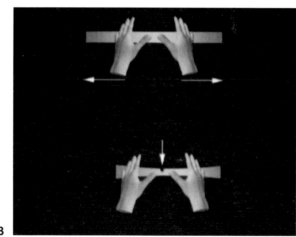

B

Fig. 9.14. Splitting & stretching forces. (A) If the forces are further away, more stretch and thus more space is required to reach break-point. (B) If the forces are applied close together very little space is required to reach the break-point.

Incorrect Direction

Correct Direction

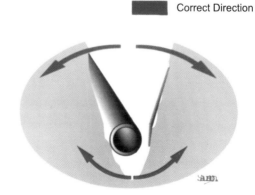

Fig. 9.15. Splitting the nucleus: Note the vertical placement of instruments in the depth and the direction of forces.

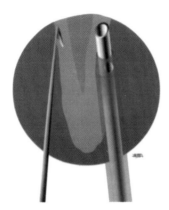

Fig. 9.16. Split extended upto the centre. Splitting forces applied at the periphery will not cause any extension of the split due to wrong placement of the instruments horizontally.

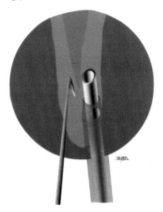

Fig. 9.17. Correct horizontal placement of the instruments.

opposite directions such that the centre tends to depress slightly and periphery of the nucleus tends to lift upwards. If the centre comes forward and the periphery is depressed then the nucleus will not crack. In this case, it means that either the trench is not deep enough or the instruments are too superficially placed. One can initiate the split at the periphery and then move both instruments towards the centre to complete the crack. In case it does not go to the opposite periphery, one can rotate the nucleus by 180 degrees to complete the split. It is essential that the split should be through & through and the two halves should be totally separated without any bridging fibres. In hard cataracts sometimes the deeper fibres may remain attached. You then need to go in deeper with both instruments and carefully separate all the fibres.

Another method of cracking the nucleus is to position the nucleus horizontally, embed the probe into the centre of the heminucleus and pull with the second instrument to achieve the crack. The settings should be those of chopping and this is only applicable for cataracts harder than grade 2.

DIVIDE AND CONQUER (Photos 9.1 to 9.20)

This technique requires trenching of the nucleus. As described earlier, trenching should be deep and wide (approx. 2 phaco tips wide). In this, the first trench is made from the centre of the nucleus, towards the cross-incisional area till the capsulorrhexis margin. It is deepened and widened as described previously. After the first trench is made, rotate the nucleus with the help of a chopper/spatula about 90 degree in a clockwise direction. Now, a second trench is made. Again, the nucleus is rotated through 90 degree and the process is initiated similarly till the third and the fourth trenches are made. It is important that each trench should be of adequate depth and width and should be in the form of '+' sign, which ensures an easy cracking of the nucleus.

The phaco probe and the second instrument (chopper/spatula) are now placed in the depth of the trench and with either a pull-push action or a cross push action, the two halves are separated till a split appears in the bottom of the trench with a bright glow shining through. No interdigitating fibres should be left which will cause difficulty during emulsification of individual quadrants.

Then turn the nucleus again through 90 degree and another split is created at the remaining intact trench. These two halves are then split till a glow appears all along the split groove. These two splits leads to four quadrants similar to the shape of pie, which are then emulsified individually.

Modified technique of Divide & Conquer

Instead of making a full cross and then dividing the nucleus, a central full length trench is made and the nucleus is divided into 2 halves. One half is divided into two after making a trench in the middle and then both pieces are phacoaspirated. The second half is also similarly divided into two and phacoaspirated.

The advantage of this is that you don't have to keep on rotating and achieving the required depth is easier. The problems faced in an imperfect cross (i.e. eccentric cross, unequal pieces) are avoided in this technique. This technique does not require vacuum seal and use of the left hand is minimal. So, till the surgeon develops ambi-dexterity, this method works well in selected cases (grade II–III cataract). However, since this technique primarily depends on trenching, it will be difficult to perform in a small CCC. In a hard cataract, the energy used will be very high and may cause corneal complications such as wound burn. If this technique is used in hard cataracts, one should take care to make a large CCC and keep cooling the tip and cornea by pouring BSS.

CHOPPING

Chopping is a term used to denote the splitting of the nucleus into smaller pieces by a chopper. Chopping may be peripheral, central or combination of the two but most essential part of all of this is stabilization of nucleus.

Stabilization of the nucleus

Before attempting to use the chopper it is important to stabilize the nucleus so that the chopper moves in the intended direction. None of the chopping techniques can work well without stabilization of nucleus which is the key to successful chopping. Stabilization involves preparing a *platform* and creation of a *vacuum seal* and a *hold* into the hardest part of the nucleus. Since the body of the nucleus provides the best grip, some route is required to reach the core of the nucleus and form the platform for holding the nucleus. This can be done with the help of a **complete trench, partial trench or no trench**.

Creating a platform

A platform for holding can be created by complete, partial or no trench at all.

Complete trench (Fig. 9.18)

A **complete trench** is made in the '*stop and chop*' technique (Photos 9.21 to 9.64). To our mind, this is the best method since it combines the advantages of the '*divide and conquer*' technique and chopping. In '*divide and conquer*', bringing the pieces into the centre is easier but more phaco energy is required whereas in direct chopping, though less energy is required, the pieces tend to get stuck together in a jigsaw fashion and may be more difficult to aspirate. In '*stop and chop*' technique, we split the nucleus into two halves as already described in 'Trenching'. The complete surface of the heminucleus now provides a good platform for holding. Also there is sufficient space for further manoeuvres. The probe can be easily embedded into the hard body of the nucleus and a vacuum seal created for chopping. Since the

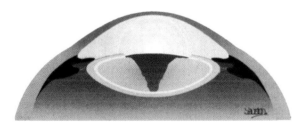

Fig. 9.18. Complete trench (stop & chop): Hemisection of nucleus provides large platform.

platform is wide, one can try an alternate site if initially a good hold is not obtained. Each heminucleus can be divided into three pieces in a safe and controlled manner.

Partial trenching (Fig. 9.19A & B)
(Photos 9.65 to 9.84)

It involves making a small trench just distal to the centre of the nucleus. Begin the sculpting just proximal to the centre and go towards the mid-periphery. Now, deepen such that you are at least a tip diameter deep; the deeper the trench, the better the platform for holding. A good platform is obtained by rotating the nucleus by 180 degrees. Phaco tip can be easily buried into the harder central nucleus for chopping. A very long and wide trench is not required for chopping as the aim is to get a good grip in the body of the nucleus.

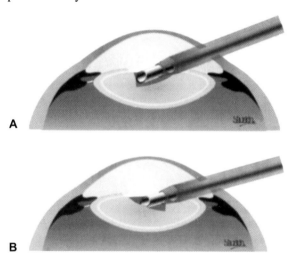

Fig. 9.19. Partial trench. (A) Platform created. (B) With rotation, larger platform created.

Chopping without a trench (Fig. 9.20A & B)

It is done in '*Direct chop*' (Photos 9.89 to 9.96). Phaco probe with **bevel down** is kept in the centre of the nucleus. High vacuum and power settings are required and a burst/panel mode is preferable. Due to the wound configuration it is not possible to go vertically down into the nucleus. To avoid going into periphery of the nucleus keep the bevel of the tip flat on the anterior surface of the nucleus proximal to the centre. With a short burst of energy, the nucleus is entered. The vacuum is allowed to build up and the nucleus may be lifted up before chopping. This technique is not advisable for beginners, as even in expert hands, there is tendency to slip into the periphery. Also, the grip is usually superficial and a complete split is not always obtained. This means that the deeper fibres remain

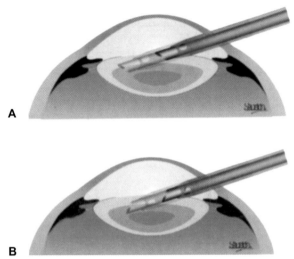

Fig. 9.20. No trench. (A) Bevel down: The tip cannot reach upto the centre of the nucleus due to occlusion occurring before that. (B) Bevel up: Note that with bevel up, the tip may go in a little deeper with repeated action.

unsplit and entangled. In a soft cataract the probe can go through and through. High vacuum settings increase the incidence of surge and therefore this technique is not ideal for second generation machines. As bevel down position of probe can injure the posterior capsule, some surgeons advocate **bevel up** position. If a good grip is not obtained in one attempt, rotate the nucleus and try again at a different site. The presumed advantage of this technique is use of less phaco energy and speed of surgery. It is only recommended for surgeons with a third generation machine and huge volumes.

Creation of vacuum seal and vacuum hold (Figs. 9.21A & B, 9.22)

Before embarking on this step, a phaco surgeon must have good understanding of the audible and tactile feedback of the foot pedal. One should be able to manoeuvre the pedal between the positions of aspiration, phaco and back to aspiration and should be able to hold on to that position for sufficient length of time to develop a vacuum hold and then chop.

As the tactile feedback of the dentation of the foot pedal is less on upward excursion, while moving from position 3 to 2, overshoot to position 1 or 0 is common. Hence it is safe to keep the machine in CIM to prevent AC collapse. If you have an overshoot, press the foot pedal back to position 2 and remain stable at the dentation.

The surgeon must also be familiar with the high pitched, fixed frequency sound that is emitted by the

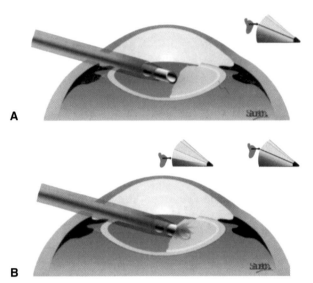

Fig. 9.21. Creation of a vacuum seal. The probe is introduced into the eye in CIM. (A) The nucleus is nudged and foot pedal brought to position 2 (IA). (B) A short burst of phaco (position 3) is given to embed the probe into the body of the nucleus. Note that the foot pedal is brought back from position 3 to position 2 (IA) to let the vacuum build up and create a hold.

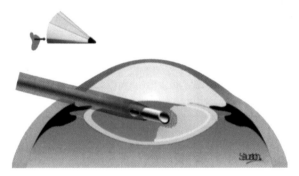

Fig. 9.22. Maintaining the foot in position 3 leads to loosening of the grip.

machine once the maximum preset vacuum is achieved. This indicates full vacuum and thus a good hold. Beginners can practise by pinching the tubing to occlude it with the probe outside the eye and listening for the sound.

Steps in vacuum hold

Foot movement	Right-hand movement
FP Pos. 1/Pos. 0 in CIM	Tip inside eye.
	Tip close to the nucleus.
FP Pos. 2	Nudge the nucleus.
FP Pos. 3	Bury the tip.
FP Pos. 2	Vacuum hold created.

If the impalement is adequate then on slight to and fro movement of the tip, both the tip and the nucleus piece will move as one unit. If, however, the grip is not sufficient i.e. adequate vacuum seal is not achieved, the nucleus piece will be set free. If impalement is not achieved in one area, move to another site and attempt again. One should carefully select the area to be impaled, trying to remain within the body of the nucleus.

Causes of poor hold include keeping the foot pedal in position 3 for too long as this leads to emulsification of the nucleus material around the tip. This loosens the grip in addition to causing milking/clouding of the AC. If the site is too superficial, complete occlusion is not achieved and therefore vacuum seal is not effective. In low or inadequate vacuum settings, the probe keeps slipping and a good hold is not obtained. In very soft cataracts, creating a vacuum seal and vacuum hold is more difficult. The cataract gets sucked even without use of phaco energy and danger of going through and through is high. In such a situation vacuum and power settings should be lower.

Settings for vacuum seal

Safe maximum vacuum and flow rate accelerates the surgery and causes less chattering by increasing the followability.The maximum settings that can be obtained depend on the type of machine, the control on foot pedal and the surgeon's anticipation of surge.

The safe limits must be found out for each individual machine. For this, the handpiece is kept 6 inches above the patient's eye and the maximum flow rate and vacuum are set. If the test chamber remains maintained and the bulb of the chamber is hard, these settings are safe. If there is collapse/flutter of the chamber, lower the settings. Handpiece must be kept 6″ above, since, as the surgery proceeds, the height of water column in the infusion bottle keeps on decreasing, thereby slowing the infusion rate.

Once a stable chamber is obtained, pinch the aspiration tube and allow maximum vacuum to build up. Once the maximum vacuum sound is heard release the pinch. This acts like creation of surge. The settings are acceptable if there is no collapse or slight fluttering of the chamber. If the test chamber collapses, reduce the settings. Collapsed chamber could occur because of inadequate bottle height, clogged infusion system or if the airway cannula is not working. TUR tubing or ACM may be used.

In standard machines, vacuum setting depends on the hardness of cataract. **Recommended vacuum settings:**

(Nucleus grade × 50) + 100 i.e. between 250 to 350. Flow rate of 26 to 36 is appropriate for beginners. In newer generation machines vacuum settings of 400 to 600 and flow rate of 36 to 50 are safe.

PHACO CHOP

There are two basic techniques of chopping, namely **peripheral** and **central**. Peripheral chopping begins from the periphery of the nucleus and proceeds towards the centre. Central chop (Karate chop) involves splitting of nucleus from mid-periphery by embedding the chopper on the anterior surface of the nucleus.

Peripheral chop (Photos 9.65 to 9.76) (Fig. 9.23A, B, C & D)

A side port incision is made between 1–2 O'clock hours to the left of the main port incision. Chamber is moderately filled with viscoelastic and continuous infusion is set. Chopper is placed on the anterior nucleus surface, close to the rhexis margin in a horizontal position. It is slipped underneath the CCC margin and positioned just to the right of the line of the phaco probe, at the delineation line. Now, with the other hand, phaco probe is impaled into the nucleus. Once the vacuum hold is obtained, the chopper is turned vertical and pulled towards the U/S tip. Just before reaching the probe, the nucleus is split sideways.

Oblique placement of the chopper leads to a rotational effect. The ideal placing of the chopper would be in the same line as the phaco probe, but this would require the entry of both chopper and the phaco probe through the main incision. Therefore, a side port incision at 1–2 O'clock instead of 3 O'clock helps in placing chopper close to the phaco line without much increase towards the rotational effect.

Problems with peripheral chop

1. Complex manoeuvrability needed for this technique. The chopper must be negotiated under the CCC margin while *simultaneously* the hold on nucleus has to be maintained.

2. There is danger of PCT while chopping. Use of a long chopper on a soft nucleus in an unstable AC can lead to peripheral capsular tear.

3. If the chopper is accidentally placed over the anterior capsule instead of underneath it and the chop is initiated, it may lead to RMT or zonulolysis.

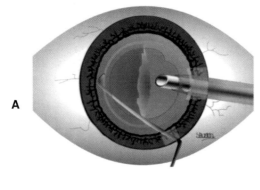

A

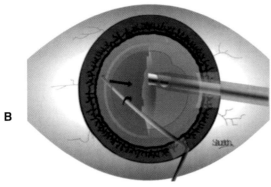

B

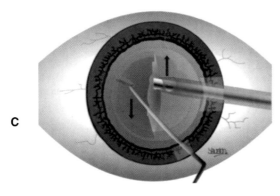

C

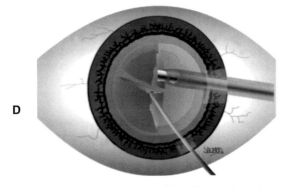

D

Fig. 9.23. Peripheral chop. (A) Place the chopper underneath CCC at the delineation line. (B) Embed the tip to create the vacuum seal. Now turn chopper vertical and pull it towards the phaco tip. (C) Once the chopper reaches the tip move it sideways to complete the crack. (D) Crack will proceed from periphery to centre.

Central chop (Photos 9.41 to 9.64)
(Fig. 9.24A, B, C & D)

Central chop entails chopping without going underneath the CCC. Instead of a blunt chopper, a sharp or thin rounded chopper or even a Sinskey hook may be used. Emphasis is essentially on *splitting* of fibres rather than on *cutting* them.

In this technique, the positioning of the chopper is all important to achieve a correct interplay of forces. The points to be kept in mind are:

- The chopper has to be very close to the phaco tip otherwise there will be rocking of the nucleus.
- At the time of actual splitting, the chopper **has** to be on the left of the tip, it **cannot** be on the right otherwise it will break the vacuum seal.

A vacuum hold is created by impaling the phaco probe with a burst of energy and withdrawing the pedal to position 2. The chopper is kept just left to or in front of the phaco tip within the CCC margin. The vertical portion of the chopper is buried deep in the nucleus in the direction of optic nerve. The chop is initiated by pulling it sideways (i.e. to your left). This can be accomplished by two methods:

1. Just pull chopper sideways while nucleus is stabilized with the phaco probe. This is easier to accomplish by beginners since concentration is only on movements of one hand.

2. Pull both the chopper and the probe in opposite directions. If the fibres do not entirely separate by the first method, the other hand can be moved to complete separation.

The break can be made full thickness by moving the chopper more central and deeper and continuing splitting if need be.

Modification

Instead of keeping the chopper centrally and embedding it vertically in the hardest part of the nucleus, chopper is kept slightly in the periphery and as you move it towards the centre, it is pushed deeper.

Problems with central chop

1. Since chopping is not started at full depth, sometimes a partial thickness chop may occur. To complete it, chopping has to be repeated twice or even thrice. In a peripheral chop, once the chop is initiated, it is usually full thickness.

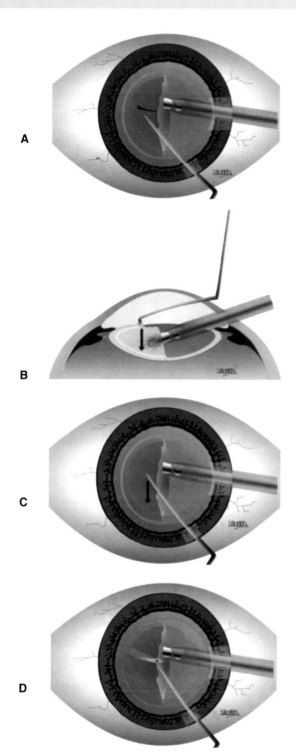

Fig. 9.24. Central chop. (A) Embed the probe into the nucleus and create a vacuum seal. Black line denotes the ideal area to embed the chopper close to and to the left of the probe. (B) The chopper is embedded close to the probe tip. Note the direction of force towards the vitreous cavity. (C) Note the direction of movement of the chopper. (D) The split starts superficially and goes deeper. One may have to move the chopper deeper to complete the crack.

2. Peripheral chop is stronger than central chop. In a hard nucleus, the chopper may not embed to the required depth. Also leathery fibres which do not split can be easily cut in the peripheral chop.

3. Central chop needs more space due to the rotational component in it.

Modified Peripheral Chop
(Fig. 9.25A, AA, B, BB & C) (Photos 9.85 to 9.88)

Negotiating the rhexis margin is the most difficult part of the peripheral chop. Benefits of both kinds of chopping are obtained using a modified peripheral chop. In this, after a vacuum seal has been created the periphery of the nucleus is brought out of the rhexis margin thus avoiding negotiating under the CCC. Following this, the method is same as in peripheral chop. However, this is only possible if:

1. The capsulorrhexis is large.
2. The nucleus is small.
3. One half of nucleus has been removed by central chopping leaving the other half for modified peripheral chop.

This is an extremely useful procedure for hard nuclei with leathery fibres.

Direct Chop (Photos 9.89 to 9.96)

In this method no trench is made and the probe is directly embedded bevel up or bevel down. Once a vacuum seal is created the chopper is used to split the nucleus. The procedure is repeated till the nucleus is split into many small pieces which are then aspirated. However, as already explained, you may not reach the core of the nucleus, as shown in the photographs, and end up chopping the exonucleus only.

Stop and Chop Technique (Photos 9.21 to 9.64)

In this technique a central complete trench is made and the nucleus is cracked into two pieces. Each heminucleus is then chopped and phacoaspirated separately.

ASPIRATION PHACO

The removal of divided nucleus segments from the capsular fornices and their aspiration in the CSZ is called aspiration phaco. In earlier days more amount of phaco power and less of aspiration was used to achieve this. This procedure was known as phacoaspiration (PA). With improvement in the fluidics of the machine, more of

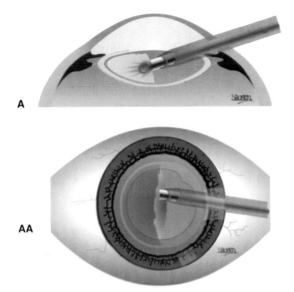

A vacuum seal is created. (A) Side view. (AA) Top view.

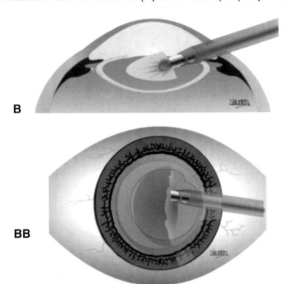

The piece is brought out of the capsular fornix into the CSZ.
(B) Side view. (BB) Front view.

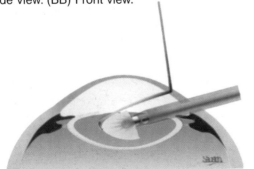

Chopper is brought from the periphery to centre to create a
split as in a peripheral chop.

Fig. 9.25. Modified peripheral chop.

aspiration and less of phaco power is used. Hence,
aspiration phaco (AP) would perhaps be a more
appropriate term.

It is essential to understand this step properly. Though
it appears technically easy, there are more chances of
complications during this step. The post-surgical
appearance of the eye depends on this crucial step. If
carefully done AP leads to bright and shining cornea and
a quiet eye. Nowadays, patients with a relatively good
pre-operative visual acuity are operated, so their
expectations for post-operative visual acuity are high.
They have to undergo tremendous amount of mental
stress for the period during which their vision is not
recovered due to keratitis.

**The aim is to perform the surgery in such a way
that there is minimal keratitis or complications,
irrespective of the hardness of the cataract, the pupil
size, anterior chamber depth and corneal health.**

Settings

• *Power settings* depend upon the grade of nucleus and
  can be further controlled by the foot pedal. A 30%
  reduction in power setting from that kept during
  trenching helps in increasing the foot gradient and
  therefore control.

• *Pulse mode* reduces the consumption of phaco energy
  by half and allows adequate time for vacuum build up
  during the interval when the phaco is off. Pulse settings
  between 2 to 6 is ideal for this procedure. The faster
  pulse settings act almost like continuous mode with
  less time for vacuum build up and, thereby, a poor grip.
  My personal choice is 3 pulses/sec.

• *Vacuum settings* depend upon the type of cataract and
  the space in the anterior chamber. For example, in
  hypermetropic eye the space in AC is less. Slight
  collapse of chamber can cause corneal probe touch and
  increase the possibility of keratitis. Therefore, low
  vacuum settings are required for such a case. While in
  myopic eyes there is enough space and high vacuum
  settings are possible. Small pupil and small CCC
  require stronger grip and higher vacuum settings to
  pull the pieces out of capsular fornices into CSZ in the
  first attempt, to avoid eating the tip away.

Types of grips (Figs. 9.26 to 9.29)

There are four types of grips for a nuclear piece: the
superficial soft skin, the firm body, pointed apex and the

Phacoaspiration

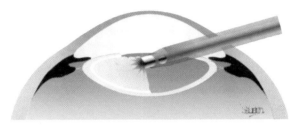

Fig. 9.26. Skin grip: Note the superficial grip.

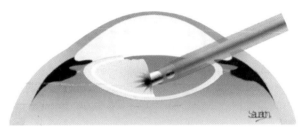

Fig. 9.27. Body grip: This grip is into the hardest part of the nucleus and is thus the strongest grip.

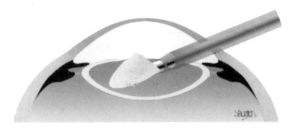

Fig. 9.28. Apex grip: The piece must be tilted up slightly to obtain an apical grip.

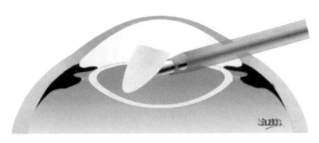

Fig. 9.29. Undersurface grip.

undersurface. The *skin* of the nucleus is soft and does not permit a firm grip as the vacuum leaks. ***The body of the nucleus provides the strongest grip***. It is not only ideal for chopping but also facilitates pulling the piece out of the capsular fornix. The **apical** and the **undersurface** grips are ideal for bringing the piece out of the fornix into the CSZ because of the direction of pull. However, these grips can be used only after the initial division has been made and the pieces have been lifted up.

Procedure (Photos 9.97 to 9.104)

For standard machine and grade III cataract the settings may be as follows:

Phaco power	50
Pulse	03
Vacuum	300
Bottle height	03 to 04 feet

AP must be done in the CSZ and the pieces must be removed from the capsular fornix (CF). Removal of the first piece from the CF is the toughest as it may be entangled with other chopped pieces, or the fibres may not be divided completely. The ideal piece to remove first is the smallest piece which has been completely separated from the rest of the nucleus.

As in chopping take the probe close to the body of the nucleus piece and embed in it with a small burst of energy. Allow time for vacuum hold to build up and then pull the piece out of CF to CSZ. Attempt to keep the piece away from cornea by angulating the probe a little downwards. Then crush or divide the piece with the help of the chopper. Phaco should be **off** while crushing i.e. FP position 2. Care should be taken throughout the procedure to avoid contact of the chopper with probe when the foot pedal is in phaco mode. After crushing, if the cataract is soft, it gets aspirated without the use of phaco energy. However, most of the time little phaco energy is required to remove the piece. Crushing not only dismantles the piece, it also increases the followability of the pieces which now get sucked in and need little phaco energy for emulsification. This procedure is repeated many times till the whole nucleus is removed. It is preferable to remove the piece by aspiration mainly, mechanical crushing may be added on as and when needed and minimal phaco must be used. Phaco should only be used when pieces are gripped by phaco probe and are not getting sucked in, i.e. the probe is fully or partially occluded.

If after removal of first piece surge is noticed, vacuum settings can be reduced as the rest of the pieces are easier to manoeuvre and remove. During removal of last piece vacuum settings can be further lowered, as at this stage there is no other piece in CF to prevent forward movement of PC. Even a small surge can cause a PCT particularly in a mature and hard cataract where the PC is not protected by the epinuclear plate. It is probably better to be closer to the cornea and run the risk of some keratitis rather than cause a PCT.

Problems

1. Inability to remove the nucleus piece

One very common difficulty that arises in phacoaspiration is the inability to remove the nuclear piece from capsular fornices. The tip of the nuclear piece is eaten away, leaving the body of the piece in the capsular rhexis. If similar treatment is meted out to rest of the pieces, a nuclear bowl is formed. The situation arises if any of the following is present:

- *Small CCC:* The widest part of the nucleus is in the periphery and the CCC can stretch to a certain limit. If the peripheral part is too big, then either the CCC breaks or the grip loosens, the latter being more common.
- *Too soft a cataract with high vacuum settings:* Here, as soon as the aspiration is switched on, the piece gets sucked in. Therefore, a good hold is not obtained.
- *Pieces entangled with each other:* The resistance offered by the entanglement causes the grip to loosen.
- *Hard cataract with low vacuum settings:* This results in poor hold, the nuclear fragments in such cases are bigger and are more prone to entanglement.
- *Unnecessary phaco:* The grip loosens due to emulsification of nuclear tissues surrounding the tip.
- *Very superficial grip:* A partial vacuum seal is created at the first place.

Management of a nuclear bowl requires phacoaspiration in the unsafe zone, i.e. the capsular fornices where the visibility is poor and the capsular bag is the shallowest.

Management of piece if tip is eaten away

Preventing the situations listed above is preferable. However, if a nuclear bowl is created, various methods can be used to deal with the piece.

One finger method (Fig. 9.30)

Phaco probe is introduced with CIM on. Chopper is horizontally placed under the rhexis margin. After taking it to the delineation line, it is turned vertically and the piece is pulled towards the CSZ for phacoaspiration. However, for beginners, it is safer to remove the probe from AC. Chamber is then filled with viscoelastic. Now the chopper is used to pull the piece into CSZ.

Two finger method (Fig. 9.31)

This method is used in a chamber filled with viscoelastic. In the vertical method, chopper is placed like in one finger method while a rounded repositor is used to lift the piece

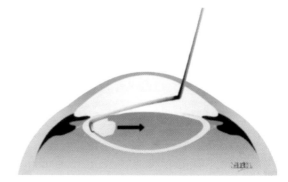

Fig. 9.30. One finger method: Chopper is placed under the capsule at delineation line to pull the piece into the CSZ.

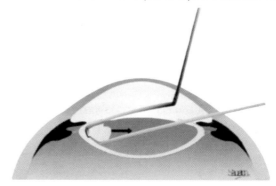

Fig. 9.31. Two finger method: Use of second instrument to take a counter-pressure.

up. In the other method, chopper can also be used with a Sinskey hook for sideways prolapse of the nuclear fragment. Alternatively, the fragment may be crushed in situ and then sucked in.

2. Burrowing of fragment (Fig. 9.32)

Continuous use of phaco energy leads to through & through emulsification of the nuclear fragment. The piece forms a ring around the U/S tip and needs to be mechanically dislodged. This is more commonly seen with large pieces. Before complete burrowing of a large fragment, it may either be cracked and crushed with a chopper and brought in front for AP.

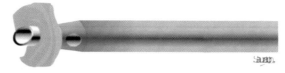

Fig. 9.32. Burrowing of fragment. Continuous use of phaco leads to through & through emulsification of the fragment.

3. Milking

This occurs due to partial or complete clogging of the aspiration system. Therefore, there is low vacuum delivery. The nucleus gets emulsified but not aspirated leading to clouding of the chamber. The blockage is usually at the junctional points. To check the system, take the phaco probe out of the eye and put on the test chamber. Now in I/A mode with highest vacuum settings, depress the foot pedal fully. Pinch the aspiration tube till maximum vacuum sound is heard and then release the tubing creating maximum surge possible. This sudden vacuum may suck the blocking piece in. This manoeuvre can be done repeatedly. Another method which can be applied is the use of reflux though it is not so effective. If these do not work then the only alternative is to detach the tubing from the handpiece and forcefully inject BSS (with a 10 cc syringe) into the tubing as well as the handpiece. One can use connecting rubber piece from IV sets as an attachment for injecting into the handpiece. At times one may have to unscrew the tip and look for clogging. After reassembling, check for the surge again to ensure that the clogging has now been cleared before you enter the eye.

4. Chattering

Chattering is more common with small hard cataract pieces. This is seen when too much power is used with a poor hold on the fragments. The hold may be poor because adequate vacuum has not built up or the vacuum settings are too low. The excursion of the tip then tends to push the pieces away, which is very damaging to the cornea.

5. Pieces lodged in no/low followability zone

Pieces lying in these zones cannot be phacoaspirated and have to be positioned in the zone of followability. In the zone of low followability, the phaco probe is taken near the piece and aspiration is attempted. If unsuccessful, this procedure should be abandoned after the first attempt. If the fragment still remains elusive and in the zones of no followability, the probe is removed. Chamber is filled with viscoelastic. The piece is brought to CSZ mechanically with the help of 1 or 2 instruments. It is then pushed below the iris plane, for phacoaspiration.

DIVIDE AND CONQUER

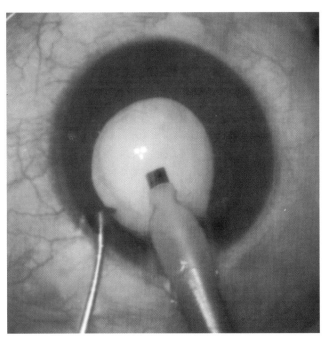

Photo 9.1. Note the bared nucleus. Epinuclear plate has been removed. Probe is placed just proximal to the centre of the nucleus for starting the trench.

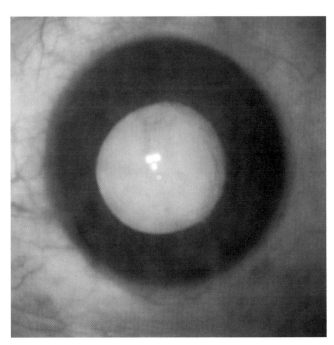

Photo 9.2. Completion of the first trench.

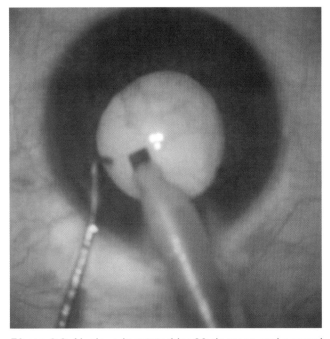

Photo 9.3. Nucleus is rotated by 90 degrees and second trench created.

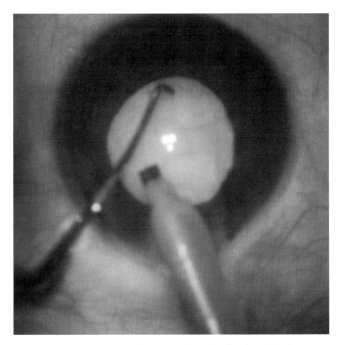

Photo 9.4. Rotation of the nucleus by further 90 degrees with chopper. Note position of chopper in most peripheral part of the groove.

DIVIDE AND CONQUER (Contd.)

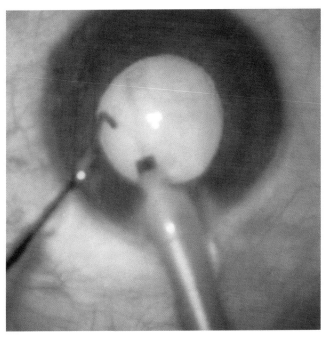

Photo 9.5. Creation of the third trench.

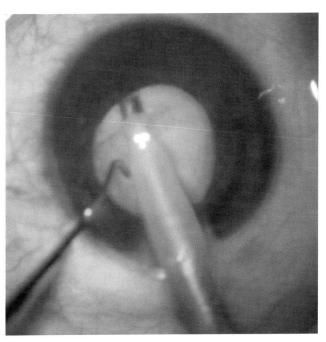

Photo 9.6. Creation of the fourth trench. Note the position of tip just short of pupillary border.

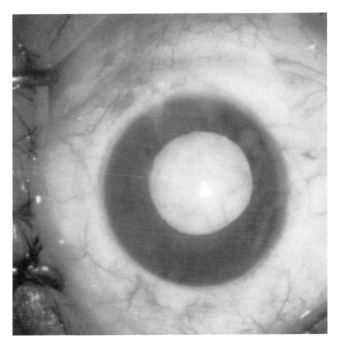

Photo 9.7. Formation of shallow Maltese cross.

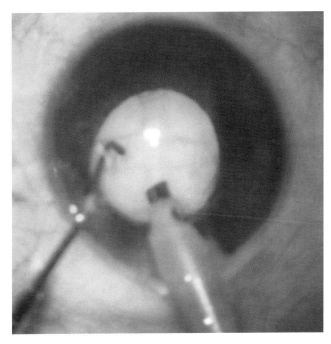

Photo 9.8. Central bump removed to deepen the cross.

DIVIDE AND CONQUER (Contd.)

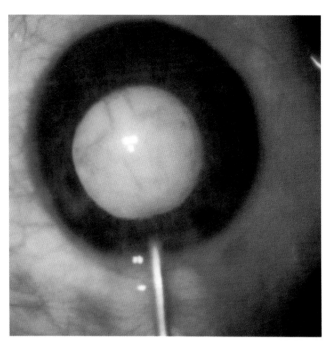

Photo 9.9. Maltese cross of adequate depth.

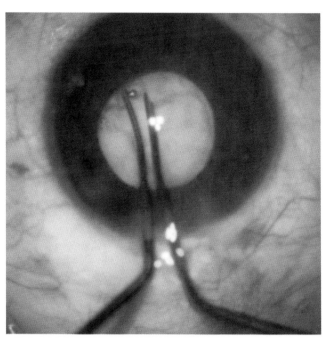

Photo 9.10. Division of the first trench by parallel placement of the instruments through the same port.

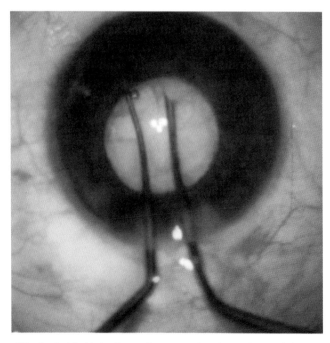

Photo 9.11. Note the split appearing from the periphery.

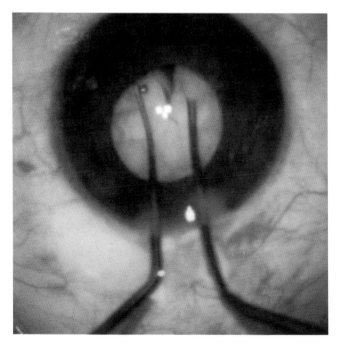

Photo 9.12. Note the split going upto the centre.

DIVIDE AND CONQUER (Contd.)

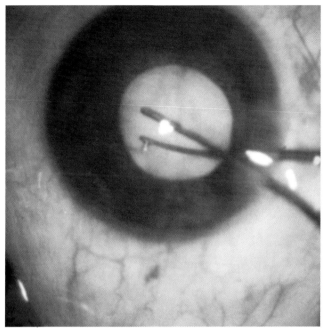

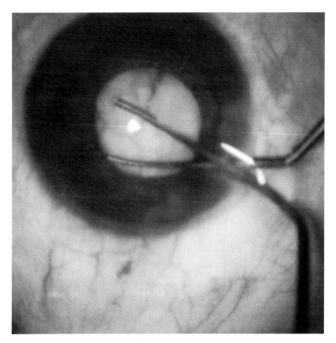

Photos 9.13, 9.14, 9.15 & 9.16. Splitting of the second trench by cross placement of the instruments from the same port.

Photo 9.14.

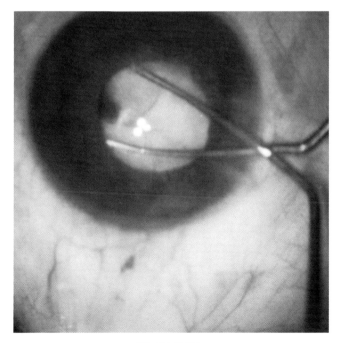

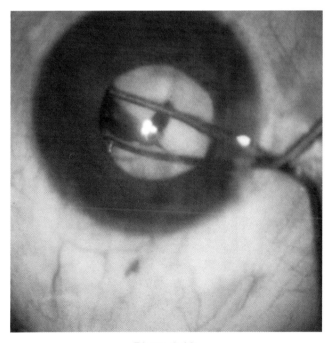

Photo 9.15.

Photo 9.16.

DIVIDE AND CONQUER (Contd.)

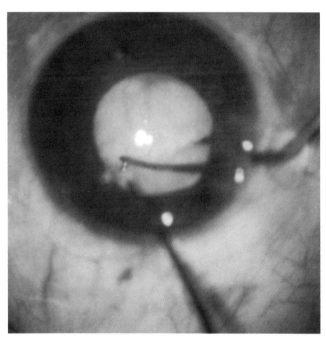

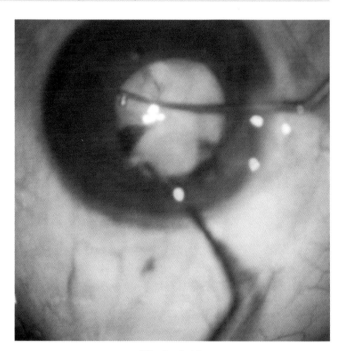

Photos 9.17 & 9.18. Splitting of the third trench by parallel placement of the instruments through the different ports.

Photo 9.18.

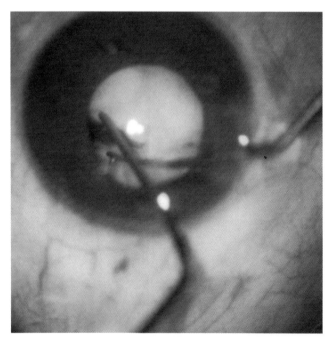

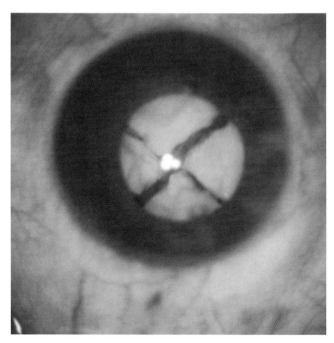

Photo 9.19. Splitting of the last trench by cross placement of the instruments from different ports.

Photo 9.20. Four separate pieces of nucleus.

STOP AND CHOP (V-Trench)

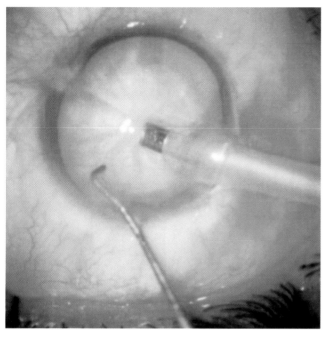

Photo 9.21. Trench is started slightly proximal to the centre of the nucleus. Note the shaving action with less than half of the tip buried.

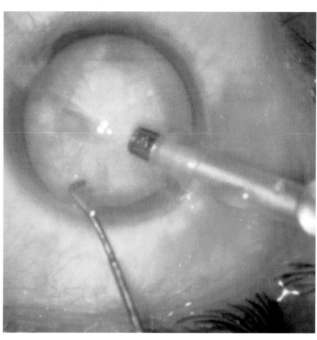

Photo 9.22. Note the formation of the first arm of the "V".

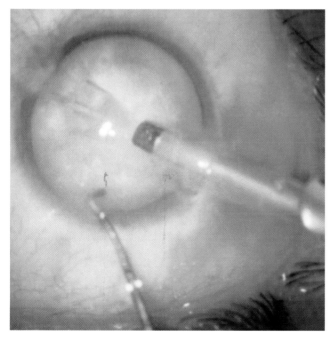

Photo 9.23. Formation of the second arm to complete the "V".

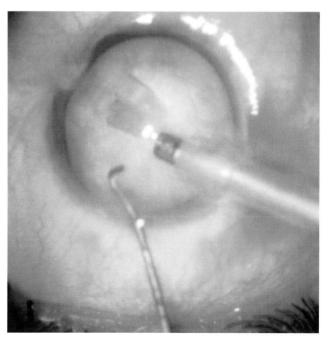

Photos 9.24 & 9.25. "V" is further deepened.

STOP AND CHOP (V-Trench) (Contd.)

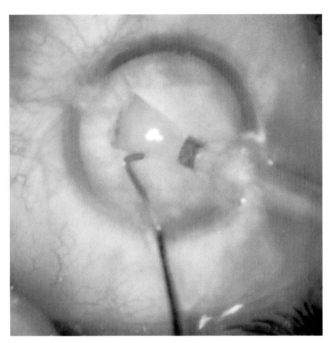

Photo 9.25.

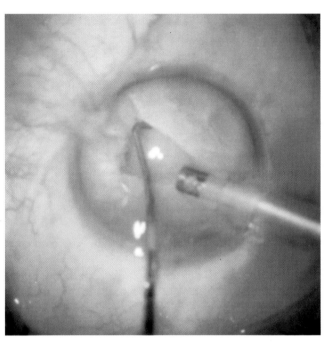

Photo 9.26. Rotation of the nucleus using the chopper (single-handed technique). Chopper is placed in the peripheral most part of trench. Nucleus is pushed to the periphery and then rotated.

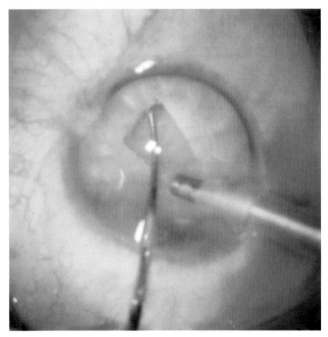

Photos 9.27 & 9.28. Note that the chopper is closer to the iris as nucleus is pushed to the periphery for counter-pressure.

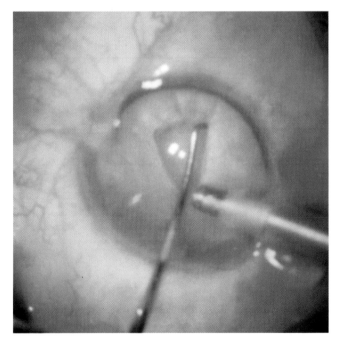

Photo 9.28.

STOP AND CHOP (V-Trench) (Contd.)

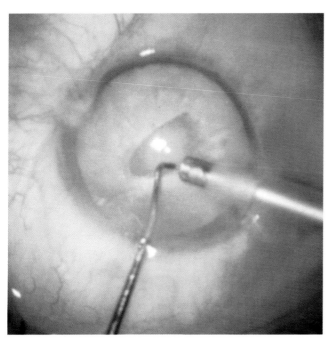

Photo 9.29.

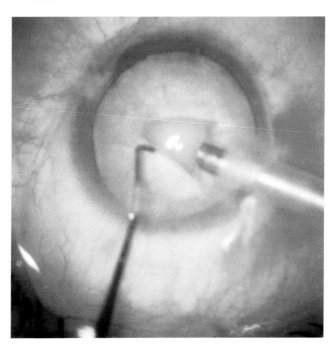

Photo 9.30.

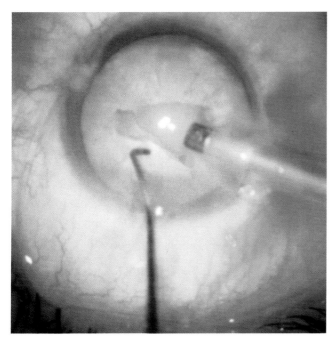

Photo 9.31. Similar shaving of the other side

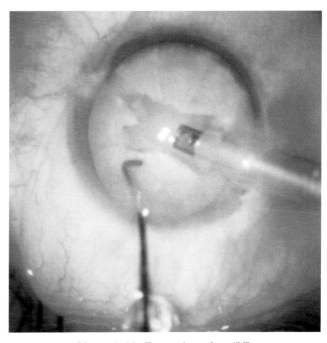

Photo 9.32. Formation of an "X".

STOP AND CHOP (V-Trench) (Contd.)

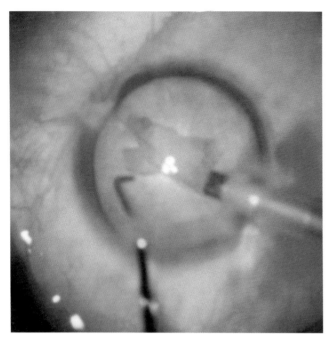

Photo 9.33. Deepening of the second arm.

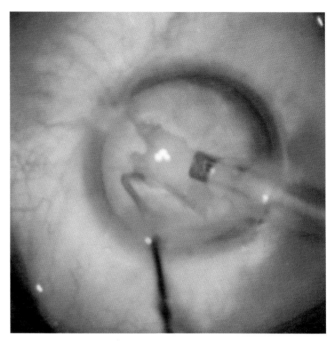

Photo 9.34. Further deepening of the first arm.

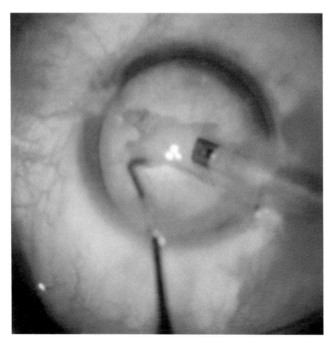

Photo 9.35. Deepening the centre.

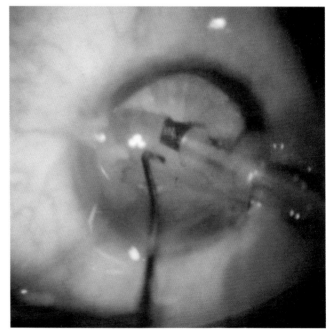

Photo 9.36. Placement of the instrument in the depth of the trench to split the nucleus.

STOP AND CHOP (Splitting)

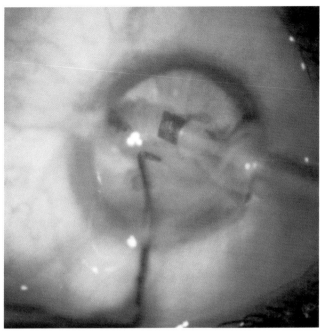

Photo 9.37. Instruments moved. Crack appears in the periphery.

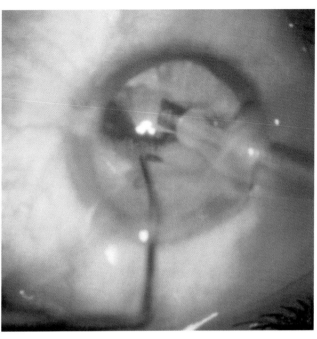

Photo 9.38. Both the instruments moved in opposite directions as far as possible.

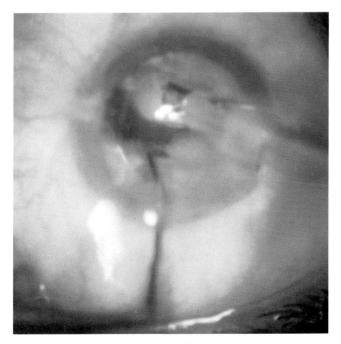

Photo 9.39. Crack still not complete.

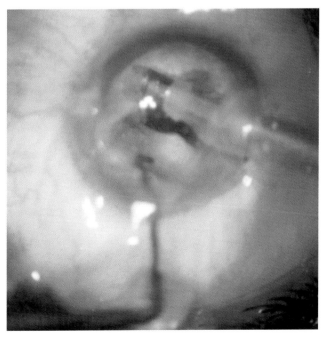

Photo 9.40. Nucleus rotated to bring the sub-incisional area to cross-incisional side and nucleus split completed.

CENTRAL CHOP

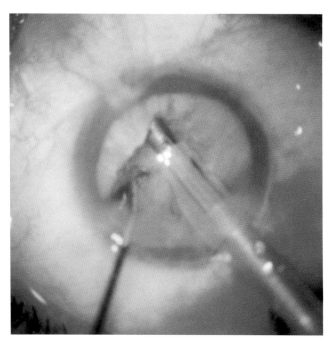

Photo 9.41. Nudging the nucleus with the probe.

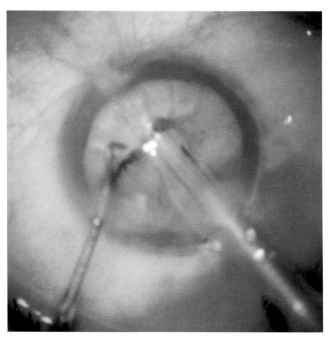

Photo 9.42. Giving a short burst of phaco to impale the nucleus.

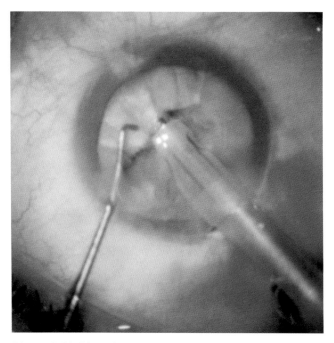

Photo 9.43. Note the position of chopper close to and just to the left of the phaco tip.

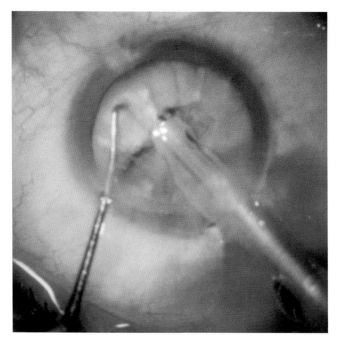

Photo 9.44. Chopper is turned towards vitreous cavity and buried into nucleus substance.

CENTRAL CHOP (Contd.)

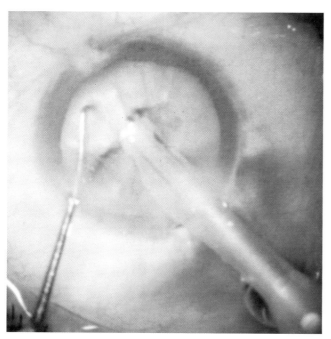

Photo 9.45. Chopper partially buried into the nucleus.

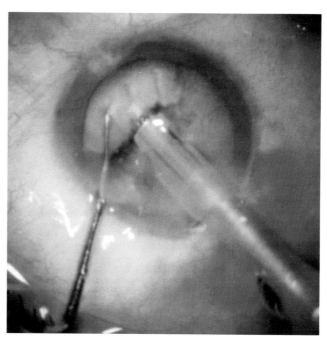

Photo 9.46. Chopper completely buried into the nucleus.

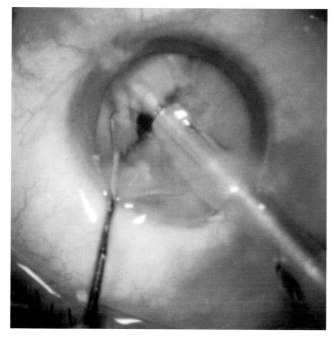

Photo 9.47. Chopper pulled towards the left to initiate the chop.

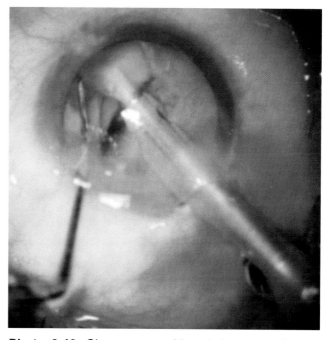

Photo 9.48. Chopper repositioned deeper and more peripheral to complete the crack. Phaco probe and vacuum seal maintained.

CENTRAL CHOP (Contd.)

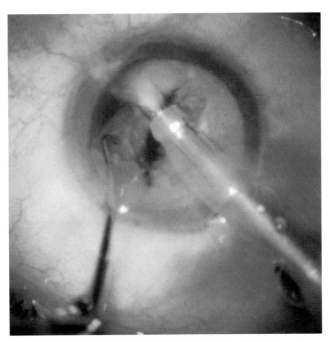

Photo 9.49. Crack completed.

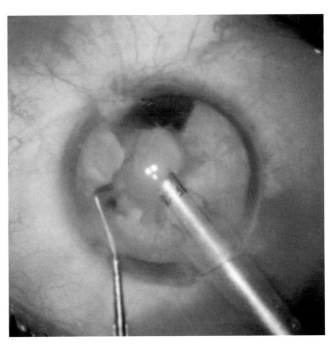

Photo 9.50. Separated piece is now phacoaspirated in CSZ.

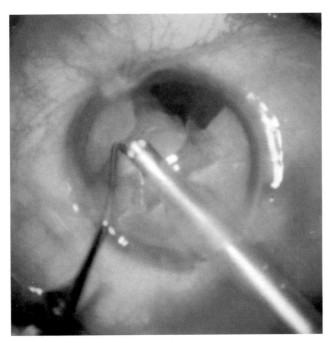

Photo 9.51. Tip brought to adjacent piece.

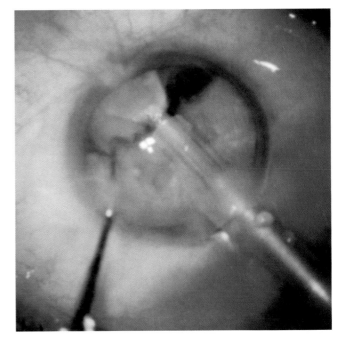

Photo 9.52. Vacuum seal created.

CENTRAL CHOP (Contd.)

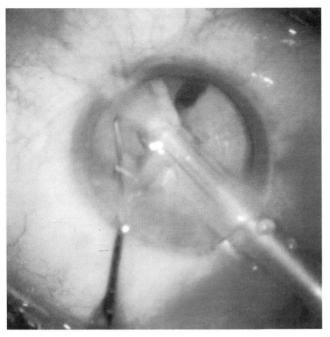

Photo 9.53. Chopper buried and chop initiated.

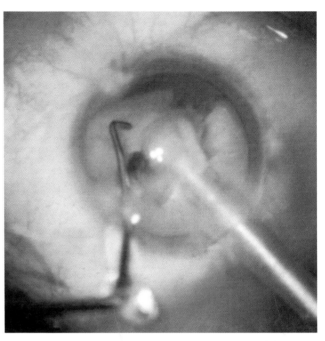

Photo 9.54. The piece is now aspirated in CSZ.

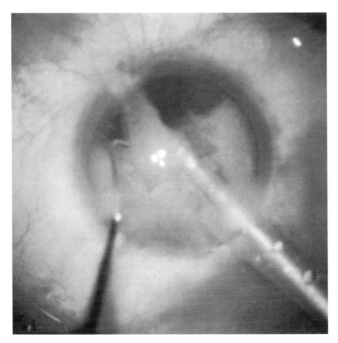

Photo 9.55. Aspiration of the last bit of the 1st heminucleus.

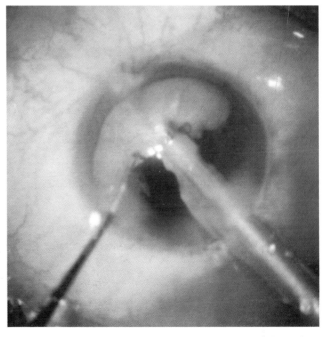

Photo 9.56. The nucleus is rotated to bring the other heminucleus into position.

CENTRAL CHOP (Contd.)

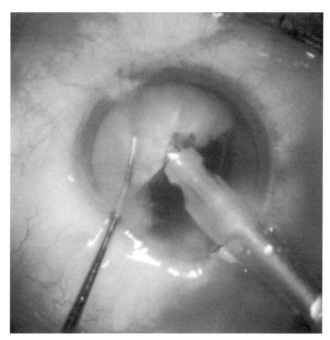

Photo 9.57. Chopper buried.

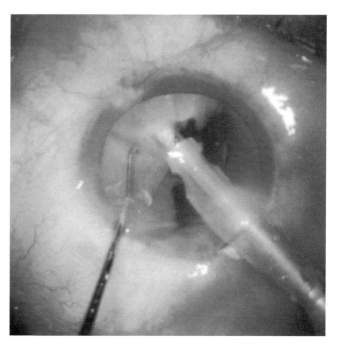

Photo 9.58. Split initiated.

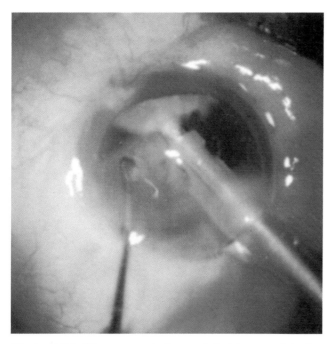

Photo 9.59. Chopper and piece rotated to complete the split. Since the space is more, chopper need not be repositioned (as was done in Photo 9.48).

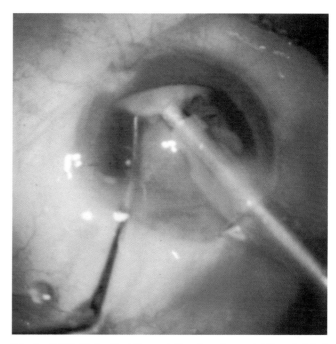

Photo 9.60. Note that the rotation has brought the divided piece in the sub-incisional area.

CENTRAL CHOP (Contd.)

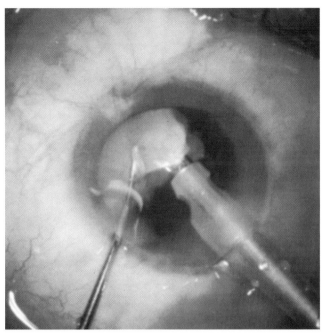

Photo 9.61. Last piece repositioned and chopping initiated.

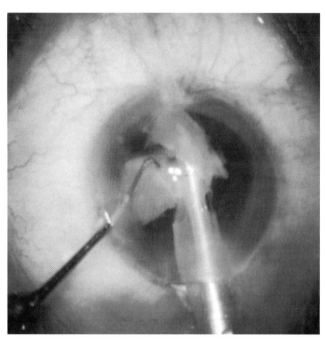

Photo 9.62. Second last piece being aspirated.

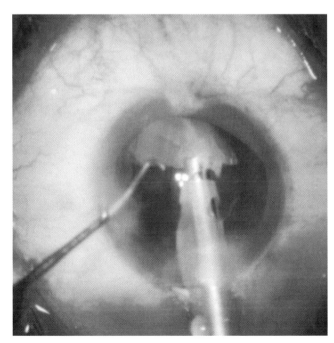

Photo 9.63. Last piece held.

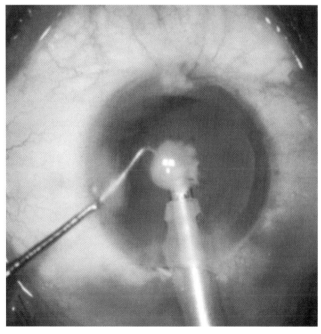

Photo 9.64. Aspiration of last piece in CSZ.

PERIPHERAL CHOP WITH PARTIAL TRENCH WITHOUT ROTATION

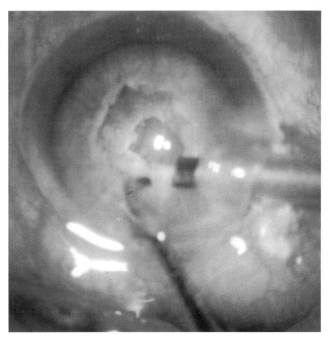

Photo 9.65. Creation of small trench.

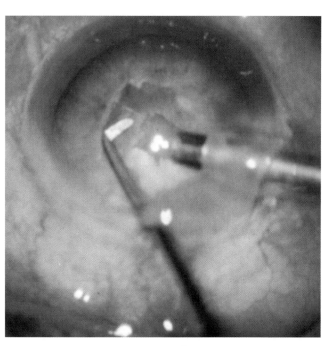

Photo 9.66. Note the position of blunt chopper. Chopper is positioned horizontally to go underneath CCC margin.

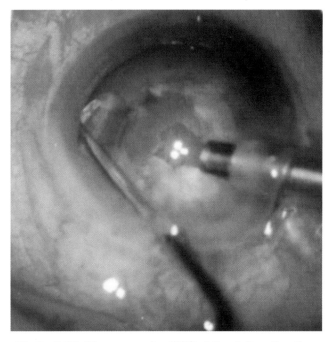

Photo 9.67. Chopper under CCC at the delineation line.

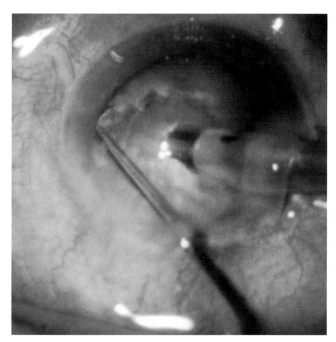

Photo 9.68. Vacuum seal created.

PERIPHERAL CHOP WITH PARTIAL TRENCH WITHOUT ROTATION (Contd.)

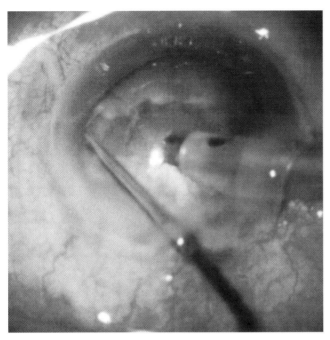

Photo 9.69. Chopper turned vertically down.

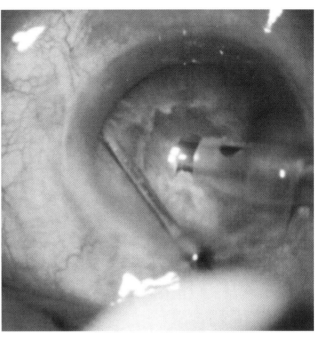

Photos 9.70 & 9.71. Chopper now pulled towards the probe cutting the intervening nuclear fibres.

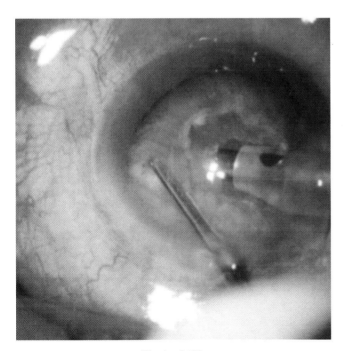

Photo 9.71.

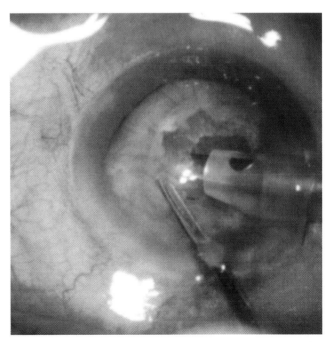

Photos 9.72 & 9.73. When the chopper reaches the probe it is pulled sideways to complete the chop.

PERIPHERAL CHOP WITH PARTIAL TRENCH WITHOUT ROTATION (Contd.)

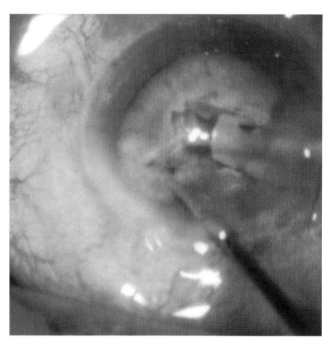

Photo 9.73.

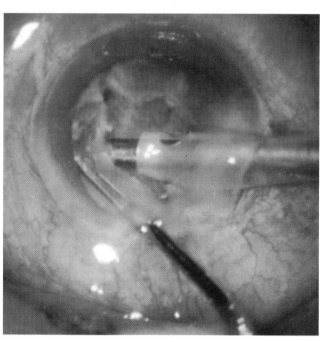

Photo 9.74. Nucleus rotated to bring next piece into position. Note that the first crack is on the right of the probe. Procedure repeated and second chop initiated.

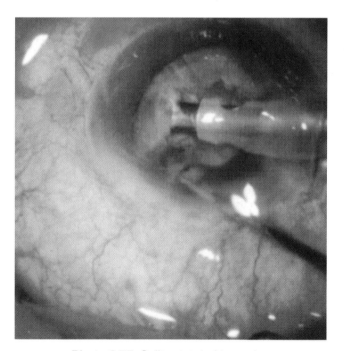

Photo 9.75. Split extended to centre.

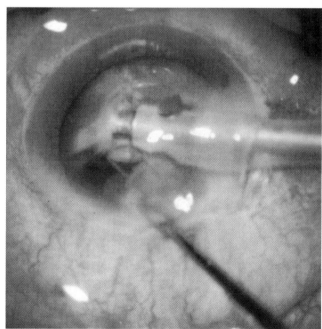

Photo 9.76. Split completed. Similarly the whole nucleus is divided into five to seven small pieces and phacoaspirated one by one.

CENTRAL CHOP WITH PARTIAL TRENCH WITH ROTATION

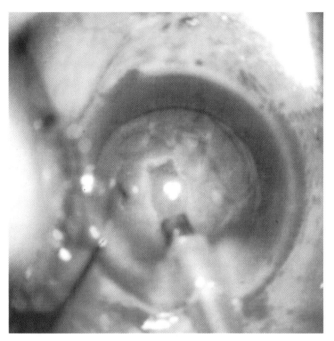

Photo 9.77. Completion of a partial trench.

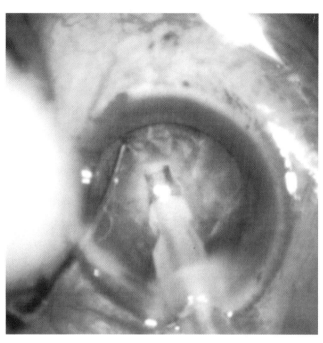

Photo 9.78. Vacuum seal can be created without rotation but tip reaches more into the periphery.

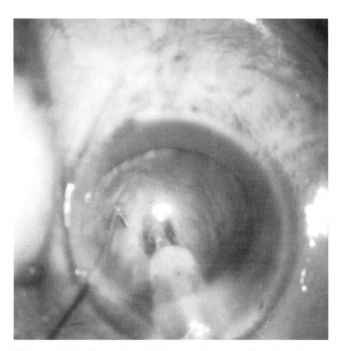

Photo 9.79. Rotation of the nucleus and using larger platform for stabilization.

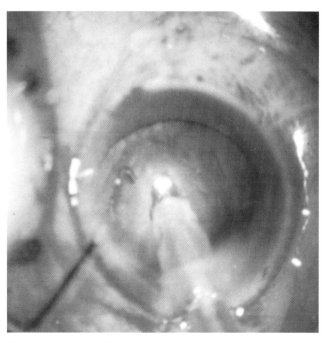

Photo 9.80. Creation of vacuum seal. Note the position of the chopper close to the tip.

CENTRAL CHOP WITH PARTIAL TRENCH WITH ROTATION (Contd.)

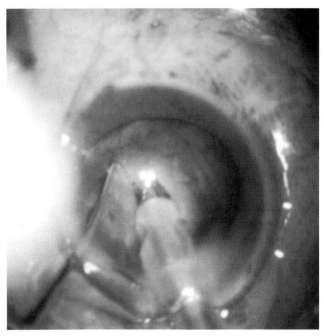

Photo 9.81. After stabilizing the nucleus with the phaco probe, burying the chopper into the nucleus for central chop.

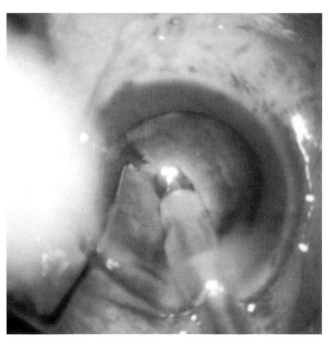

Photo 9.82. Splitting by moving the chopper to the left.

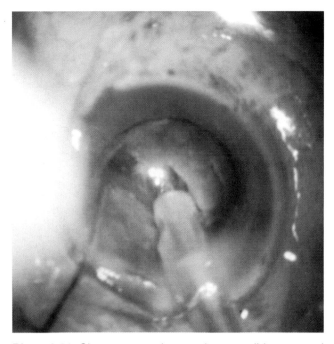

Photo 9.83. Chopper moved as much as possible to extend the split.

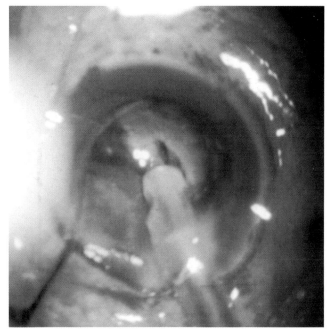

Photo 9.84. Extending the split to centre by moving the probe in the opposite direction.

MODIFIED PERIPHERAL CHOP

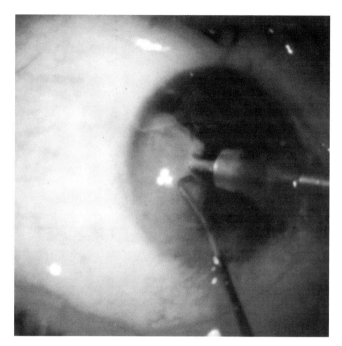

Photo 9.85. Creation of vacuum seal.

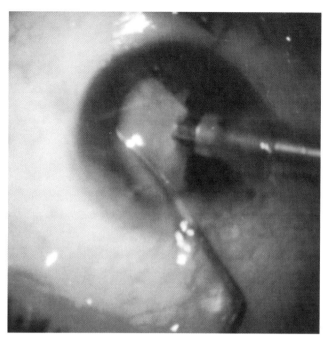

Photo 9.86. Pull the piece out of the CCC margin till the peripheral edge is visible. Note the position of the chopper at the peripheral edge.

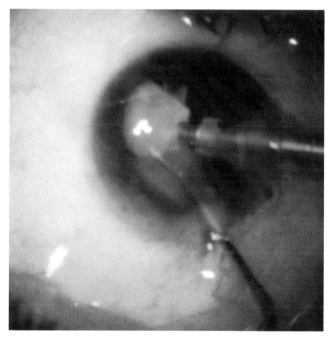

Photo 9.87. Pull the chopper towards the tip to create a crack.

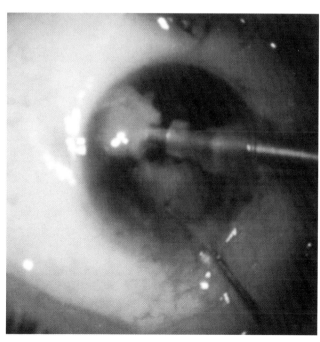

Photo 9.88. Chopper pulled sideways to complete the crack.

DIRECT CHOP

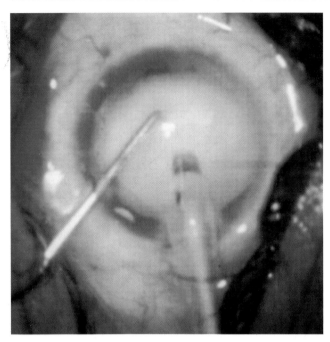

Photo 9.89. Note the bevel down position of the phaco probe. Bury the tip and create a vacuum seal. Chopper is buried close to the tip.

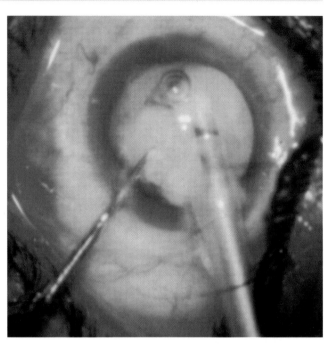

Photo 9.90. Chopper pulled towards the side to create a crack.

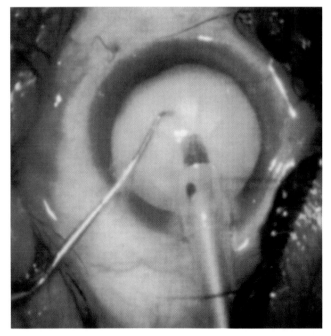

Photo 9.91. Repeat the manoeuvre. Note the position of the tip at the centre of the nucleus.

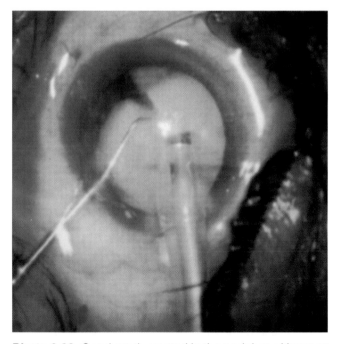

Photo 9.92. Good crack created in the periphery. However note that the tip has reached to the mid periphery.

DIRECT CHOP (Contd.)

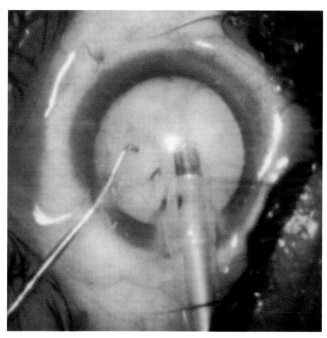

Photo 9.93. Nucleus is rotated and procedure is repeated all around at 4 to 5 places.

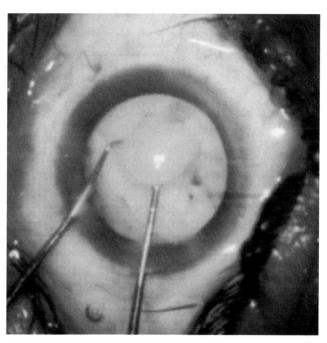

Photo 9.94. Note the creation of endonucleus because of inadequately buried probe. The chops were created in the exonucleus sparing the hard endonucleus.

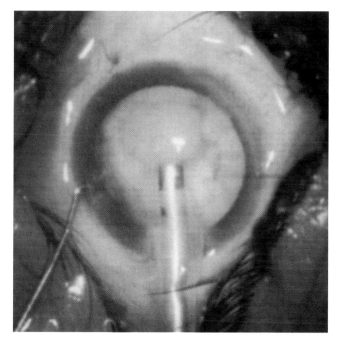

Photo 9.95. Endonucleus being aspirated.

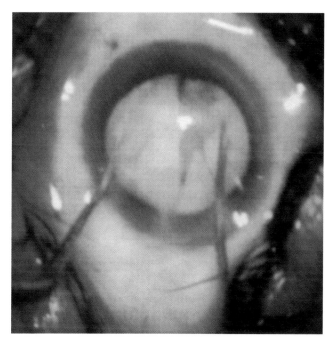

Photo 9.96. Completing the cracks in the posterior exonucleus to facilitate phacoaspiration.

PHACOASPIRATION

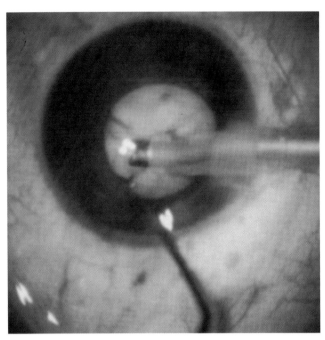

Photo 9.97. Nudge the nucleus in the body of the piece.

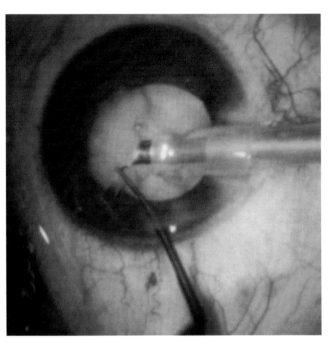

Photo 9.98. Body grip—see the triangular piece going upto the sleeve.

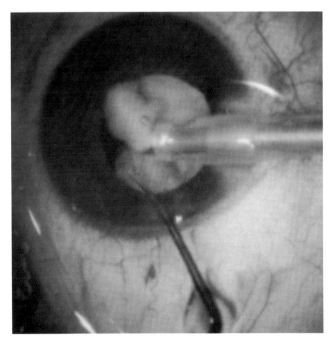

Photo 9.99. Body grip—Aspiration in CSZ.

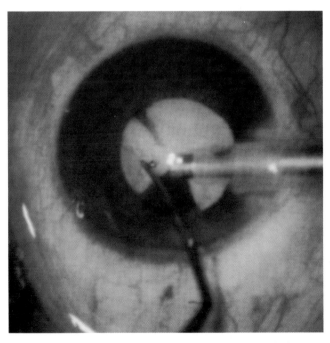

Photo 9.100. Apex grip—Note probe positioned close to the apex. Dumbbell pushing periphery down to lift the apex.

PHACOASPIRATION (Contd.)

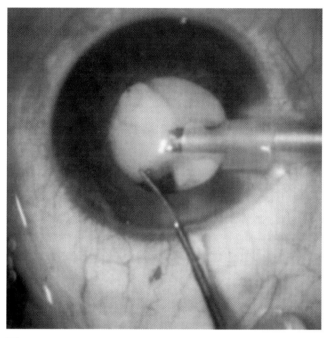

Photo 9.101. Apex grip—Probe buried into the apex and pulling into CSZ.

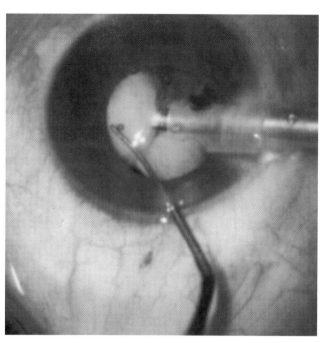

Photo 9.102. Undersurface grip—Dumbbell lifting the piece further to expose the undersurface.

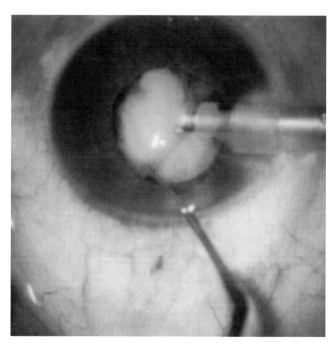

Photo 9.103. Undersurface grip—Piece pulled out into CSZ for aspiration. Note the rough surface facing the cornea.

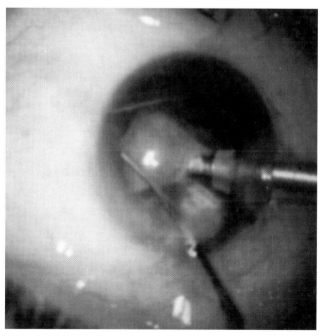

Photo 9.104. Chopper can be used for crushing if the chopped piece is still too big. Note phaco should be off when using the chopper to mechanically crush.

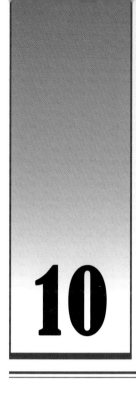

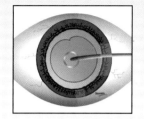

10
Epinuclear Plate Removal

Somehow the step of epinuclear plate (ENP) removal has not been given due importance with the result that many good surgeons struggle at this stage after successfully completing nucleotomy. Rather than the hit and trial methods followed by some, a reproducible and effective technique is required. A very safe, simple and effective technique for epinuclear plate removal is the flip and chip method which was initially described for nucleotomy.

APPLIED ANATOMY (Figs. 10.1 & 10.2)

Two important aspects of the epinuclear plate need to be discussed. One is that the size of epinuclear plate is very large vis-à-vis the CCC. Therefore any attempt to prolapse it intact into the AC will invariably fail. For practical purposes the plate consists of 3 parts, i.e. anterior (beneath the anterior capsule), equatorial (at the capsular fornices) and posterior (along the posterior capsule). The central part of the anterior epinuclear plate is already partially removed before nucleotomy. As is with the nucleus, the epinuclear plate also varies in its hardness depending upon the type of cataract. The hardness of the ENP usually corresponds with the grade of nucleus. However, in few cases, a disproportionately hard yellowish-brown ENP may be found in cases with a relatively softer nucleus. The thickness of the ENP is related inversely to the size of the nucleus. The thickness of ENP also depends upon where the delineation line is created by the surgeon. If inadvertently two delineation lines are created, double

Parts of the Epinuclear Plate
Note the anterior (pink), equatorial (blue), posterior (green) epinuclear plate.

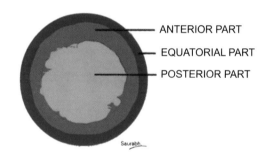

Fig. 10.1. Top view.

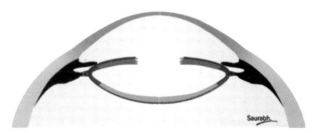

Fig. 10.2. Side view.

ENP may be created which may be partially or completely separated from each other. Some ENPs have a weak equatorial zone where they tend to break off easily. Few plates have division along the 'Y' sutures into 2 or 3 pieces. This is more common in hard cataracts. ENP may be absent in hypermature cataracts and grade V cataracts where ENP gets merged with the nucleus.

INSTRUMENTS

Rounded iris repositor/Rod-shaped iris repositor

This instrument is very important for the rotation of epinuclear plate. It can be manipulated through the side port and is atraumatic.

Phaco settings

The settings depend upon the hardness of the epinuclear plate. Phaco power is kept between 10% to 30% at the lowest to get a better foot gradient. Flow rate need not be low as the CSZ has been increased in size due to nucleus removal and there is adequate space in the eye. Vacuum, however, can be lowered, as bombardment of the ENP with phaco will not be needed and so a very firm grip is not required. In fact, higher vacuum may result in biting of the ENP and loosening of the grip especially in a soft cataract. The vacuum should be adequate to help pull the ENP into CSZ without aspirating it. In a soft cataract a setting of 80 mmHg is sufficient which can be increased upto 120 mmHg in a hard ENP.

TECHNIQUE: FLIP & CHIP METHOD
(Photos 10.1 to 10.20) (Figs. 10.3 to 10.9)

The objective of **chipping** is to reduce the size of the ENP by removing most of the anterior and equatorial ENP and some of peripheral posterior ENP. For this purpose, the phaco probe is placed under the anterior ENP with bevel up to occlude the port with the ENP. The foot pedal is depressed between positions 1 and 2 and a vacuum seal is created. Once a firm grip is obtained, you should try to pull it into the CSZ. If the grip appears to loosen, one can allow the vacuum to build up further. Note that no phaco is used to create vacuum seal in this step. Once the ENP is in the CSZ give a burst of energy to aspirate the part which is occluding the port. Before the plate falls back, you should simultaneously move the probe forwards and then sideways in an 'L' shaped manner. This manoeuvre allows for wider removal of the equatorial ENP which has a larger circumference. This sideways movement also helps you to grip the adjacent part of the ENP. Now the tip is disengaged by bringing the foot pedal to position I (or position 0 if in CIM). The ENP is then rotated with the help of a rounded repositor to bring the adjacent site into the line of attack and the procedure is repeated. This is continued (may be upto 6 to 8 times) till the last 2 to 3 clock hours of anterior ENP are left.

At this point, you are left with most of the posterior ENP attached to a tongue-shaped extension of equatorial and anterior ENP. This now has to be flipped. The tongue-shaped area should be sufficient to allow for two attempts of flipping. Vacuum seal is created as described earlier at the tongue-shaped area, and the rounded repositor is placed at the centre of posterior ENP. The anterior plate is pulled towards the CSZ with the probe and, simultaneously, the rounded repositor is used to slide the posterior plate towards the capsular fornix facilitating the flipping. In case the grip loosens or the ENP breaks, repeat the procedure from another site. Once half of the posterior ENP is pulled out of CCC or flipped over, it does not go back easily and now phaco can be used to aspirate the plate. Most of the times ENP gets sucked without use of phaco energy. It should be noted in this step the PC cannot be visualized as the entire ENP lies in the AC in a zig-zag manner. Therefore, the rounded repositor should be kept below the tip to prevent PCT in case of inadvertent surge. The soft ENP is less damaging to the cornea so this aspiration can safely be performed a little more anteriorly to safeguard the posterior capsule.

PROBLEMS

1. **Hemisected/trisected plate** (Photos 10.21 to 10.23): In such an ENP usually one piece is lying over the other. Identify the piece on the top and remove it first. These pieces are usually pulled easily to CSZ and there is no need to use flip and chip. Sometimes the pieces are partially separated. In such a situation pressurize the eyeball with VES and try to mechanically separate the pieces with two instruments. Always keep the split line vertically, since it is easier to flip the ENP fragment on the left side. For a triangular piece also grip the edge on the right side. This both improves the visibility and permits easy flipping with rounded repositor.

2. **ENP with a wedge in posterior ENP without anterior extension** (Fig. 10.10A & B): The commonest problem encountered in ENP removal is when only the posterior plate is left without any anterior extension. This problem is so common that the surgeon must prepare himself from the beginning to manage it. For this, an attempt should be made to create a wedge in the posterior plate during chipping. Once the first few chips have been made, the plate tends to prolapse easier. Then, along with the anterior and equatorial parts, you should try to remove a small piece of the posterior ENP as well. Even if you haven't created a wedge, there may be an inadvertent

Flip & Chip Method

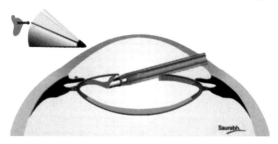

Fig. 10.3. Creation of vacuum seal. (Note: No phaco power is used for creation of vacuum seal. Cf. nuclear vacuum seal.)

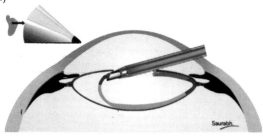

Fig. 10.4. Pull ENP into CSZ. FP intermittently taken to position 3 for emulsification. Simultaneously tip advanced toward and under the CCC making sure that the ENP does not fall back.

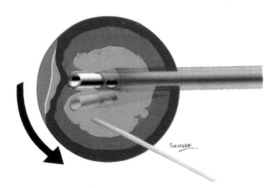

Fig. 10.5. After reaching the CCC margin the tip is moved to the left to remove wider area of equatorial ENP. Note that the tip is now closer to the RR in the figure.

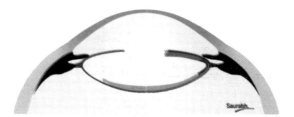

Fig. 10.6. Efficient removal of ENP where anterior, equatorial and part of posterior ENP have been removed.

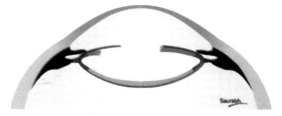

Fig. 10.7. Inefficient removal: only part of anterior ENP is removed.

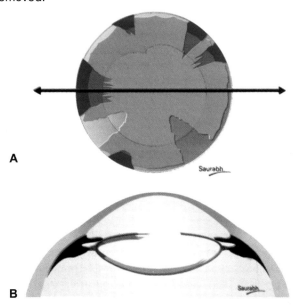

A

B

Fig. 10.8. Pre-flip ENP. Note that most of the anterior ENP and parts of the equatorial and posterior ENP have been removed. Only tongue-shaped extension of anterior ENP remains for flipping. (A) Top view. (B) Side view.

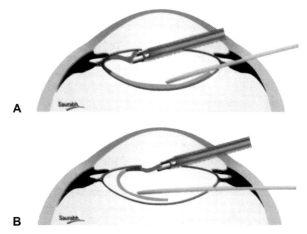

A

B

Fig. 10.9. Flipping. (A) Note the position of RR on centre of posterior ENP. Create a vacuum seal on anterior ENP before flipping. (B) ENP is pulled in to the centre by tip and simultaneously posterior ENP is pushed towards the periphery to facilitate flipping of ENP into CSZ.

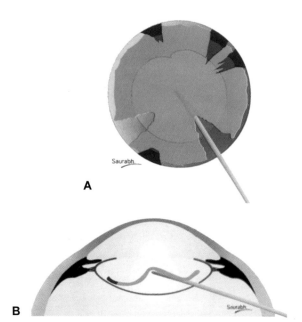

Fig. 10.10. Removal of ENP when no anterior extension is left and there is a chink/wedge in the posterior ENP. In a pressurized eye, RR is slipped through the chink under the ENP and it is lifted up into the CSZ for phacoaspiration. (A) Front view. (B) Side view.

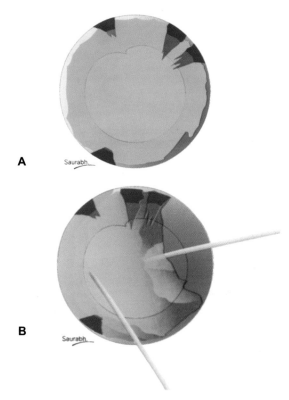

Fig. 10.11. ENP when no anterior extension and no wedge is present. (A) Note the position of two instruments, one from main port and one from the side port. (B) Side port instrument pushes ENP to the periphery and the second instrument now introduced under the edge of ENP and lifted up (artificially creating a chink).

wedge created which can be used. Once only the plate is left, pressurize the eye with VES. Now engage the rounded repositor between the ENP and posterior capsule at the wedge and lift the ENP. Repeat the process till the whole plate is prolapsed into the AC.

3. **ENP without anterior extensions and without a wedge in posterior ENP** (Fig. 10.11A & B): Rounded repositor pushes the EPN till one end of ENP plate appears close to CCC. Now second instrument is introduced underneath it for lifting it up.

4. If these methods fail to mobilize the plate, you can remove the probe and start irrigation-aspiration. Aspiration of the cortical fibres situated posterior to the plate usually result in its prolapsing into the AC. You can then either mechanically crush it and remove with IA itself or else re-introduce the probe for removal.

5. A method followed by some surgeons is to decompress the AC by sudden depression of the posterior wound lip. This results in forward movement of the EPN and injection of viscoelastic below it can further elevate it. Some surgeons also hold the EPN plate directly with the bevel down—this is **not** recommended especially for beginners.

EPINUCLEAR PLATE REMOVAL (FLIP & CHIP TECHNIQE)

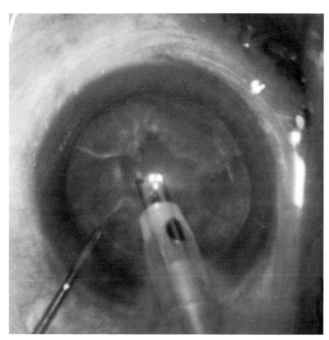

Photo 10.1. Note the position of rounded repositor. Enter with infusion on. Foot position 1 or CIM.

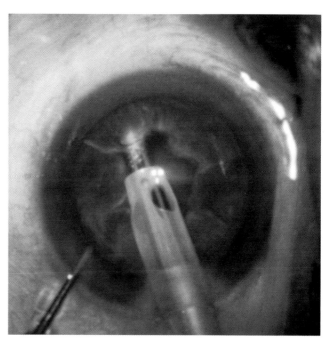

Photo 10.2. Go under CCC and create vacuum seal on anterior ENP.

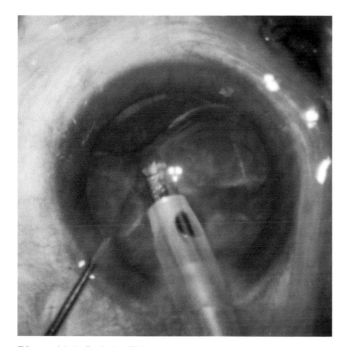

Photo 10.3. Pull the EN plate out of the rhexis margin. Take the tip towards the rhexis margin with FP between 2 and 3. As soon as emulsification takes place, go back to FP2 and advance to hold before the EN falls back. Keep on oscillating your foot, advancing till the CCC margin and then leave removing part of anterior epinuclear plate, equatorial epinuclear plate and posterior epinuclear plate as far as possible.

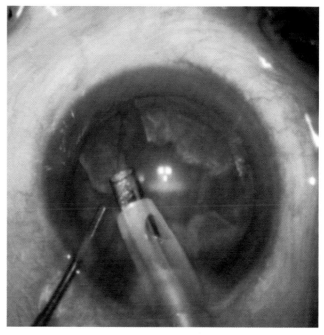

Photo 10.4. Go to the adjacent site and repeat the procedure.

EPINUCLEAR PLATE REMOVAL (FLIP & CHIP TECHNIQE) (Contd.)

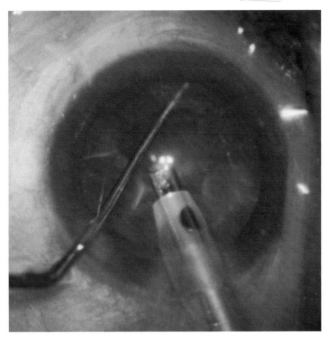

Photo 10.5. Place the rounded repositor at the equator to rotate the epinuclear plate.

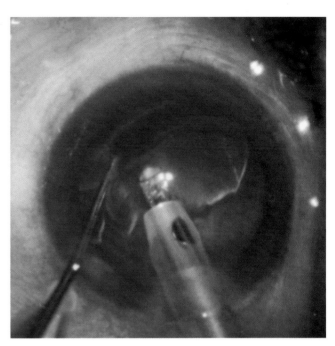

Photo 10.6. Removal of epinuclear plate continues.

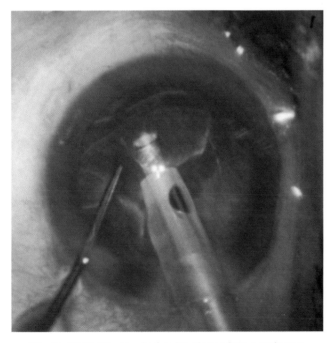

Photo 10.7. Removal of epinuclear plate continues.

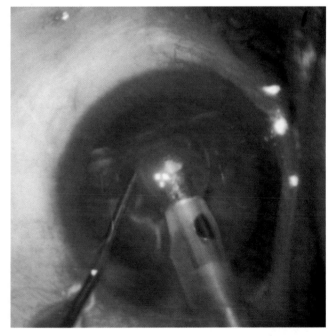

Photo 10.8. Note the position of the rounded repositor with respect to the tip.

EPINUCLEAR PLATE REMOVAL (FLIP & CHIP TECHNIQE) (Contd.)

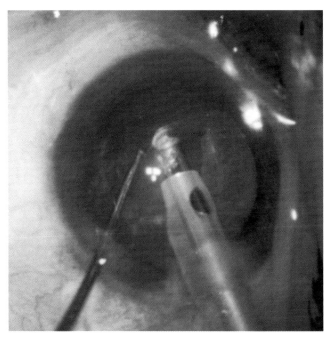

Photo 10.9. ENP is widest at the equatorial region. Move the tip to the left to remove more of the equatorial plate. Note that tip has come nearer to the rounded repositor.

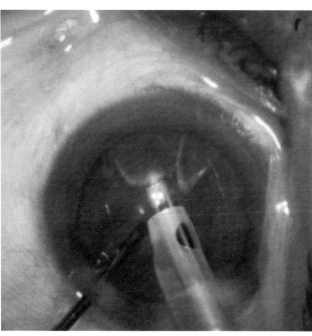

Photo 10.10. Keep on emulsifying till 1–2 clock hours of tongue-shaped anterior ENP remains attached to the posterior epinuclear plate. Take the tip under anterior ENP and create a vacuum seal. Note position of rounded repositor on posterior EN plate.

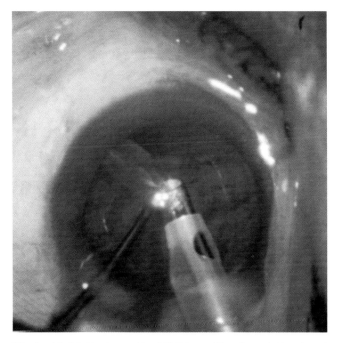

Photo 10.11. Prolapse the ENP by pulling from in front and pushing from behind with rounded repositor.

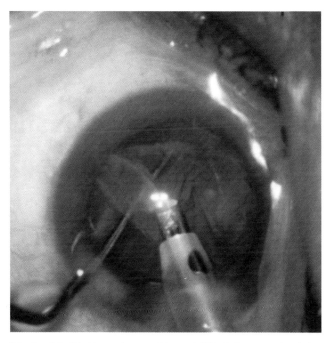

Photo 10.12. Note the position of RR, it has pushed the central part of ENP towards periphery for flipping.

EPINUCLEAR PLATE REMOVAL (FLIP & CHIP TECHNIQE) (Contd.)

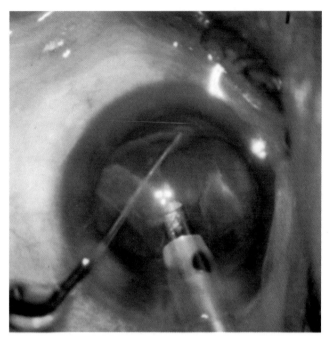

Photo 10.13. The rounded repositor is slid further into the periphery pushing the ENP out into the CSZ by taking counter-pressure from anterior capsule.

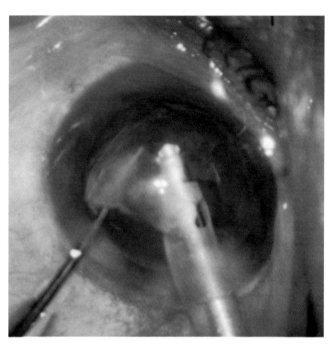

Photo 10.14. Note the RR outside the CCC margin lifting the epinuclear plate further for completion of flipping.

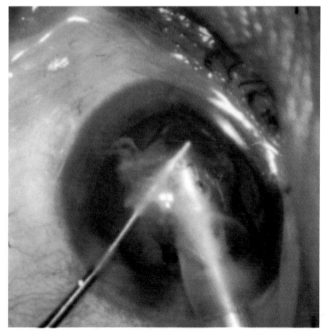

Photo 10.15. Emulsification of the flipped ENP in the AC keeping the RR below (as AC cannot be visualized) the tip to prevent PCT.

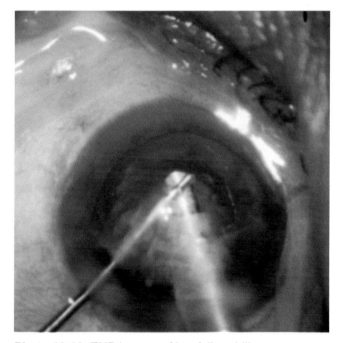

Photo 10.16. ENP in zone of low followability.

EPINUCLEAR PLATE REMOVAL (FLIP & CHIP TECHNIQE) (Contd.)

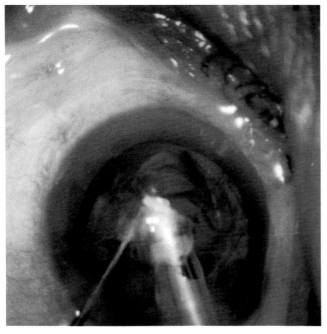

Photo 10.17. ENP pushed mechanically by RR into the zone of followability (in front of the tip).

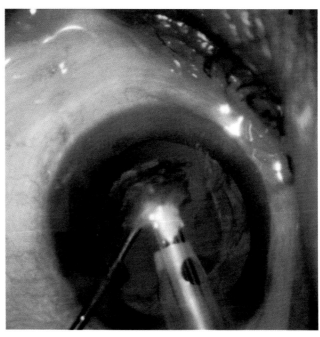

Photo 10.18. Mechanical crushing by RR to assist the aspiration of epinuclear plate.

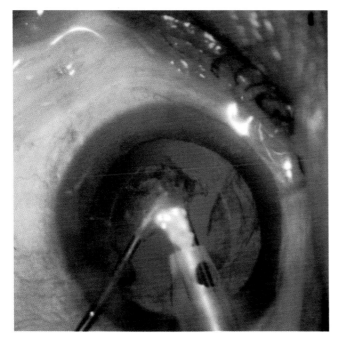

Photo 10.19. Last part of ENP in CSZ.

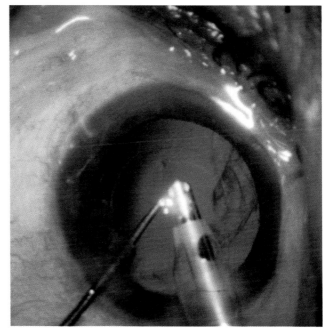

Photo 10.20. Completion of ENP removal at CSZ.

REMOVAL OF ALREADY DIVIDED EPINUCLEAR PLATE

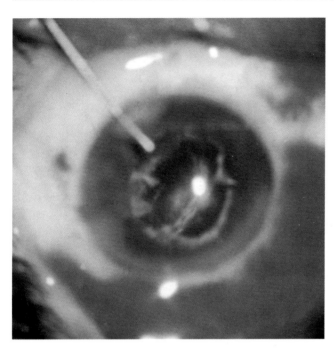

Photo 10.21. The visible "Y" line on the epinuclear plate. RR pushing one of the pieces towards the periphery to look for and break any adhesions between the three pieces of epinuclear plate.

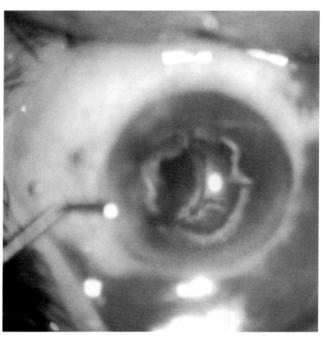

Photo 10.22. Check for complete separation of rounded repositor. If separation is incomplete it can be mechanically separated by two instruments. Note that RR is pushing the piece towards the periphery.

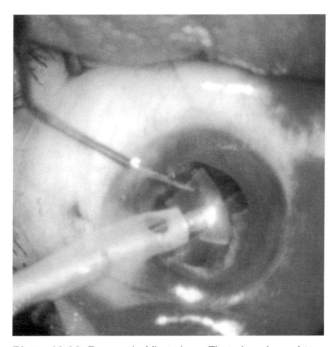

Photo 10.23. Removal of first piece. First piece brought up in the CSZ for removal.

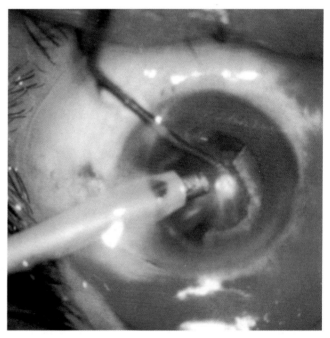

Photo 10.24. Rotation and removal of second piece. Second piece rotated and brought into the cross-incisional area for aspiration. Similarly all three pieces are removed.

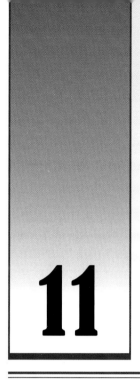

11 Cortical Aspiration

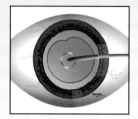

A complete cortical clean up is essential to decrease the incidence of early and late uveitis and posterior capsular opacification (PCO). With the increasing use of foldable acrylic and silicon lenses, performing YAG capsulotomy has now the risk of pitting of the IOL and even dislocation of plate haptic IOLs into the vitreous, especially in patients with the capsular contracture syndrome. So, it is better to take extra care during cortical aspiration and decrease the PCO rate as much as possible to avoid complications later. Inadequate cortical aspiration can cause opacification of both anterior and posterior capsule which can interfere with posterior segment evaluation and vitreoretinal surgery.

INSTRUMENTS

1. Co-axial irrigation-aspiration system

This has an aspiration orifice in front and the tip may be straight or angulated. The angulation may vary from 45° and 90° and also may be steerable or U-shaped. The aspiration tip may be fixed or detachable. The size of the orifice varies from 0.2 mm to 0.7 mm, 0.3 mm being the one commonly used. A smaller orifice will have better vacuum seal and prolonged aspiration time. The reverse is true for a large orifice.

Irrigation sleeve

This may be detachable (silicon) or fixed (metallic), with two openings 180° away from each other. The silicon sleeve has the advantage of less leakage since it takes the contour of the wound. One needs to carefully negotiate the sleeve while entering the eye to avoid Descemet's tears. There is more wear and tear of silicon sleeves, which need to be replaced more frequently as compared to steel ones which need no replacement.

2. Bimanual irrigation-aspiration (IA) system

Aspiration and infusion cannula with attached tubings.

Aspiration cannula

This is usually curved and has an opening 1 mm away from the tip. The port size may vary from 0.2–0.7 mm, 0.3 mm being the one commonly used. These cannulas may be available with a handle. Any cannula can be used for aspiration if a connecting piece (from an IV set) is utilised to connect it to the aspiration line.

Infusion cannula

May be used from the main port or side port. A thick, flat or rounded cannula, connected to the infusion line usually serves the purpose for providing infusion through the main port. An infusion cannula with two orifices on either side (0.5 mm) can also be used from the side port.

TECHNIQUES OF IRRIGATION AND ASPIRATION

CO-AXIAL IRRIGATION AND ASPIRATION
(Photos 11.1 to 11.16) (Figs. 11.1 to 11.4)

Entering a partially filled or fully formed chamber prevents a Descemet's tear. Entering with the infusion

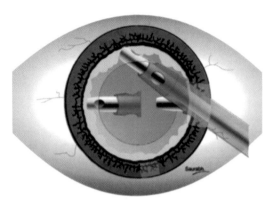

Fig. 11.1. Direction of orifice for coaxial irrigation-aspiration. Note, orifice is anterior for cross-incisional, turned sideways for the side and turned posterior for sub-incisional cortex.

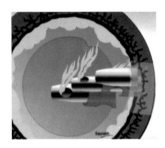

Fig. 11.2. Sub-incisional cortex removal. Note the position of orifice is posterior initially. As a grip on the fibres is obtained, the orifice is turned more anteriorly for aspiration in CSZ.

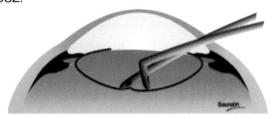

Fig. 11.3. Note the 90° tip is safer for sub-incisional cortex as the orifice is further away from the posterior capsule.

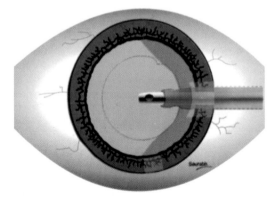

Fig. 11.4. Area of reach with coaxial handpiece. Green area denotes accessible area and gray denotes inaccessible area.

on may disturb the visibility so one can enter with the infusion off and put it on when inside the AC. This may result in the introduction of an air bubble which may then be sucked out. One should also aspirate any air bubbles or fluffy material that is lying loose in the AC. Keeping the aspiration orifice facing forward, go close to and underneath the anterior capsule and create a **vacuum seal** by occluding the port with the cortical fibres, pressing the FP between positions 1 & 2 (Note: in IA mode, there is no position 3, for further explanation, refer to **Phacodynamics**). Once a firm grip is formed, try to pull the fibres into the CSZ. If successful, a triangular piece of anterior and posterior cortical fibres will be visible. If the fibres are not peeling, the vacuum seal may be only partial. You may need to get a better grip by occluding the tip more (by either moving it deeper or sideways). You can depress the FP further and increase the vacuum and try to peel again. If you fail again, make a 3rd attempt, this time with full depression of the foot pedal. You may go up to the capsular fornix to get a better grip, even if you cannot see what you are holding. Striae on the capsule is an indication of inadvertent holding of the capsule and the foot pedal should be released immediately. If you are still unsuccessful, try at another site. **DON'T** try to hold the posterior cortical fibres or turn the aspiration orifice posteriorly.

After creating the first triangle, peel off the fibres in an area just adjacent to the one aspirated. It is better to completely clean up one area before moving onto the next. For the cross-incisional area, the orifice is on top, but as you come to the sides you will have to turn the orifice sideways and then upwards to get a better grip. It is easier to get a grip when the fibres are prolapsing out of the CCC and more difficult when they are recessed into the CCC.

The straight IA cannula is excellent for the cross-incisional area but worst for the sub-incisional area. The 90 degree tip is more suitable for the sub-incisional area but not so for the cross-incisional. The 45 degree tip is a good compromise for all areas.

Problems with co-axial IA

1. Sub-incisional area: This is difficult to reach with any co-axial handpiece. U-shaped cannulas have been made for the sub-incisional area but have not been found to be so useful due to being bulky and difficult to manoeuvre.

2. The co-axial IA tip is thinner than the phaco tip and so wound leak is more leading to an unstable chamber.

BIMANUAL IRRIGATION AND ASPIRATION
(Photos 11.17 to 11.28) (Fig. 11.5A & B)

For this, 2 side port incisions are made approximately **150** degrees from each other; one for infusion and the other for aspiration. These side ports should allow for a smooth fit of the 2 cannulas so that there is no wound leak. The procedure remains the same i.e. go under the anterior CCC margin, press FP and create a vacuum seal, hold the fibres and pull into CSZ for aspiration. By interchanging the irrigation and aspiration cannulas one can ensure that all areas are cleaned up especially the sub-incisional area. Another advantage of *Bimanual IA* is that irrigation cannula can be used for crushing the fibres if they are not getting aspirated easily. The only disadvantage is that one has to create another side port and these may need to be a little larger to accommodate the cannulas. Also the surgeon needs to be ambidextrous.

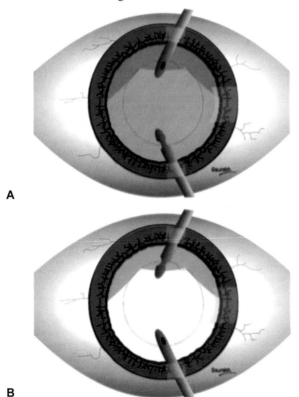

Fig. 11.5. Bimanual irrigation aspiration. Note 2 orifices on either side of infusion cannula and one orifice on top in aspiration cannula. (A) Green area denotes accessible area and gray denotes inaccessible area. (B) By interchanging the cannulas now no area is inaccessible.

BIMANUAL MODIFIED TECHNIQUE OF IRRIGATION AND ASPIRATION
(Photos 11.29 to 11.40) (Fig. 11.6A & B)

In this, we use the main wound for inserting the irrigation cannula using a thick cannula which may be rounded or flat. This cannula is placed obliquely into the section to prevent wound leak. The only area difficult to access in this method is the side port sub-incisional area. For this one can introduce both cannulas from the main port. One can also make another side port if the cortical matter is still not getting aspirated. It provides a large quantity of fluid and the creation of another larger side port is avoided. This is our preferred method of cortical aspiration, though we have nothing against creating another side port.

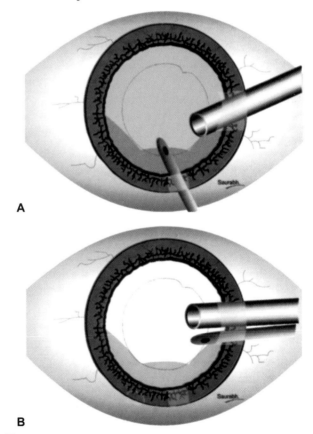

Fig. 11.6. Bimanual modified technique—Area of reach. (A) Green area denotes accessible area and gray denotes inaccessible area. (B) By placing both instruments through main port all areas can be reached.

MANUAL IRRIGATION AND ASPIRATION

Surgeons, specially trained in SICS, still prefer manual IA with a Simcoe cannula. However, removal of the sub-incisional cortex is even more difficult.

SUB-INCISIONAL CORTEX REMOVAL
(Photos 11.13 to 11.16, 11.24 to 11.26, 11.30 to 11.40)

The sub-incisional cortex removal is the most difficult for a number of reasons. Firstly, this area has decreased visibility since it is directly under the tunnel. Incomplete hydrodissection can add to the problem. One must keep in mind that leaving some cortex behind is less problematic than creating a PCT. Sub-incisional cortex removal is easier in a large CCC or in a rhexis that is decentred upwards. The sub-incisional area is difficult to aspirate with all types of co-axial handpieces due to disturbed visibility. While using the *co-axial handpiece* it is best to inflate the bag with viscoelastic and switch over to a 45 degree/90 degree handpiece. *Bimanual aspiration* is better for this area since no area remains underneath the incision. Another method that can be tried is the "*suck and spit method*". In this the bag is inflated with viscoelastic. The aspiration cannula (26/27 G) is introduced under the CCC through the side port. A vacuum seal is created and the fibres dragged to the centre and spit out there. Do not try to aspirate completely with the 27 G cannula as the AC may collapse. This is repeated till all the fibres are in the CSZ and then are aspirated with the aspiration cannula. One can also use the side port for the manual Simcoe cannula after enlargement.

Removal of cortical matter after IOL insertion
(Photos 11.37 to 11.40)

Sometimes sticky fibres don't peel so well in spite of repeated attempts and you may need to repeatedly try to get a grip. There is less chance of damage to the PC after the IOL has been inserted. The dialing of the lens can result in dislodging of some of the sticky stubborn fibres in the periphery. For this one needs to pull the IOL towards the side where the fibres need to be dislodged, squeezing the fibres between IOL haptics and capsular fornices, while at the same time dialing the IOL. This manouvre must be performed in a well-pressurized eye.

Move to Bimanual IA; it will be smooth, safe and make your life comfortable.

CAPSULAR POLISHING

Capsular polishing is not required in most cases, if the peeling of the cortical fibres has been good. Beginners can avoid this step especially if central 5 mm (sub-optic) area is clear. However, there are certain situations in which capsular polishing becomes important. These include hypermature cataract with vacuolated fibres. These fibres are virtually impossible to peel as they break wherever they are held. Sometimes there may be thin, flimsy fibres in no particular arrangement. Polishing is also required when a central PC plaque is present. In a small CCC, there is more chance of development of a PCO, so polishing of the capsule should be done. Younger patients and complicated or traumatic cataracts form the other group at high risk for PCO where polishing should be done. Also, in patients with posterior segment pathology, who may require further intervention, a good cortical clean-up is essential.

TECHNIQUE
Central PCC polishing (Fig. 11.7)

A rounded repositor, sand-blasted or ring capsular polisher may be used. There are high chances of PCT, so, it must be done very carefully. The bag is inflated with VES to make the PC stretched and concave. The IOP should be about 30 mmHg. The magnification is increased and one should focus on the PC while gently scrubbing. Folds on the PC imply that the eyeball is not well pressurized. Sometimes the capsule is so loose that despite inflating the eye with VSD, the folds remain. In such a situation it is better to leave it alone.

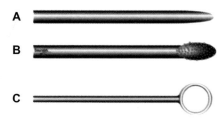

Fig. 11.7. Capsular polishers. (A) Rounded repositor. (B) Sand-blasted capsular polisher. (C) Ring capsular polisher.

If there is a fibrous opacification or plaque, one can try to lift the edge with rounded repositor and then peel with Utrata forceps. However, if any difficulty is felt this procedure should be abandoned. Alternatively, a PCC can be undertaken.

Polishing beyond the optical zone

With the rounded repositor, try to lift the fibres off the PC, i.e. mechanically dislodge them so that a sufficient grip is possible with the aspiration handpiece at low vacuum for easy aspiration. However, if the cornea is getting hazy or the block is wearing off or you are losing patience it is better to leave those fibres alone.

Polishing of anterior and equatorial zone

This is best done with the help of aspiration cannula. As there is not much counter-pressure on anterior capsule, rounded repositor cannot be used—use low vacuum (controlled by foot pedal) and clean all around. Using the bimanual aspiration technique facilitates all round cleaning.

'Cap vac' mode (Fig. 11.8)

Some machines have a **'cap vac'** mode. In this, a variable amount of vacuum is used by different surgeons, ranging from 0 to 40 mmHg. This can be done either by keeping the orifice down or keeping it up.

Orifice facing downwards

While keeping it down, capsule is gently held with the cannula with a force sufficient to bring it to the orifice for scrubbing but not enough to tear it. This is not recommended for beginners because of the unstable chamber and decreased visibility and danger of rupturing the capsule.

Orifice facing upwards

The undersurface of the bimanual aspiration cannula can be used as a polisher to scrub the posterior capsule. Since

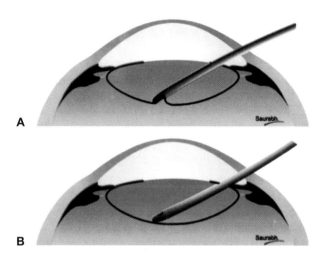

Fig. 11.8. 'Cap vac'. (A) Orifice facing downwards. Note danger of PCT. (B) Orifice facing upwards.

the orifice is facing upwards a higher vacuum can be maintained for suction of the scrubbed material.

Capsular polishing is a step that needs to be performed with great care. We feel that the use of a rounded repositor in a viscopressurized eye is the safest method for capsular polishing.

CO-AXIAL IRRIGATION-ASPIRATION

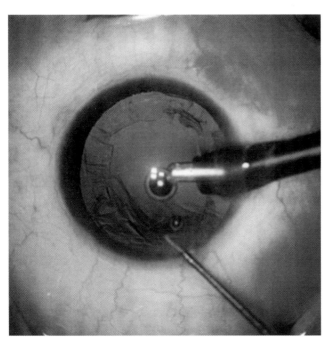

Photo 11.1. Entering without the infusion on may result in introduction of an air bubble, which should be aspirated first.

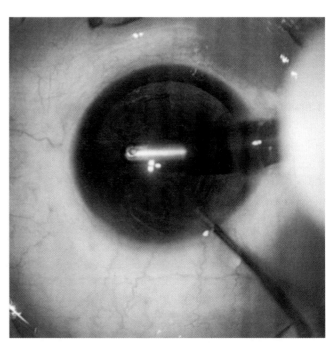

Photo 11.2. Go under the CCC margin below the cortical fibres and create a vacuum seal. Note the stretch on the fibres and gap on the sides, indicative of creation of vacuum seal.

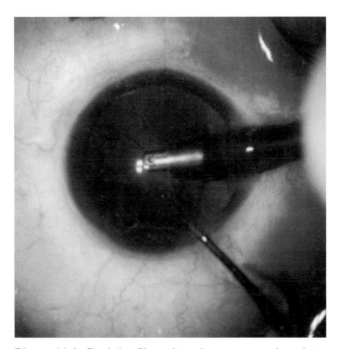

Photo 11.3. Peel the fibres into the centre and aspirate there.

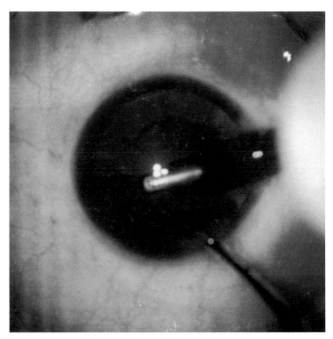

Photo 11.4. Now take handpiece to fibres adjacent to those removed, and create a vacuum seal. Note: There should be no fibres left in between.

CO-AXIAL IRRIGATION-ASPIRATION (Contd.)

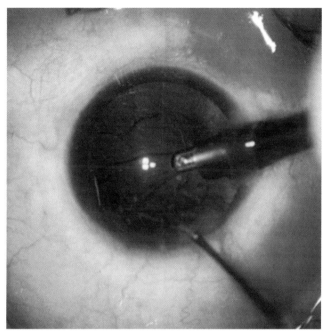

Photo 11.5. Peel off the fibres and aspirate.

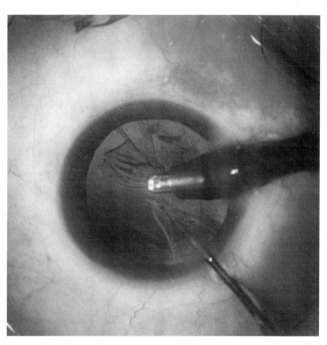

Photo 11.6. Similarly keep moving to the next site, aspirating 1–2 clock hours each time.

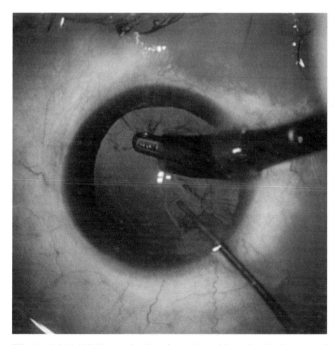

Photo 11.7. While aspirating from the sides, the tip is turned sideways to create the vacuum seal.

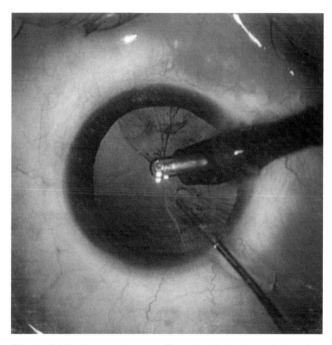

Photo 11.8. As you start peeling, the tip is turned anterior. Note that the aspiration orifice is now facing forwards.

CO-AXIAL IRRIGATION-ASPIRATION (Contd.)

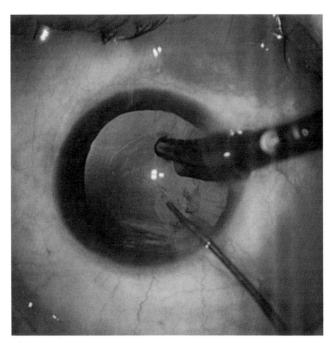

Photo 11.9. As you come closer to the sub-incisional area, the tip needs to be tilted (posterolateral) more.

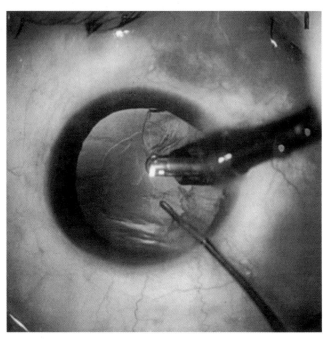

Photo 11.10. Once the peeling is initiated, start turning the tip forward.

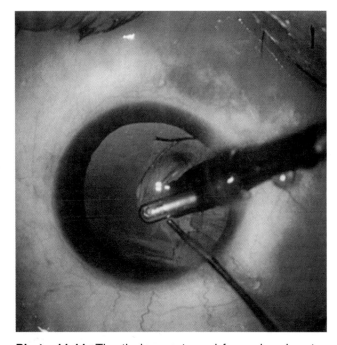

Photo 11.11. The tip is now turned forward and cortex aspirated in central safe zone.

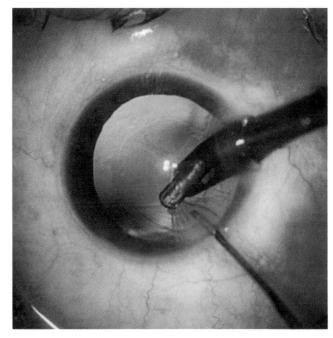

Photo 11.12. Repeat the same on the other side of the incision.

CO-AXIAL IRRIGATION-ASPIRATION (Contd.)

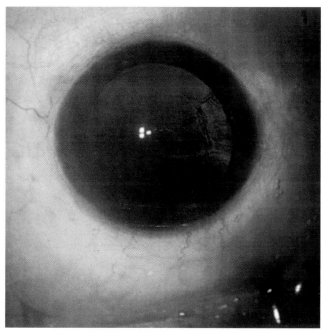

Photo 11.13. Note the remaining sub-incisional cortex.

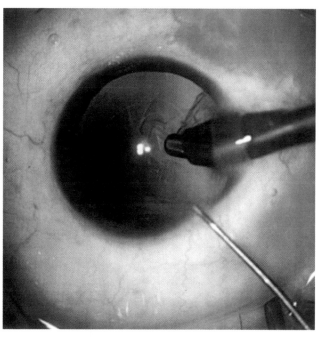

Photo 11.14. Sub-incisional cortex removal: turn the tip posteriorly and create a vacuum seal on the anterior fibres.

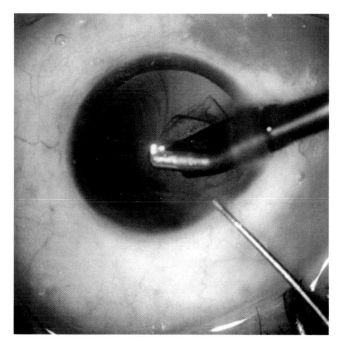

Photo 11.15. Start peeling and turning the tip forward.

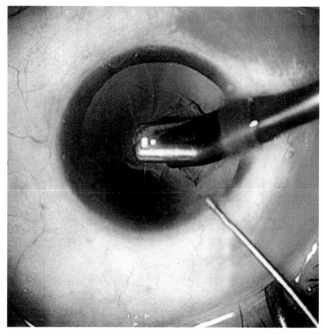

Photo 11.16. Aspirate in the central safe zone with the tip facing forward.

BIMANUAL CORTICAL ASPIRATION

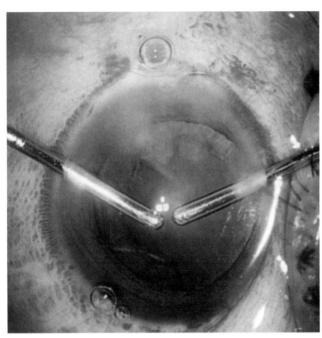

Photo 11.17. Note two side port incisions 2–3 clock hours from the main incision. The two cannulae are making an angle of 150° at the centre of the eye. The infusion cannula has two orifices and the aspiration cannula has one orifice on top.

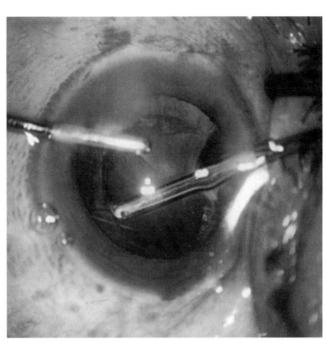

Photo 11.18. Aspiration cannula is introduced under the CCC and vacuum seal created.

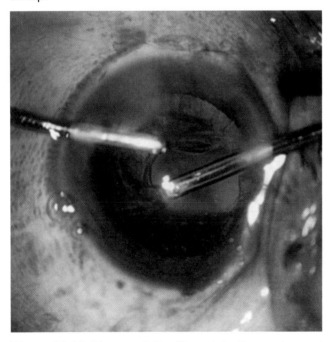

Photo 11.19. Now peel the fibres into the centre and aspirate. The cross-incisional area is aspirated.

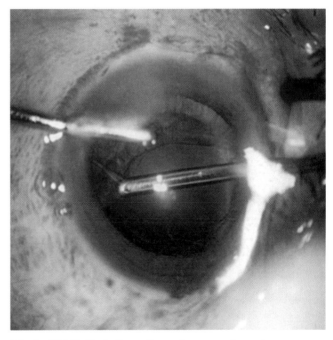

Photo 11.20. Go to the adjacent area and create a vacuum seal. Note that for the cortical matter on the side, the tip remains anterior.

BIMANUAL CORTICAL ASPIRATION (Contd.)

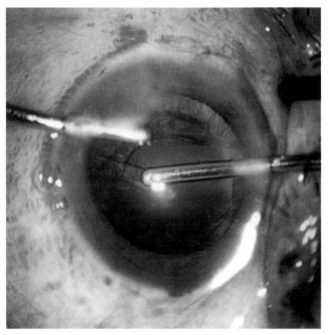

Photo 11.21. Note: No rotation of tip is required, tip is always facing forwards.

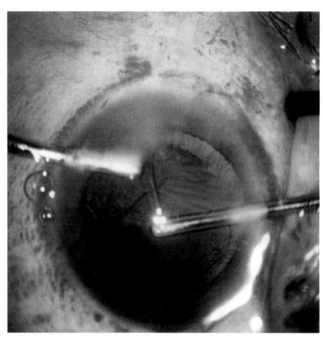

Photo 11.22. Peeling the side port sub-incisional area.

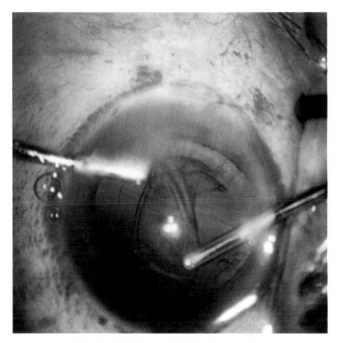

Photo 11.23. Aspirate in the centre.

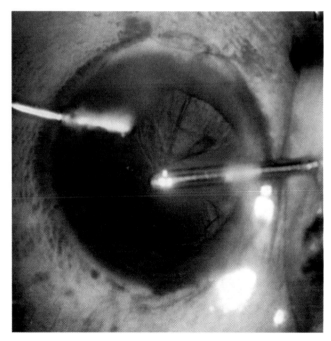

Photo 11.24. Aspiration of main port sub-incisional area. Note the easy access, stable chamber and better visibility due to use of bimanual technique.

BIMANUAL CORTICAL ASPIRATION (Contd.)

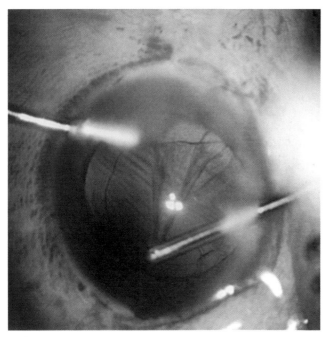

Photo 11.25. Sub-incisional cortex easily brought into centre. There is no need for cumbersome torsional rotation of the tip.

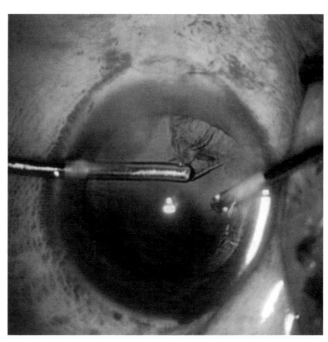

Photo 11.26. Note the exchange of infusion and aspiration cannulae to reach the other side of the eye, particularly the sub-incisional area.

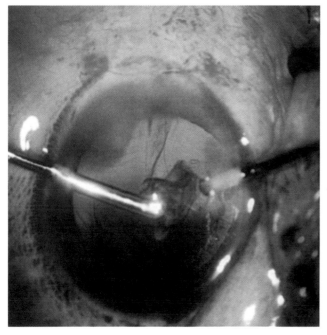

Photo 11.27. Large amount of cortex not getting aspirated.

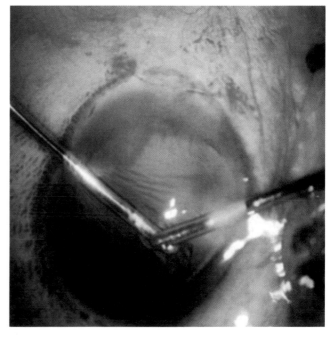

Photo 11.28. Using the aspiration cannula for mechanical crushing.

MODIFIED BIMANUAL CORTICAL ASPIRATION

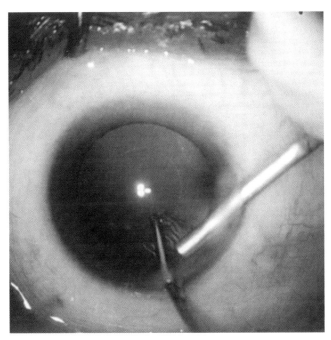

Photo 11.29. Note the rounded infusion cannula placed obliquely to avoid wound leak. Rest of cortex removed, side port sub-incisional cortex remaining.

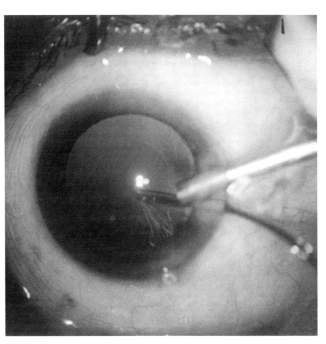

Photo 11.30. Introduction of both instruments from the main port.

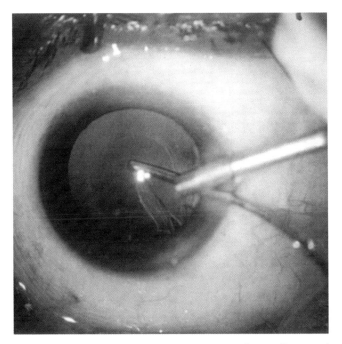

Photo 11.31. Creation of vacuum seal, peeling and aspiration in central safe zone.

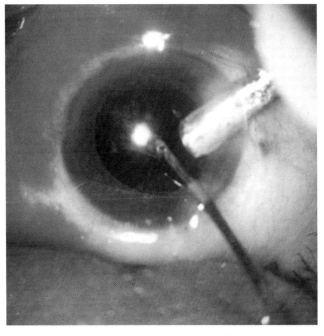

Photo 11.32. Note the use of thick flat infusion cannula in the main port to decrease the wound leak.

SUCK & SPIT (SUB-INCISIONAL CORTEX REMOVAL)

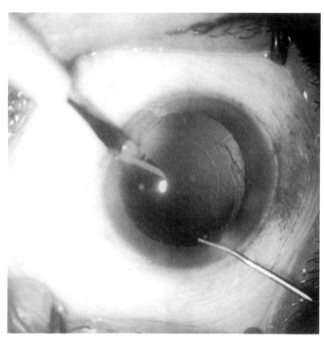

Photo 11.33. Sub-incisional cortex remaining. Note creation of another side port 4 clock hours from the main incision for better access.

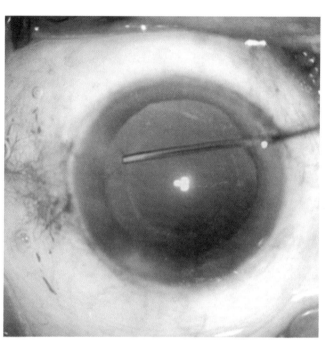

Photo 11.34. Introduction of 26/27 G cannula on a visco-elastic filled syringe, engaging the anterior fibres and creating a vacuum hold.

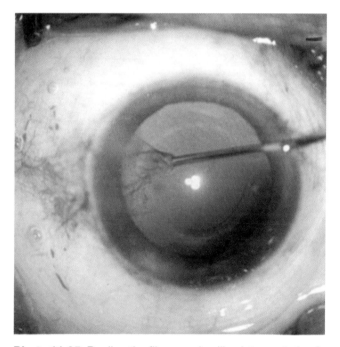

Photo 11.35. Peeling the fibres and pulling into central safe zone.

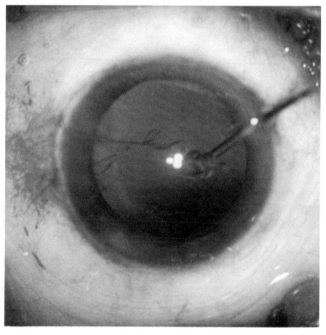

Photo 11.36. Expelling into the centre. DO NOT try to aspirate as aspiration may cause shallowing of chamber. Keep repeating the procedure till all the cortical fibres have been brought to the centre and then remove by irrigation-aspiration or viscoexpression.

REMOVAL OF CORTEX BY DIALING THE IOL

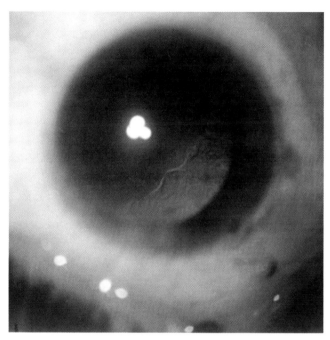

Photo 11.37. Removal of cortex by dialing the IOL. Sub-incisional thin cortical fibres remaining.

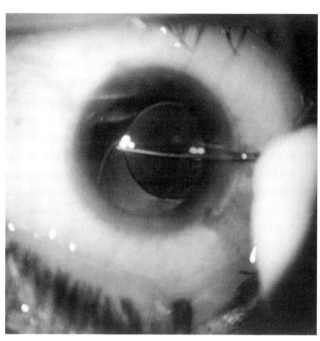

Photo 11.38. Pull the IOL towards the side of remaining cortex causing pressure on the capsular fornix by the haptic.

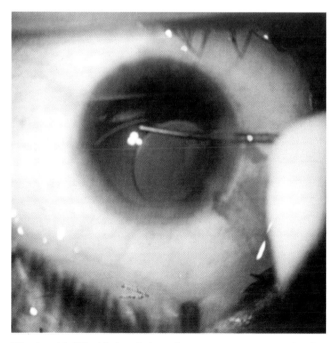

Photo 11.39. Maintaining the pressure towards the periphery, start rotating.

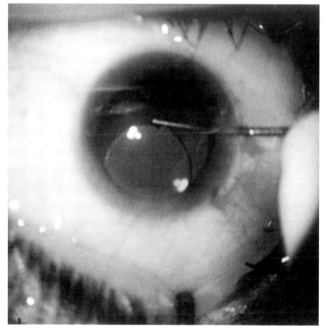

Photo 11.40. Note that 90° rotation has taken place while maintaining pressure on the periphery. This will dislodge the cortical fibres. The procedure can be repeated if need be. Loosened fibres can now be removed by irrigation-aspiration.

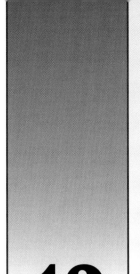

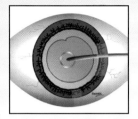

12 | Insertion of IOL

The insertion of the intraocular lens (IOL) is a step that, if well done, will hardly take any time. However, it can be very time-consuming if the proper technique is not followed. There are 2 types of IOLs available—the non-foldable or single-piece PMMA lenses, and the foldable lenses

Phaco profile IOLs

With the advent of small incision cataract surgery, the IOLs have been modified too. The commonest phaco profile lenses available are single-piece PMMA lenses with an optic size between 5–6 mm. These are preferred over the 3-piece lenses with polypropylene loops due to the better stability and memory of PMMA loops.

Foldable IOLs

There are a wide variety of foldable IOLs now available. Essentially, all can be inserted through an incision ranging from 1.8 to 3.5 mm. The technique of insertion depends on the material of the IOL and the method used i.e. injection system, holder/folder, etc. Three types of IOL material used in the order of preference are:
1. Hydrophobic Acrylic
2. Hydrophilic Acrylic
3. Silicone

INSTRUMENTS

• **McPherson forceps** – for lifting the lens from cartridge.

• **Holder:** The IOL holder has a concavity in the centre to accommodate the central thickness of the IOL.

• **Folder:** The folder has a handle, arms and a folding element. The folding element further has a ledge to go under the optic, a socket in which the IOL gets folded and a vertical part, which makes a flank with the holding forceps. The two arms should be flat and should not touch completely even when closed.

• **Injector systems** are designed for particular IOLs and are supplied by the manufacturer. They may be reusable or disposable.

PRE-REQUISITES

Viscopressurized eyeball (Fig. 12.1)

After the completion of cortical aspiration, the AC and bag is full of BSS. This BSS needs to be nearly totally replaced with VES. Take the cannula of the viscoelastic filled syringe to the opposite pole (at the angle) and inject to create a bolus. As soon as the bolus reaches the CCC, inject underneath the CCC posteriorly, to push the PC back. Now direct the VE into fornices of the bag and start injecting to get a well-formed capsular bag. You may see small rings of BSS getting pushed into the periphery which will not cause any problems. Now bring the cannula into the centre and deepen the AC.

Alternatively if AC is flattened completely, then start forming it by injecting VES from the wound itself. After forming the AC, inflate the bag with viscoelastic. Admixture of VES and BSS decreases the visibility and

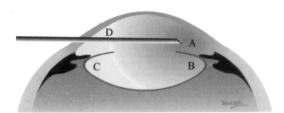

Fig. 12.1. Replacement of BSS with VES before insertion of IOL. First inject into cross-sectional angle 'A', then into cross-incisional fornix 'B', then in sub-incisional fornix 'C' and lastly in sub-incisional angle 'D'.

it may leak out as soon as you start putting in the IOL. The posterior capsule should be well posterior and concave and the eyeball well pressurized (IOP should be in the range of 30–35 mmHg). You can focus on the PC to ensure that it is well stretched.

Adequate incision size

The incision size should be adequate for the IOL, particularly the inner lip. The outer incision can be stretched but the inner lip, if small, will get torn. This will cause astigmatism and interfere with the valvular function. The size of the incision for a PMMA IOL needs to be slightly longer to accommodate the thickness of IOL and the forceps that goes along. For example, for a 5.25 mm optic IOL you will require a 5.5 mm incision. For foldable lenses, most injecting systems require 1.8 to 3.00 mm of incision. The injector should go in easily without pushing. With the holder/folder, the incision size will depend on the size of the optic of the lens and thickness of the lens, which varies according to the refractive index of the material and the power of the IOL. *The lower the power, the thinner the lenses and they are easier to fold. They require a smaller incision.* However, beginners may need to give themselves an extra 0.25 mm of space to accommodate poorly folded/eccentric folded IOLs.

TECHNIQUE FOR SINGLE-PIECE PMMA LENSES
(Photos 12.1 to 12.16) (Figs. 12.2 & 12.3)

Before inserting the lens one can wash it with BSS in the container itself. A drop of methyl cellulose can be put on the leading haptic and optic. Lens is gripped with the McPherson either transversely (10–2 O'clock) or longitudinally. The transverse grip is stronger but you need to release the lens once the optic is in the AC. Holding the IOL in the transverse grip, it is introduced into the section. When the centre of the optic crosses the internal lip,

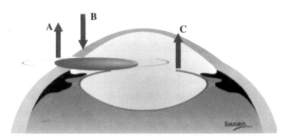

Fig. 12.2. Insertion of leading haptic under CCC. Lift the IOL by trailing haptic or optic in direction 'A'. 'B' denotes the fulcrum for increasing the tilt of the IOL. 'C'—the CCC margin can be lifted by a rounded repositor to facilitate the loop going into the bag.

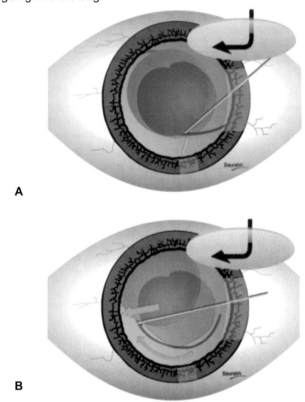

A

B

Fig. 12.3. Dialing the trailing haptic. (A) Dumbbell dialer is placed at optic-haptic junction. Note the direction of force denoted by arrows—the dialer is pushing both into the periphery and downwards. (B) The haptic is pushed against the CCC margin. Note the deformation of the CCC margin denoting adequate resistance. Now, on rotating the IOL further, the haptic will slip in.

release the grip (1 mm of the optic will still be outside the wound). The loop of the leading haptic will be close to the CCC margin but because of the direction of the tunnel, it will not be pointing down. With the McPherson forceps, hold the lens at the section and lift it up using the internal lip as a fulcrum, so that the leading haptic goes into the CCC. If it does not go in, use a RR to press on the external surface of the cornea at the site of the internal lip, to increase the tilt of the IOL. You should be able to see the haptic slipping under the CCC. You can also introduce a RR from the side port to lift the CCC margin and guide the haptic in. This is useful in cases of corneal edema/small rhexis. After the leading haptic has gone under the rhexis, push the IOL in such that part of the optic also slips in behind the CCC. The trailing haptic will now be in the section, but optic haptic junction will be in the AC. This optic-haptic junction is engaged with a dumbbell dialer or a 'Y' shaped dialer. The instrument should be perpendicular to the haptic (the dialer slips if it is kept oblique). Now push this junction downwards (i.e. towards the vitreous) and towards the periphery. The trailing haptic should come and touch the CCC margin 90° away from the incision. Maintaining the same force, now slightly rotate the optic clockwise (stretch on the CCC will be visible). The haptic will slip in by the time you rotate by 30–40°.

The dialing force has to be applied such that the maximum resistance is felt from the CCC margin, i.e. try to tear the CCC margin with the trailing haptic—it will slip in automatically. Once you see the peaking of CCC margin it means that enough force has been generated and now on rotation, the haptic will slip into the bag.

If the trailing haptic has not gone into the bag and has moved beyond 180° from the incision, applying these forces is more difficult. It is better to rotate the IOL over the capsule, so that the haptic comes to the original position, i.e. just to the left of the incision and then make a second attempt. In case the AC becomes shallow, re-inflate the bag with viscoelastic.

Alternatively, the IOL can be inserted by holding it longitudinally. Though this grip is not so strong, the forceps and the IOL are introduced into the section so that the leading haptic can be directly placed under the CCC margin. The disadvantage is that the viscoelastic and the IOL tend to come out of the section in this grip. This manoeuvre is more difficult in a scleral tunnel. Once the leading haptic is under the CCC margin, the rest of the insertion is as described above.

Putting the trailing haptic by forceps
(Photos 12.13 to 12.16)

After inserting the leading haptic and the optic, hold the free end of the trailing haptic with a McPherson forceps. Push it towards the cross-incisional area till the peripheral

most part of the loop is at the CCC margin. Now pronate your hand so that the loop of the trailing haptic points posteriorly, and leave it. It will slip under the CCC. Since sometimes the visibility in the sub-incisional area is poor, to overcome this, while releasing the loop, one can rotate the IOL by 30–40° to enhance visualization.

FOLDABLE IOLs

Foldable IOLs are inserted by a holder-folder method or an injector system method.

Holder-folder method
(Photos 12.17 to 12.24) (Fig. 12.4)

Various types of holders and folders are available, the description of which is beyond the scope of this book. The IOL may be folded *longitudinally* (along the long axis) or *transversally* (perpendicular to the long axis). Transverse technique is nowadays no longer popular as it requires a larger incision and is more cumbersome.

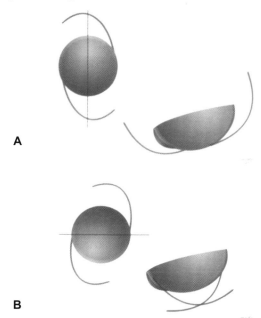

Fig. 12.4. Types of fold. (A) Longitudinal—the IOL is folded along the longitudinal axis. (B) Transverse—the IOL is folded along the transverse axis.

Technique (Figs. 12.5 to 12.10)

The technique being described is the one used for acrylic IOLs. Put a drop of viscoelastic on the container. Lift the IOL out of the socket and dab the undersurface on the VES. Place on the edge of the container for folding. The folder is held in the left hand. For a longitudinal fold of the IOL the folding forceps should be placed such

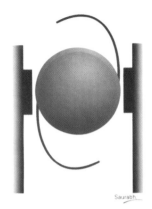

Fig. 12.5. Placement of folder. Note that the 2 arms are parallel to the long axis and placed in the centre of the optic.

Fig. 12.6. Folder is placed such that the ledges slip under the IOL. The arms are pushed together so that the IOL folds centrally.

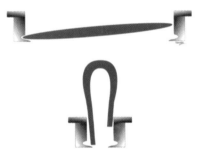

Fig. 12.7. Incorrect placement of the folding forceps will result in an eccentric fold.

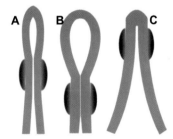

Fig. 12.8. Vertical placement of holder. (A) Correct placement, slightly above the centre of the IOL. (B) Holding the IOL close to the free end makes it bulky and difficult to insert. (C) Holding the IOL too close to the folded end results in fishmouthing.

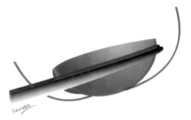

Fig. 12.9. Horizontal placement of holder. The correct position is such that the tips meet just beyond the folded optic.

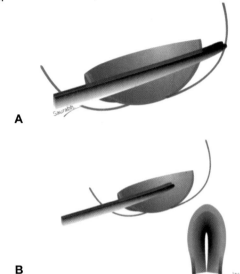

Fig. 12.10. Incorrect horizontal position. (A) The holder is placed too far outside the margin of the folded optic. (B) Placement of the holding forceps too much within the margin of the folded optic causing fishmouthing.

that its two limbs are parallel to the haptics and in the middle of the periphery of the optic. These two arms of the forceps must be kept flat on the surface for getting a good grip on the IOL. If both the arms are not flat, you may get an eccentric fold and the hold will be unstable. Now start closing the arms such that the ledges slip under the edge of the optic. If the IOL is not flat, then use a RR to flatten it. Press the 2 arms together and the IOL will start folding. Don't compress fully otherwise the lens may jump out. Now drop the IOL container and take the holder in the right hand. You can either use the holder to complete the fold or complete the folding with the folder and hold immediately by positioning the holder just above the folder. The vertical position of the arms of the holder is just above the centre of the folded lens. If positioned closer to the folded side, the IOL will be 'V' shaped and tend to slip out. However, this will unfold easily in the eye. If the grip is closer to the free end, the IOL is thicker and more difficult to insert. The horizontal positioning of the holder should be such that the tip protrudes just beyond the optic edge.

Position the leading haptic close to the external incision and push it inside the AC with a dumbbell dialer, simultaneously pushing the IOL into the section such that the folded optic enters the section after the leading haptic is inside the AC (if the leading haptic is not introduced into the AC first, it will get stuck with the optic in the section, causing a tear or needing a larger section). Once the leading haptic is near the CCC, guide it under the rhexis margin and then push the optic into the AC. Now pronate the hand to make the optic vertical. Place a second instrument between the lens and the cornea and then open the holding forceps. Usually the lens slips out easily. In case of Acrylic IOLs you may have to push it down with second instrument. The holder and second instrument are withdrawn and the trailing haptic is inserted as for the PMMA lenses.

To position an IOL in the bag after it has accidentally opened in AC, the technique is followed as described in Photos 12.45 to 12.48.

For *Silicon IOLs* the basic technique is the same. Keep in mind that Silicon IOLs cannot be folded if they are wet.

INJECTING SYSTEMS (Photos 12.25 to 12.44)

Injector systems are designed for particular IOLs and are supplied by the manufacturer. One should familiarize oneself with the particular system by reading the literature provided by the company. While injecting the IOL, one should ensure that the leading loop opens in the capsular bag. Leading loop needs to be kept horizontal all the time by appropriately rotating the cartridge. Inability to do so may lead to posterior capsular tear, more so with 3-piece IOLs and high powered IOLs. High powered IOLs, being tight in the barrel, have a tendency to get injected with sudden force and speed in the eye, which may lead to posterior capsular tear. Trailing loop can be dialled as PMMA IOLs but more often is guided under the CCC by pushing the optic-haptic junction down. Wound-assisted injection of single-piece IOL is possible in expert hands. The presumed advantages of an injector system are:

- Smaller incision
- Disposable cartridge
- Trailing haptic may be inserted without coming in contact with the external ocular tissues.

Procedure for injecting IOL in the bag has been illustrated in Photos 12.49 to 12.53.

PMMA LENS

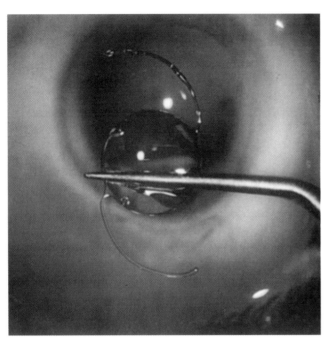

Photo 12.1. Transverse grip. Note that forceps is perpendicular to the long axis.

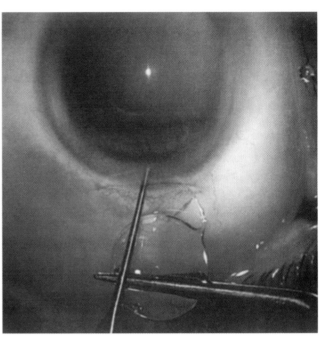

Photo 12.2. Push the leading haptic into section by dumbbell dialer, simultaneously advancing the optic.

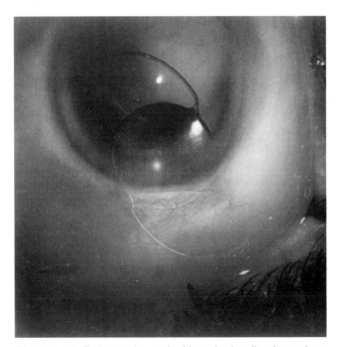

Photo 12.3. Release the optic. Note the leading loop close to CCC.

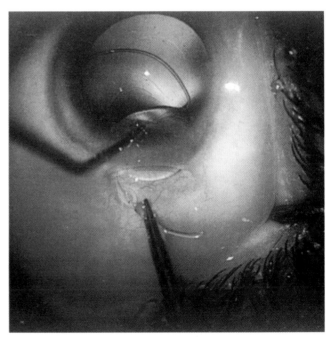

Photo 12.4. Lift the optic edge or trailing haptic to tilt the IOL downwards. Simultaneous use of dumbbell dialer on the surface of cornea further tilts the IOL downwards and helps push the leading haptic under the CCC margin.

PMMA LENS (Contd.)

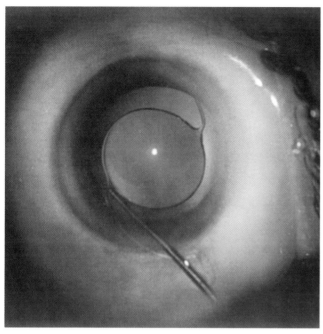

Photo 12.5. For insertion of trailing haptic, position the dumbbell at optic-haptic junction.

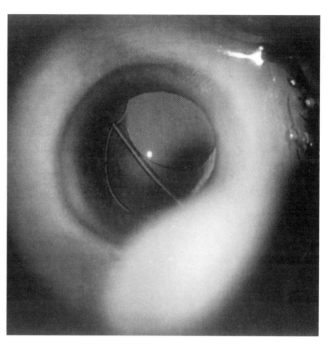

Photo 12.6. Note the direction of push and dialing.

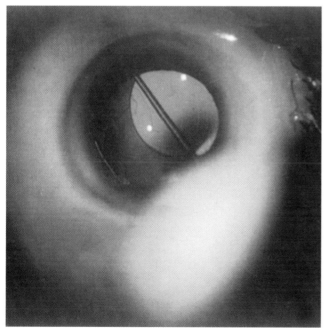

Photo 12.7. Note the stretch on CCC margin due to the trailing haptic.

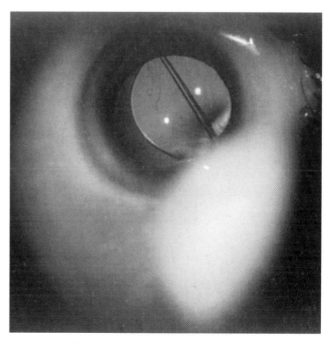

Photo 12.8. Trailing haptic slips in.

PMMA LENS (Contd.)

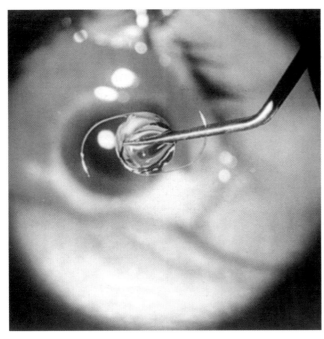

Photo 12.9. Longitudinal grip. Note that forceps is parallel to the long axis.

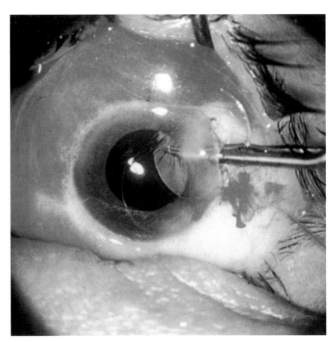

Photo 12.10. Insert both the forceps and optic into AC.

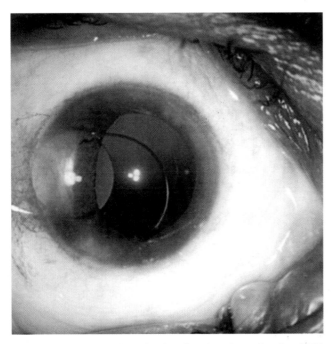

Photo 12.11. Negotiate the leading haptic under the CCC margin.

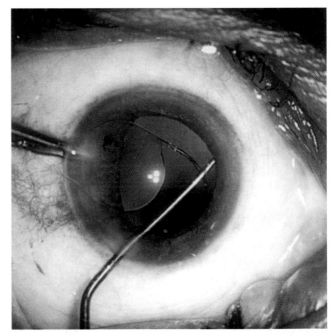

Photo 12.12. Rounded repositor on top of the leading haptic and under the CCC to facilitate haptic entry in the bag.

INSERTION OF TRAILING HAPTIC WITH FORCEPS

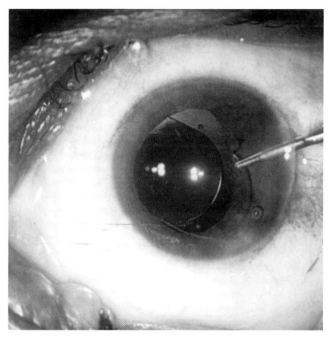

Photo 12.13. Hold the trailing haptic with McPherson's forceps.

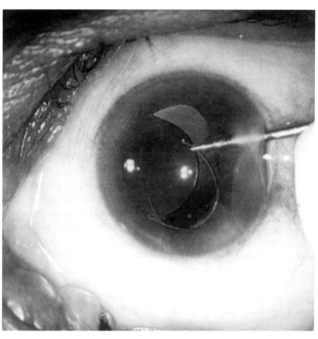

Photo 12.14. Push the IOL so that the knee reaches CCC and passes under the CCC margin.

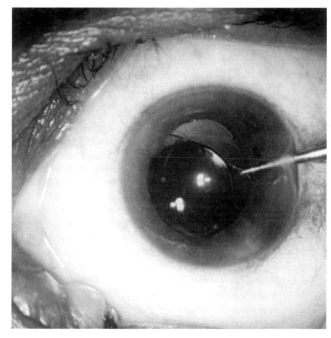

Photo 12.15. Pronate your hand so that the knee points backwards.

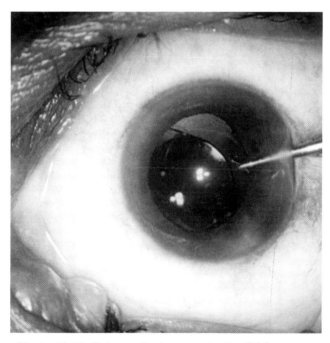

Photo 12.16. Release the knee under the CCC margin.

FOLDABLE LENS (HOLDER-FOLDER METHOD)

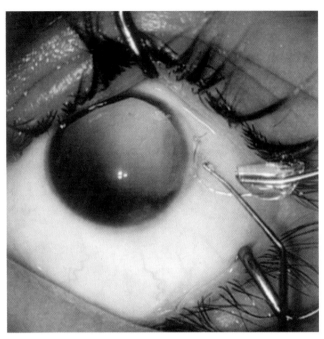

Photo 12.17. Ideal position for holding a folded lens. Leading haptic close to the external wound.

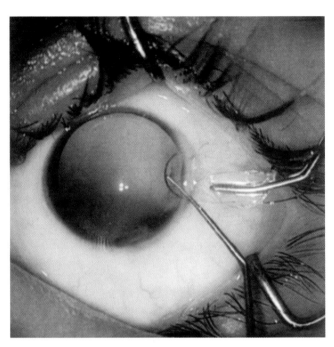

Photo 12.18. Leading haptic being pushed in by dumbbell dialer and simultaneously lens is advanced.

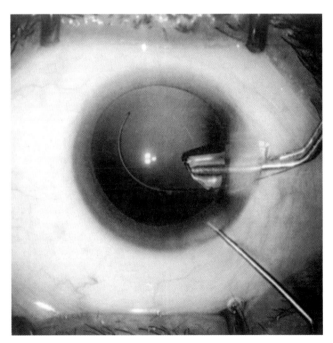

Photo 12.19. Leading haptic negotiated under the CCC margin. Dumbbell positioned at the side port.

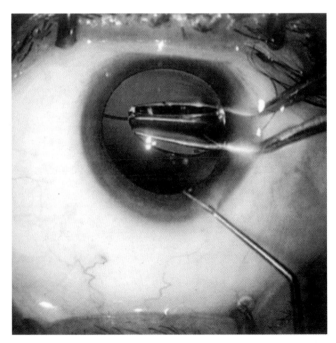

Photo 12.20. Once the whole optic is in the AC, pronate your hand to make the optic vertical.

FOLDABLE LENS (HOLDER-FOLDER METHOD) (Contd.)

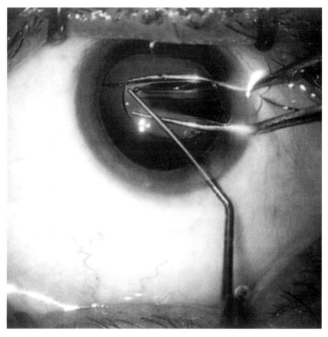

Photo 12.21. Unfold the lens by releasing the holder. Depress the lens with the help of dumbbell dialer.

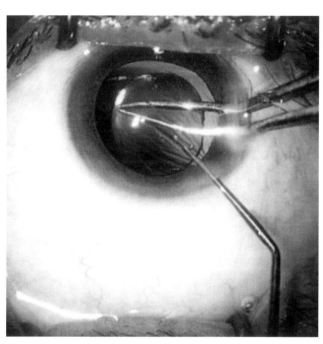

Photo 12.22. Lens unfolded in the bag. Gently remove the holder and dumbbell dialer.

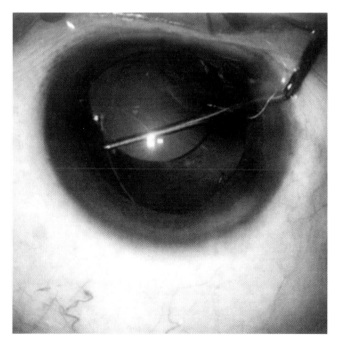

Photo 12.23. Dial the trailing haptic in as for PMMA lens.

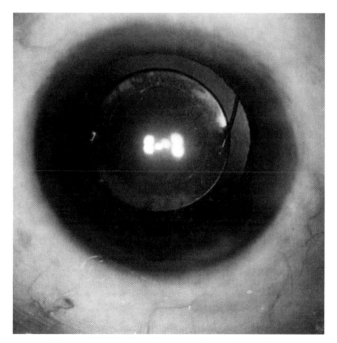

Photo 12.24. A well-centred lens in the bag.

INJECTOR SYSTEM

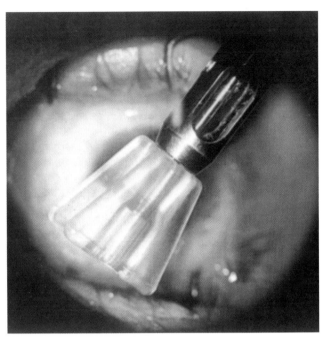

Photo 12.25. Putting the silicone sleeve.

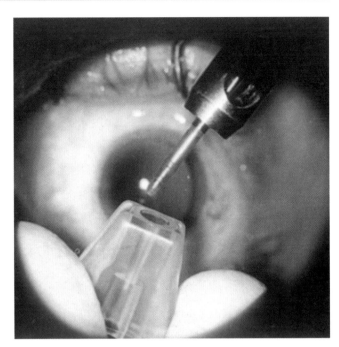

Photo 12.26. Injector with silicone sleeve on.

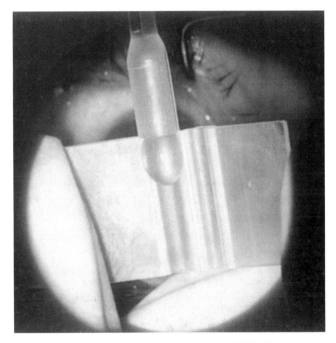

Photo 12.27. Fill the cartridge barrel with VES till it appears in the groove.

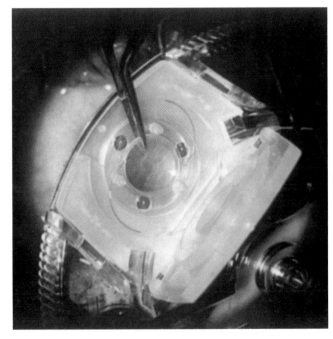

Photo 12.28. Lift the lens from the container.

INJECTOR SYSTEM (Contd.)

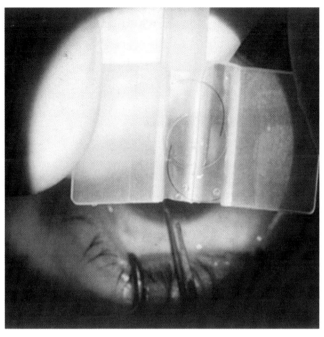

Photo 12.29. Place the lens in the cartridge. The position of the IOL should be same as the diagram on the flap of the cartridge.

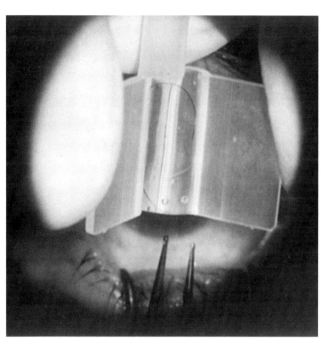

Photo 12.30. Start to fold the cartridge.

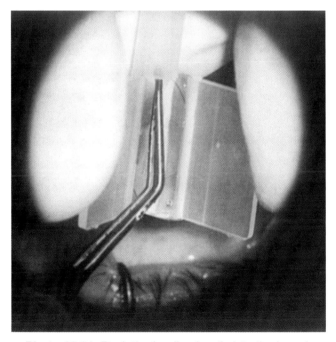

Photo 12.31. Push the leading haptic into the barrel.

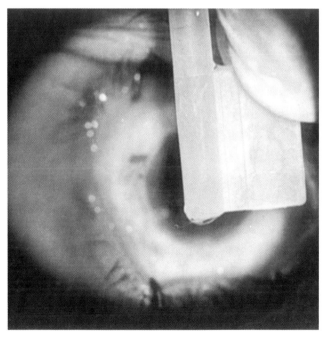

Photo 12.32. Fold completely. The optic should be concave. If need be press with forceps on the top. The trailing haptic should protrude out and to the left.

INJECTOR SYSTEM (Contd.)

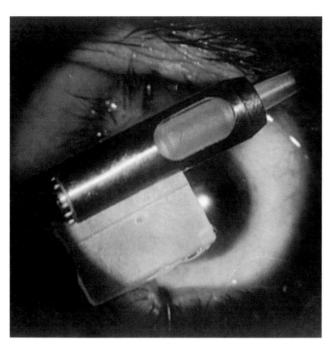

Photo 12.33. Cartridge loaded into the injector system.

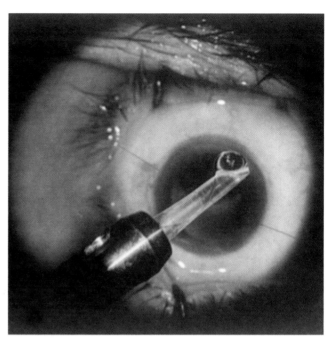

Photo 12.34. Rotate the lever of the injector so that the leading haptic reaches the bevel of the cartridge barrel.

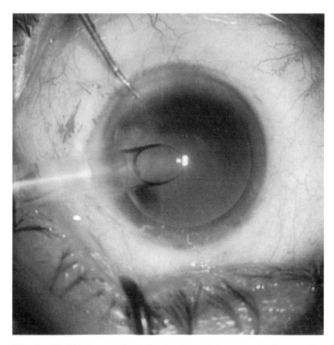

Photo 12.35. Insert the injector bevel down upto the centre of the eye.

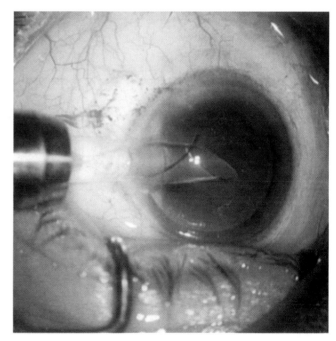

Photo 12.36. Turn the bevel to the left and start rotating the lever.

INJECTOR SYSTEM (Contd.)

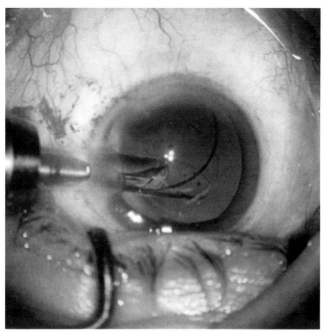

Photo 12.37. Leading haptic guided under the CCC margin.

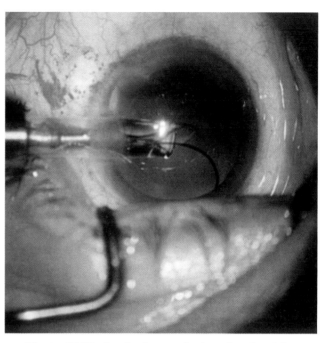

Photo 12.38. Gradually turn the bevel to the right.

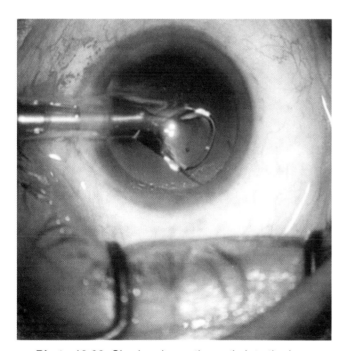

Photo 12.39. Slowly release the optic into the bag.

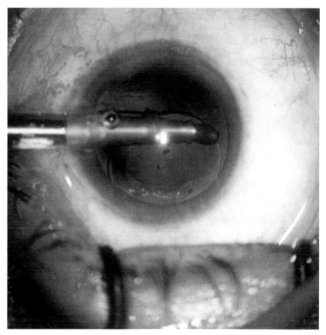

Photo 12.40. Unfolded optic in the bag.

INJECTOR SYSTEM (Contd.)

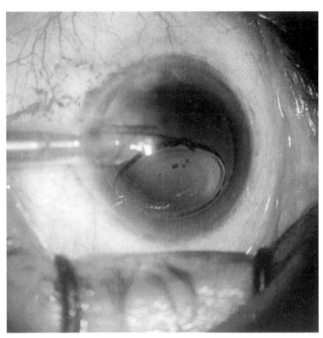

Photo 12.41. Withdraw the injector tip behind the knee of the trailing haptic.

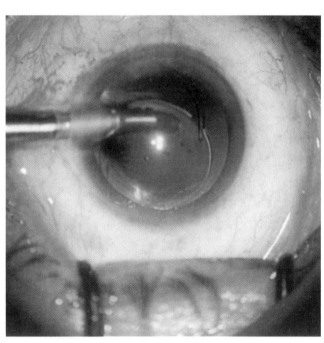

Photo 12.42. Now turn the bevel down or to the left and try to push the trailing haptic under the CCC margin by rotating the tip.

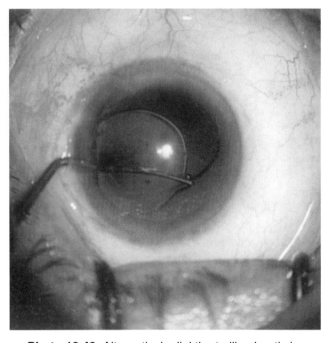

Photo 12.43. Alternatively dial the trailing haptic in.

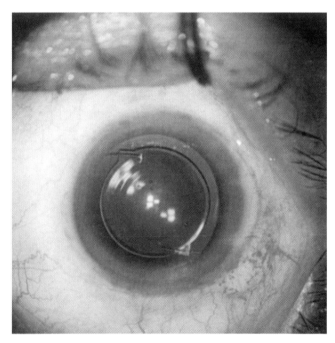

Photo 12.44. IOL in the bag.

CAPSULAR PLACEMENT OF ACCIDENTALLY OPENED IOL IN AC

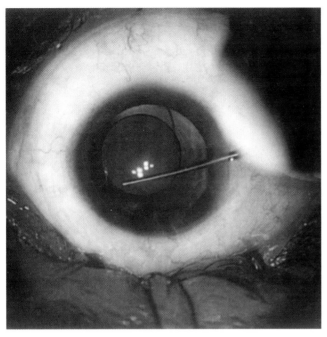

Photo 12.45. Unfolded IOL into the AC. Note the position of the haptic on right side on the top of the iris.

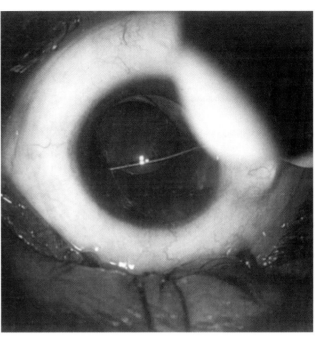

Photo 12.46. Presume that one loop is inside capsular fornices and dial the other loop as for trailing haptic.

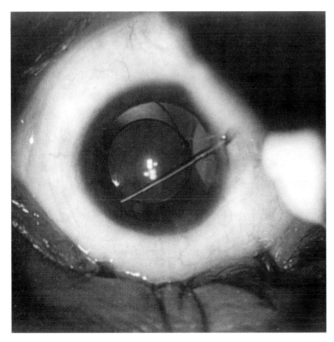

Photo 12.47. Note that one loop has gone in the bag. The lens is dialed to place the other haptic in position for dialing.

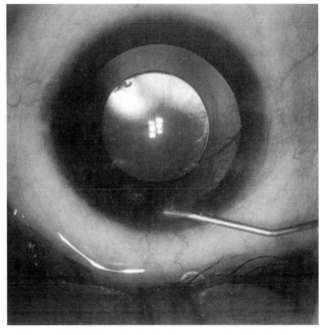

Photo 12.48. Note both the loops are inside the bag.

PROCEDURE FOR INJECTING IOL

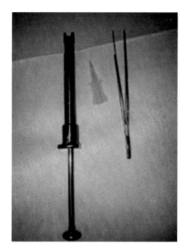

Photo 12.49. Injector system with cartridge and forceps.

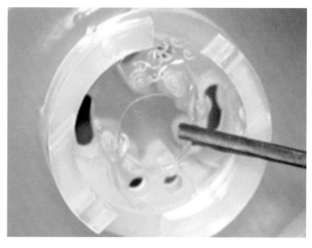

Photo 12.50. Lift the IOL from the container.

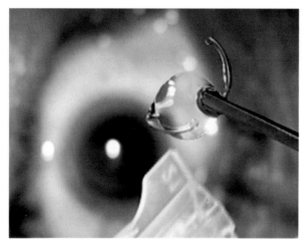

Photo 12.51. The leading haptic of the IOL is folded before inserting into the cartridge.

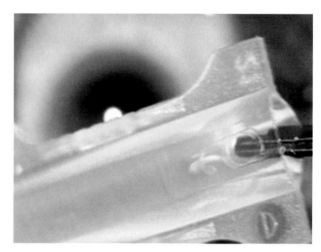

Photo 12.52. IOL inserted into the cartridge.

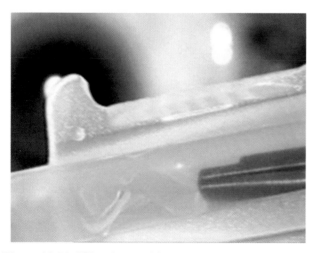

Photo 12.53. IOL advanced further into the cartridge, with the help of forceps.

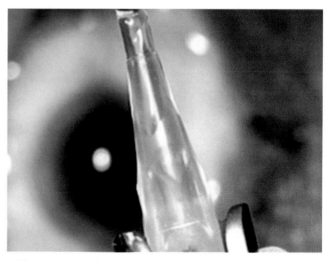

Photo 12.54. Cartridge loaded into the injector system.

PROCEDURE FOR INJECTING IOL (Contd.)

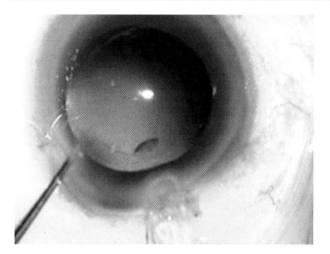

Photo 12.55. Inserting the IOL. Injector placed at corneal main wound and dialler placed at the side port to stabilize the eye.

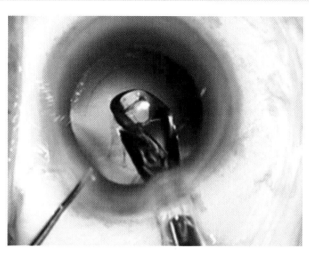

Photo 12.56. IOL being released into the AC.

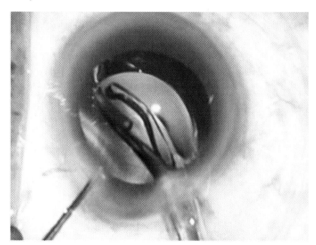

Photo 12.57. IOL released into AC. Leading haptic placed below the CCC margin.

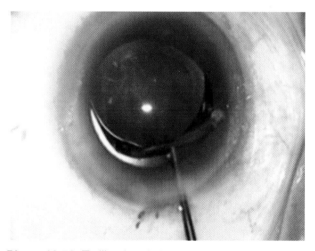

Photo 12.58. Trailing haptic being positioned in the bag.

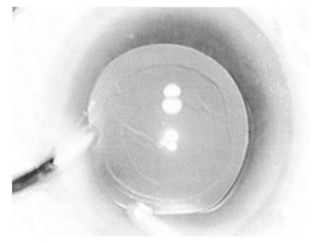

Photo 12.59. Final position of IOL in the bag.

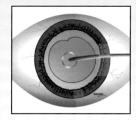

13 Our Preferred Technique for Phacoemulsification and Settings in Different Situations

As soon as a patient comes to us, we assess the patient and rate him on the difficulty score given below. Patient is well educated about the procedure and reassured that, if need be, the surgery would be safely converted to a conventional procedure.

ASSESSMENT OF THE PATIENT

The factors considered while deciding on the type of surgery are as shown in the box.

The patient should be re-assessed in the operation theatre. I am of the opinion that if the difficulty score is more than 5, then beginners should not attempt phaco. It also acts as a guidance to whether topical phaco should be done.

Anaesthesia

I usually perform all cases under topical anaesthesia. Majority of my patients are administered 4% xylocaine drops just two minutes prior to the operation. However, if the surgery is being performed under block, and if the eyes are rolled up or the exposure is poor, then we do not hesitate to put inferior and superior rectus bridle sutures.

Draping

Before draping, the skin should be cleaned 4–5 times with betadine. Draping should be done in such a way that the drape does not come beyond the eyebrow. Operating microscope light should not fall on the drape to avoid reflexes. Steridrapes should be applied over open eye. Cut the drape in the middle and turn it to cover the

eyelashes and meibomian gland orifices completely, for it to be effective.

Betadine cleaning

Eye is next washed with a swab-stick dipped in betadine while the assistant keeps pouring BSS. This should be carried on till the lipid layer is thoroughly removed. Usually 2 to 3 washes are enough. Scrubbing of lid margins while cleaning is debatable. Some believe that this releases bacteria into the conjunctival sac while others believe that this eliminates lipid layer. I believe in the latter. Presence of meibomitis warrants an extra betadine wash.

Incision

All my phacoemulsification surgeries are performed from the temporal side until and unless a refractive surgery is planned along with it. I make a uniplanar incision for foldable and biplanar for non-foldable lenses.

I first make a straight groove (500 micron deep) of 1.8–2.75 mm length for foldable lens and 5.5 mm length for non-foldable IOLs as close to the posterior limbus as possible, without disturbing the conjunctiva in the centre. After the initial groove, I make a side port incision with the same blade and aqueous is replaced with VES to pressurise the eyeball. Now, with 2.8 mm keratome, a biplanar tunnel is made.

However, I modify this incision depending upon the case. In case of hard cataracts, I make a deeper groove

Difficulty Score for Phacoemulsification

1. Corneal status
- Clear   1
- Minimal corneal guttate   2
- Moderate to severe guttate   3
- Additional 1 for corneal opacity/large arcus/prominent pannus

2. Density of cataract
- Upto grade III   1
- Upto grade IV   2
- Upto grade V   3
- Hypermature   3
- Brown/black grade V   4

3. Pupil
- 5 to 6 mm   1
- 4 to 5 mm   2
- < 4 mm   3

4. Other factors
The following factors are assigned one point, if present.
- Shallow anterior chamber
- Deep anterior chamber
- VIP
- One-eyed
- Age more than 70 years
- Deep set eye
- Small palpebral fissure
- Inadequate performance of the machine
- Below average microscope

(i.e. thicker upper flap) placed more posteriorly onto the sclera to avoid corneal burns. In a small pupil, the initial groove is more corneal to avoid iris prolapse. In deep chamber syndrome, my tunnel is shorter for easy access into the deep area. A slightly leaky wound may be advantageous in this condition. For PMMA lenses the tunnel is larger (2 mm long).

CCC

Before starting the CCC, I repressurize the eyeball with VES and put a drop of VES on the centre of cornea. As this fluid moves peripherally it takes all the debris away. Then the magnification and illumination of the micro-scope is increased. Focus is on the anterior lens capsule. My ideal CCC is 5 mm, keeping the pupillary border as guide. I prefer to err on the side of large CCC for easy phacoemulsification. However, if the CCC has become small, further management depends upon the type of cataract. If the cataract is soft I proceed. If the cataract is hard I prefer to enlarge the CCC especially in the cross-incisional area.

If pupil is small (< 4 mm) I always put adrenaline diluted in BSS 1:10 for further dilatation. If this fails I either use iris hooks or I resort to multiple small sphincterotomies. In these cases CCC is performed all along the pupillary border. In the cross-incisional area CCC can be taken beyond the pupillary border.

In *paediatric cataracts* I plan a 3 mm CCC, which usually turns out to be 5 mm finally. In *phaco trab* I prefer to have a small CCC, larger CCC is performed in *hard cataract, deep chamber syndrome, zonular dialysis and posterior polar cataract.* Anterior capsule with trypan blue staining is done in hypermature cataract.

The anterior capsule flap is always removed either by viscoexpression or Utrata forceps after completion of CCC. If the flap is left behind, it can lead to confusion with a Descemet's tear.

Hydroprocedures

VES is partially removed so that AC depth is normal or slightly less than normal before performing hydro-dissection. Hydroprocedure is performed as described earlier followed by modified compression hydro-dissection. I use 27 G cannula provided with Healon on 2 cc syringe, preferably glass. I always check for the patency, flow and tight fit of cannula and resistance of the system.

In *posterior polar cataract* hydrodissection is not done as there is a risk of a PCT. In *hypermature*, milky cataract any hydro removes the milky cortical material. The nucleus then becomes so mobile that trenching becomes very difficult. In *small CCC, small pupil, thin posterior capsule*, I resort to multiple mini hydrodissections. In most of the cases even after delineation ring appears I mechanically lift/delineate the anterior epinuclear plate. If the area lacking delineation is sub-incisional, the nucleus is rotated and delineation is completed.

Eye is again pressurized with VES to check for nucleus rotation. Single-handed or bimanual technique is tried. If mobility is not there hydrodissection is repeated after partial removal of VES. Rotation is again repeated. Before proceeding I ensure that the nucleus is rotating by looking at the pattern of cortical fibres. I do not attempt rotation in a very soft cataract. In moderately soft cataract gentle rotation is attempted. In case this fails the cataract is left alone. After removal of nucleus if ENP does not rotate, hydrodissection can be attempted again at that stage. In the case with zonular dialysis either no rotation is attempted or minimal rotation is attempted after implanting the endocapsular ring. In grade 5 cataract, do not attempt phaco till you are sure of rotation, as some fibres are strongly adherent to the PC. Little reverse rotation is done to reduce the stress on the zonules. If the nucleus prolapses out during hydro, replace the nucleus back. The displaced cortical matter is detached from their posterior extensions by sweeping the rounded repositor over the CCC. This cortical matter is then viscoexpressed.

Nucleotomy

We usually prefer the *Stop and chop* technique for nucleotomy.

For baring of the nucleus, I use the following settings:

Power   Same as for trenching
Flow rate   Same as for trenching
Vacuum   70 mmHg

Enter with irrigation on in partially pressurized eye. Baring is done as described before. Vacuum settings are kept high to facilitate aspiration.

Trenching

Kelman tip is my preferred tip for trenching. It is particularly useful in deep chamber syndromes, mature and hard cataracts. This tip permits trenching closer to sub-incisional area. This is especially useful in soft cataract as rotation can be then avoided. Our preferred mode of trenching is 'V' trench. I always enter in *CIM*. Relaxing nucleotomy is done in cases of soft cataract to facilitate splitting. Trench is made wider and longer in hard cataract, so as to allow one to reach the depth easily.

Splitting

I do the splitting under CIM with phaco probe and chopper in the centre of the trench. If the split fails to reach the periphery sub-incisionally, nucleus is rotated 180° and splitting is attempted again. In hard cataract, sometimes deep leathery bridging fibres are present. I

break these by placing the instruments deeper and close to fibres by using rotational motion.

Chopping and phacoaspiration (Fig. 13.1)

After splitting the nucleus, it is rotated by 60° to 80° to bring the heminucleus into correct position for chopping. Each heminucleus is divided into 3 parts. First heminucleus is divided using central chop or if possible modified peripheral chop. For second heminucleus, it is always possible to do a modified peripheral chop because of available space in the eye. If a burrow is created it can be used as a trench in 'divide & conquer' technique and I split it here. This is common in soft cataract. If a burrow is created in hard cataract, I go deeper to an adjacent site and repeat. If I fail again, I try third time. After chopping one should release the nucleus piece and phacoaspirate the smaller piece first. If this attempt also fails I chop and phacoaspirate the other heminucleus first. Once the space is more in the eye the previous heminucleus is tackled. This loosening of grip may be because of low vacuum in hard cataract and high vacuum in soft cataract. If one heminucleus lies over the other in the centre, I handle the part on the top first.

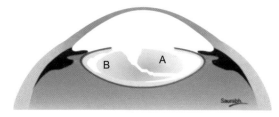

Fig. 13.1. When one heminucleus is lying on top of the other, remove the one on top (A) first and the one below (B) afterwards.

Sometimes when it is not possible to get a vacuum seal and to get the nucleus out of fornix, then a chopper is introduced at the delineation line and the nucleus is pulled into the CSZ mechanically for aspiration. This technique is very useful in a soft cataract where vacuum hold is poor and nucleus is sticky but easily amenable to mechanical pulling and crushing. If there is a small nucleus piece lying at the capsular fornix, then instead of venturing into the peripheral unsafe zone to create a vacuum seal, I viscopressurize the eye taking counter-pressure from the anterior capsular rim and the piece is prolapsed into the CSZ by a rounded repositor.

In case of paediatric cataract or very young patient, just irrigation-aspiration may be sufficient. No trenching is required by phaco probe.

Settings for Phaco in Various Machines						
	STANDARD			**NEW GENERATION**		
	Power (%)	Flow rate (cc/minute)	Vacuum (mmHg)	Power (%)	Flow rate (cc/minute)	Vacuum (mmHg)
Grade I						
Trenching	40	28	100	30	32	100
Phacoaspiration	30	28	200	20	32	300
Grade II						
Trenching	55	28	100	40	32	100
Phacoaspiration	40	28	250	30	32	350
Grade III						
Trenching	70	30	100	55	32	100
Phacoaspiration	50	32	300	40	36	400
Grade IV						
Trenching	85	30	100	70	32	100
Phacoaspiration	60	34	350	50	36	450
Grade V						
Trenching	100	30	100	85	32	100
Phacoaspiration	70	36	400	65	36	550

Epinuclear plate settings			
	Flow rate (cc/min)	Vacuum (mmHg)	
		Standard	New Generation
Soft	28	200	300
Medium	32	250	400
Hard	36	300	500

Epinuclear plate removal

Once the nucleus has been emulsified completely, keeping the phaco tip in a CIM inside the eye, replace left-hand chopper with the rounded repositor. I remove the EN plate by *flip and chip* method as described earlier. I reduce the phaco power to 30%, keeping rest of the settings same as for phacoaspiration. However, if the EN plate is too soft and biting of the EN plate is taking place, then vacuum and flow rate settings can be lowered. If surge is a problem and chamber is unstable, then in such a situation vacuum settings are lowered instead of flow rate, because we do not need a strong grip but we do need a good followability.

Cortical aspiration

Withdraw the left-hand instrument first and then remove the phaco tip leaving the AC formed. If the AC collapses, then partially form the chamber by viscoelastic before putting irrigation-aspiration cannula inside the eye. My preferred mode of cortical aspiration is *modified bimanual technique*. However, if there is any cortical matter in the sub-incisional area or side port or main port which is not getting aspirated, I do not hesitate to make a second side port to tackle it.

Capsular polishing

I viscopressurize the eye and under high magnification, I polish the capsule by a rounded repositor. No attempt is made to aspirate it now. It can be done at the time of viscoelastic substance removal.

IOL insertion

Incision is enlarged to the appropriate size before IOL insertion.

Hydration of the wound

Both main port and side port incisions are hydrated. A 27 G cannula is placed close to internal wound into the stroma and a small amount of fluid is injected till a whitish area appears on the cornea.

IOP at the time of leaving the eye

After IOL insertion, viscoelastic substance is thoroughly

washed and removed. IOP should be around 15 mmHg. If the valves are not well constructed, one may pressurize the eye more (25–30 mmHg) to have a better valve action. In a patient where optic nerve is compromised, one may leave the eye as soft, but do inject air bubble. If valve action is poor, one can use intracameral pilocarpine to constrict the pupil or one can inflate the eyeball with an air bubble. Sometimes the AC becomes shallow after removal of wire speculum. It can be inflated again.

If operation is performed under topical anaesthesia, no pad is applied and the patient gets up and goes seeing.

If done under block, subconjunctival injection of Gentamicin, Decadron and Xylocaine is given. If keratitis is suspected, Hypersol 6 eye ointment is given. Finally, pad is applied which is opened after 6 hours.

In conclusion, one should aim for perfection in every step of the surgery if one is to be a successful phaco surgeon. Each step should be 100% reproducible regardless of the type of cataract or machine, etc.

You should keep in mind that the war is won by winning many small battles!

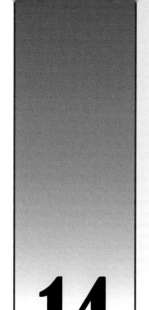

14

Correction of Pre-existing Astigmatism: LRIs, OCCIs & Toric IOLs

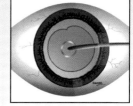

Phacoemulsification, in recent years, has changed the fundamental aim of cataract surgery, that was, the replacement of an opacified crystalline lens with an artificial lens. Now the aim of modern cataract surgery is to have uncorrected visual acuity (UCVA) as good as best corrected visual acuity (BCVA). To achieve this one needs to address the issue of **Preexisting Asitgmatism** (PEA) at the time of planning cataract surgery.

Incidence of astigmatism

- About 36–45% of patients have astigmatism of > 1 D, out of which 78% have < 1.5 D, 20% have 1.5–3.0 D and 2% have > 3.0.
- The 3-year incidence rate of astigmatism was 33.6% (cylinder power of 0.5 D or worse) or 11.5% (cylinder power of 1.0 D or worse) when measured in children age 7–9 years. Myopic children had a higher incidence rate of astigmatism than nonmyopes.
- The incidence of astigmatism in adult Navajo population was found to be 4% of with the rule astigmatism of at least 2 diopters or more in at least one eye.
- Astigmatism was found to exist in about 63% of the eyes when studied in 1112 patients from a military optometric clinic. It was found that with-the-rule (WTR) and against-the-rule (ATR) astigmatism were the predominant types of astigmatism, and that approximately 70% of astigmatism found required 1.00 D of correcting cylinder power or less.

The chief methods of correcting preexisting astigmatism during cataract surgery are:

1. Limbal/corneal relaxing incisions (LRIs)
2. On axis cataract incision & Opposite clear corneal incisions(OCCIs)
3. Toric intraocular lens (Toric IOLs)

LIMBAL / CORNEAL RELAXING INCISION

Astigmatic keratotomy was a routine procedure for correction of astigmatism for patients undergoing radial keratotomy for myopia. These incisions were made parallel to the limbus, in between the radial incisions of the radial keratotomy and had a depth of about 90% of the corneal thickness. Various surgeons, Muller-Jensen et. al (2000), Budak et. al (2000), Gills et. al (2002), Wang et. al (2003), Shen et. al (2004), Kaufmann et. al (2005) have established the effectiveness of limbal relaxing incisions in correction of preexisting astigmatism.

Correction depends upon the *length of the incision* (4 to 8 mm), *the number of incisions* (single, doubled, paired doubled), *the type of the incision* (uniplanar, biplanar, triplanar and hinged), *the distance from the centre of the cornea* (the nearer the relaxing incision to the centre of the cornea, the greater the relaxing effect), *the depth of the incision* (about 600 microns depth gives good results) and *the age of the patient* (more the age of the patient, the greater will be the effect).

It is advisable to use a diamond knife with a guard for more predictable results. Every surgeon needs to establish his own nomogram, however the following nomograms may be helpful, and can serve as a useful guide.

Gills Nomogram

Amount of astigmatism	Number of incisions	Length of incisions
1 D	1	6
2 D	2	6
3 D	2	7
4 D	2	8
> 4 D	2	10
		2 mm for every D over 4 D at 8 mm OZ (Optic Zone)

The NAPA nomogram (Nichamin Age and Pachymetry Adjusted Intralimbal Arcuate Astigmatic Nomogram)

Pre Op Cyl (Diopters)	Paired incisions in degrees of arc 50–60 years of age
With the rule astigmatism (10 degrees arc = 1 mm)	
0.75	30
1.00	35
1.25	40
1.50	45
1.75	50
2.00	55
2.25	60
2.50	65
2.75	70
3.00	80
Against the rule astigmatism (10 degrees arc = 1 mm)	
0.75	35
1.00	40
1.25	45
1.50	50
1.75	55
2.00	60
2.25	65
2.50	70
2.75	75
3.00	80

Donnenfeld Nomogram (1 clock hour = 30 degrees)

Pre-operative astigmatism	Number of incisions*	Length of incisions, Clock hours†
0.50 D	1	1.5
0.75 D	2	1
1.50 D	2	2
3.00 D	2	3

* All incisions are placed 0.5 mm from the limbus in the correct axis.
† Patients who have against-the-rule astigmatism or who are less than 45 years old may benefit from slightly longer incisions. Shorter incisions may be indicated for patients older than 65 years.

Limbal relaxing incisions can treat upto 4.0 D of astigmatism; however outcomes are less predictable with higher levels of astigmatism due to variable tissue healing.

Limitations

- Regression: The higher the astigmatism, the greater is the regression. Most regression occurs in eyes with more than 3.5 D of astigmatism and maximum regression can be seen between 1 to 3 months. Regression also causes changing refraction.
- Diamond knife is preferable.
- Mechanical instability: LRIs may lead to weakening of the globe which is prone to rupture or trauma.
- Ocular surface discomfort: Post-operative tear film instability is seen.

ON AXIS CATARACT INCISION AND OPPOSITE CLEAR CORNEAL INCISIONS

Phaco-incision is considered to be astigmatically neutral. Typically, a 3.2 mm incision induces 0.25 to 0.50 D of astigmatism. If we were to place this incision on the steep axis, it can be used to lower the PEA. If one incision corrects 0.25 D then two incisions (Fig. 14.1) will correct more than 0.5 D. It is nearly 30% more than the addition of the two, i.e. the correction will be around 0.65 D.

In phacoemulsification, adding an identical, penetrating CCI opposite the initial CCI can be used to reduce the preexisting astigmatism. The paired opposite CCIs are placed on the steepest meridian axis to flatten it. One CCI is used to perform cataract surgey and the opposite CCI is made to enhance the flattening effect on the cornes to modulate PEA.

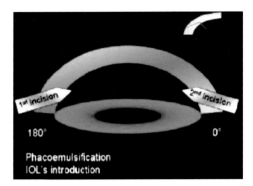

Fig. 14.1.

It is possible to correct about 1.0 to 4.0 D of astigmatism by this method so that majority of the patients are able to achieve UCVA as good as BCVA. In the patients desirous of going in for accommodative or multifocal IOLs, using on axis incision, the PEA can be brought down to within 1.0 D which is mandatory for the use of these IOLs.

The biggest advantage of this technique is the *stability* of the cornea which is achieved in 2 weeks time. Also, post-operatively, there are minimum fluctuations in vision and minimal regression.

Additional point in favour of this method is that no extra instruments or training is required. The surgeon has to learn to mark the axis correctly and he may have to shift the position of the operating chair depending upon the site of incision.

The amount of correction depends upon:
- Types of incisions
- Site of the incision
- Wound construction
  - Length
  - Width
  - Location
- Amount of astigmatism
- Number of incision

Types of incisions (Figs. 14.2 to 14.5)

The incisions may be:

1. Uniplanar
2. Biplanar
3. Triplanar
4. Hinged

If all the parameters remain the same, then as one progresses from uniplanar to hinged incision, the amount of astigmatism corrected will be nearly doubled.

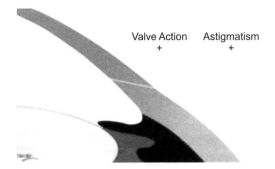

Fig. 14.2. Uniplanar incision.

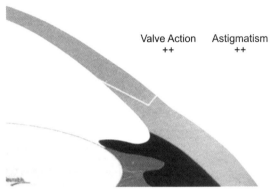

Fig. 14.3. Biplanar incision.

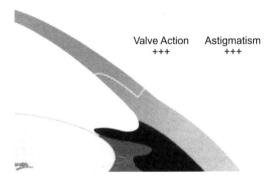

Fig. 14.4. Triplanar incision.

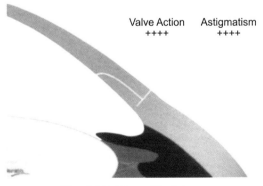

Fig. 14.5. Hinged incision.

Site of the incision

A superiorly placed incision gives more correction than a superotemporal or a superonasal incision which in turn provides more correction than a temporally placed incision (Superior > superotemporal/superonasal > Temporal). This may be because of more slippage of the wound and more importantly the superior incision is more central in location as the vertical diameter is less than the horizontal diameter of the cornea.

Wound construction (Fig. 14.6)

- **Length**
- **Width** – The lesser the width of the incision, the more will be the correction.
- **Location** – Central the incision more is the correction, i.e. a corneal incision will correct more than a limbal incision.

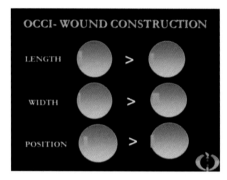

Fig. 14.6. Wound construction.

Number of incisions

Paired double incisions will correct more. For doing double incision keratotomy second incision is made 1 to 1.5 mm central and parallel to the initial incision either on one or both sides.

Amount of astigmatism

The more is the preexisting astigmatism, the greater is the correction achieved.

NOMOGRAMS

Lever and Dahan (2000) corrected astigmatism of 2.06 D using incisions ranging from 2.8 to 3.5 mm. Zemaitiene R et. al (2003) used incision sizes ranging from 3 to 4 mm to achieve an astigmatic correction of 0.67 D. Tadros A, Habib M et. al (Feb 2004) corrected astigmatism of 1.3 D using incision size of 2.85 to 3.5 mm. Abid Mahamood Qamar et. al (2005) used incision size of 3.2

mm to correct astigmatism upto 1.25 D. Khokar et. al (2006) corrected astigmatism of 1.66 D using 3.2 mm paired OCCI.

The following nomograms can be used as a guideline:

Pre-op astigmatism (D)	Age (Y)	Number	Length (Degrees)
With-the-rule			
0.75–1.00	< 65	2	45
	≥ 65	1	45
1.01–1.50	< 65	2	60
	≥ 65	2	45 (or 1 × 60)
> 1.50	< 65	2	80
	≥ 65	2	60
Against-the-rule/Oblique*			
1.00–1.25†	–	1	35
1.26–2.00	–	1	45
> 2.00	–	2	45

* Combined with temporal corneal incision
† Especially if cataract incision is not directly centred on steep meridian.

J Cataract Refract Surg 2003; 29: 712 –722[10]

Nomogram devised by Dr. Harbansh Lal based on his experience	
Type of incision	Amount of astigmatism corrected
Single steep axis	< 0.50 D
OCCI 3.2 mm incision	0.5 to 1 D
OCCI 3.5 mm incision	1 to 1.5 D
OCCI 4.0 mm incision	1.5 to 2 D
OCCI 4.5 mm incision	2 to 2.5 D
OCCI 5.0 mm incision	2.5 to 3 D

The amount of astigmatism corrected depending upon the type of incision:

Hinged > Triplanar > Biplanar > Uniplanar

The amount of astigmatism corrected depending upon the site of incision:

Superior > Oblique > Temporal

The lower value of the astigmatic correction (for OCCI with a 3.2 mm incision, this value is 0.5 D) is achieved with a uniplanar + temporal incision and the higher value of correction (for OCCI with a 3.2 mm incision, this value is 1 D) is achieved with a superior + hinged incision.

DO I NEED TO CHANGE IOL POWER?

No, I do not need to change IOL power due to the coupling effect.

Coupling Effect

Cravy has described Gauss's law of elastic domes: "for every change in curvature in one meridian there is an equal and opposite change 90 degrees away". This phenomenon of corneal behaviour is known as the coupling effect.

Corneal coupling is ratio of magnitude of corneal flattening or steepening in axis of surgery divided by magnitude of flattening or steepening 90 degrees away.

$$\text{Coupling ratio} = \frac{\text{Amount of flattening in the incision meridian}}{\text{Induced steepening in the opposite meridian}}$$

Coupling ratio =1, indicates that the spherical equivalent is unchanged.

Limitations of OCCI

The major limitation of OCCI is the variability of correction. Aiming the post-op astigmatism below 1 D is more realistic than aiming zero astigmatism. Another point to ponder is that we are moving towards a smaller and smaller incision while in OCCI we need to make a larger incision which may theoretically increase the incidence of endophthalmitis. But in spite of all this, I will still prefer to do an OCCI in low astigmatism patient and try to have post-op astigmatism less than one diopter in my patients.

TORIC INTRAOCULAR LENS

The advantages of toric IOLs are that they do not require the additional surgical skills needed to create clear corneal incisions and they can be implanted using standard cataract surgical techniques.

One major drawback of toric IOLs is that rotation of these IOLs following implantation can decrease the efficacy. For this reason, proper alignment of a toric IOL during surgery is critical. It is also important that the toric IOL shows rotational stability post-operatively to maintain the full intended effect.

Surgical Pearls

- As in all patients, marking of the axis should be done in the sitting position first and then in the supine position.

- Incision should be placed on the steep axis. As a result, the corneal astigmatism will be partially corrected and the cylindrical power required in the IOL will be less. One degree of off-axis rotation can result in a loss of up to 3.3% of the IOL's cylinder power. This means that approximately one-third of the astigmatic correction is lost if the toric IOL is rotated 10 degrees off-axis. Similarly, two-thirds of the effect is lost with a rotation of 20 degrees off-axis. From this, one can infer that if the cylindrical power used in the IOL is less, the loss of effect will be less, if by chance the IOL gets misaligned. Steep axis incision should be performed until and unless one needs to give an incision, which is technically difficult. For example, an inferotemporal/superonasal incision will be difficult for a right-handed surgeon.

- The capsulorrhexis should be smaller in size than the size of the IOL optic, should be well-centred and should cover the optic equally on all side so that IOL misalignment is reduced. If the capsulorrhexis is eccentric or irregular, it can cause decentration and misalignment of the IOL. It is always better to err on the side of a smaller CCC. An ideal size would be about 4.5–5.5 mm.

- Cohesive viscoelastics should be used for IOL implantation as they can be removed completely from the capsular bag at the end of surgery, thus preventing rotation of the IOL. Dispersive viscoelastics should be avoided as they cannot be removed completely from the capsular bag, which may result in rotation and misalignment of the IOL.

- Toric IOL should be placed 20–30 degrees away from the desired position and then rotated clockwise. After removing all the viscoelastic, final positioning of the IOL should be done. Irrigation port of the bimanual or coaxial system is used as an anterior chamber maintainer, through the side port while doing the final positioning of the IOL. Before withdrawing the irrigation port, air should be placed in the anterior chamber so that the IOL is pushed back into position.

- Any doubts in the positioning of the IOL, it is advisable to correct the misalignment, then and there before closing the eye.

- Post-operatively, one should attempt to determine the correction of corneal astigmatism by measuring the axis of keratometry readings and the refraction.

- If the astigmatism left is > 1 D and if this is due to misalignment of the lens realignment should be done within 1–2 weeks. Alternatively, if the patient is very demanding, corneal procedures for correcting residual astigmatism may be used.

The results of corneal procedures like LRIs and OCCIs are variable as they depend upon a large number of factors like site, size, number, length, depth of the incision, age of the patient, amount of astigmatism and many other factors. The correction obtained by a Toric IOL is much more predictable, if aligned correctly.

TECHNIQUES OF CORRECTION

Treat only corneal astigmatism

Astigmatism is of three types: Corneal, lenticular and retinal. The amount of astigmatism contributed by the retinal slope cannot be assessed. Lenticular astigmatism is treated by removal of the crystalline lens and implantation of an IOL. However, the contribution of the IOL to astigmatism cannot be predicted. Corneal astigmatism is the only astigmatism which can be assessed and corrected. Also, DO NOT TREAT THE REFRACTIVE ERROR. For example, if a patient has 2.5 D of astigmatism, but keratometry shows only 0.5 D of astigmatism, then treat only 0.5 D.

For correct assessment and treatment of corneal astigmatism, following are important:

1. Keratometry

Keratometry can be done by the following methods:

• Manual keratometry
• Automated keratometry
• IOL Master
• Topography

MANUAL METHOD IS THE GOLD STANDARD. Certain points should be kept in mind while proceeding with manual keratometry:

1. The patient should be asked to look into the barrel of the machine. Measurements should be taken of the central part of the cornea.
2. The instrument should be clean.
3. There should be no play in the instrument.
4. Standardisation should be done regularly either with an artificial eye or with a calibration sphere.
5. The instrument should be properly centred.
6. Patient's eyelashes should not come into the view.
7. If the patient's tear film dries up , topical lubricants may be used.

8. Inter-operator differences should not be there; if differences are present, it means that either operators are not trained or instrument is not correct.
9. If the operator has any refractive error, it should be corrected.
10. Tonometry should always be done after keratometry.

Any of the above mentioned methods may be used , however the most important point is to maintain consistency of readings. Also, same method should be used post-operatively for analytical purposes.

2. Marking of the axis of astigmatism

It is the most important step and should be done accurately. There may be torsion in the supine position of 5–6 degrees in majority of the patients. So, initially the 6 O'clock axis should be marked with the patient in the sitting position and then in the supine position.

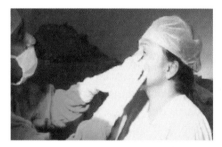

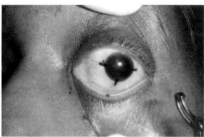

Fig. 14.7. Marking of the axis of astigmatism in the sitting position.

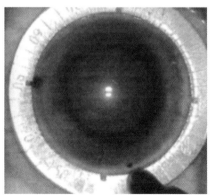

Fig. 14.8. Marking of the axis of astigmatism in the supine position.

Other more accurate methods, such as air bubble, pendular and electronic, can be used for marking the axis. This needs expensive instrumentation. Marking on a slit-lamp or with a pen in sitting position is equally effective.

CONCLUSION

- OCCIs and LRIs both correct astigmatism and can be combined together for better effect. Because of better post-operative stability of refraction, OCCI seems to be a better option.
- TORIC IOLs are more predictable than LRIs and OCCIs for correction of PEA but the cost, the exact operative positioning and the post-operative rotational stability remains an issue.

- OCCI can also be clubbed with toric IOLs to increase the range of astigmatism corrected. It can also be safely used with multifocal and accommodative IOLs. The patients who are left with < 1.0 D of astigmatism remain comfortable, particularly if the astigmatism happens to be against the rule (ATR), as the patient will experience increased depth of focus due to pseudo-accomodation. Probably, better nomograms for OCCIs is the need of the day.

Thus, with a little extra effort of marking the axis correctly and changing the operating chair according to the site of incision, the pre existing astigmatism may be tackled. This proves to be a rewarding experience for the surgeon and a highly satisfactory experience for the patients.

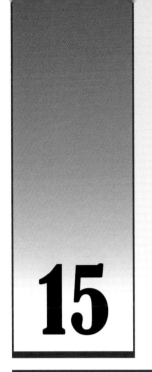
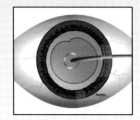

15 | Complications of Phacoemulsification

WOUND-RELATED COMPLICATIONS

There are many wound-related complications, of which some like torn edges, premature entry, and scleral disinsertion, have been earlier described in **Chapter 6: Incisions and Wound Construction.**

Scleral / corneal burn (Photos 15.1 & 15.2)

The primary cause of scleral/corneal burn is heat generated by the phaco tip. The irrigating silicone sleeve cools the tip and helps to prevent burns. *Tight wound and uninterrupted excessive use of high phaco energy* are the major causes of the burn. The sclera, and a thicker superior flap can withstand the burn better. This implies that a uniplanar corneal incision will have more chances of burns rather than a triplanar corneal or scleral incision. Lifting the handpiece up causes stoppage of fluid from top; to avoid this, always make conscious attempt to rest handpiece on scleral bed.

To prevent corneal burns, BSS cooled to 4°C can be used. This also protects the corneal endothelium. Using just adequate and intermittent phaco energy also facilitates prevention of burn. The assistant must keep putting fluid at the incision site to dissipate the heat generated.

Luckily, most of these burns do not reach the internal opening and the valve action remains intact. An area of corneal thinning can be seen post-operatively at the burn site. If the burn is enough to cause a wound leak, one should give a horizontal mattress suture on the sclera or a shoelace suture on the cornea to seal the wound.

Descemet's detachment (Photo 15.3) (Fig. 15.1)

This occurs when instruments are not introduced in a proper direction particularly in a softer eye or partially collapsed AC. Descemet's detachment should be recognized and care should be taken that it does not get into the suction port of any instrument. To differentiate this from a capsular tag, if the detachment is spread to one side, an area of a similar contour will be seen as a mirror image on the other side of the base.

Pressurize the eye from another site, e.g. for Descemet's detachment of the main port, introduce the

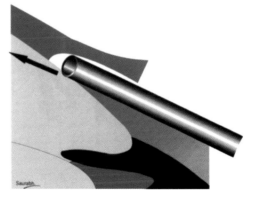

Fig. 15.1. Descemet's detachment is caused by incorrect advancement of the instrument through the sclera. To prevent this, the instrument should be tilted up to turn the tip down while entering.

fluid through the side port. Now depress the lower lip of main port. As the BSS leaks, the Descemet's fold unrolls. Now pressurize the chamber again either with BSS or air from the side port.

CORNEAL COMPLICATIONS

Apart from the corneal wound-related complications, endothelial damage may be a potentially dangerous complication.

Endothelial damage

Endothelial damage may be *chemical, thermal or mechanical*. As far as *chemical* toxicity is concerned, every fluid is potentially toxic to the endothelium, depending upon the extent to which its composition and pH differs from that of aqueous. BSS plus has a composition and pH that is closest to that of aqueous. Drugs such as adrenaline, xylocard and pilocarpine should be diluted with BSS and used at the lowest possible dilution. *Do not use distilled water for dilution* as it is very toxic to the endothelium. *Thermal* damage is caused by high temperature generated due to the vibrations of the phaco tip. This heat can damage the cornea if phaco is performed very close to cornea; otherwise it does not play a very significant role.

The commonest cause of endothelial damage is mechanical. Mechanical damage may be caused by instruments, lens matter or shock waves due to fluid turbulence. The excessive use of fluids washes away the endothelial cells and the surge can cause corneal dimpling with or without instrument touch. *The rubbing of a hard nuclear fragment against the endothelium is often responsible for endothelial injury.* This happens during inadvertent chattering of nuclear fragments or phaco-aspiration in the AC close to the cornea. Sometimes even small innocuous pieces can be damaging. In cramped chamber syndromes small pupil, a small CCC or a large CCC, the chances of endothelial damage increase.

Prevention is better than cure

To prevent endothelial damage the surgeon must be careful from step one of the surgery. Wound construction should be proper. VES should be used frequently. An attempt should be made to divide the nucleus mechanically into small pieces so as to facilitate judicious intermittent use of phaco energy in CSZ. Conscious effort to emulsify the fragment away from the cornea will go a long way in reducing the endothelial cell loss.

IRIS COMPLICATIONS

Iris chaffing

Iris chaffing is caused by inadvertent aspiration of the iris by the phaco probe. It is more common in a small pupil. Once the iris has been caught in the probe it becomes floppy and tends to repeatedly get sucked in. Post-operatively it may be seen as an atrophic patch.

Iridodialysis

Catching the iris and pulling can lead to iridodialysis. This should be prevented as it will lead to a disabling glare post-operatively.

Scleral wall fixation of iris with the help of prolene sutures can be done. Scleral flaps/pockets (Fig. 15.1A) can be made as explained during scleral fixated IOL.

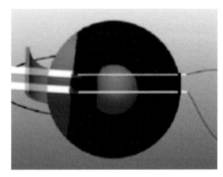

Fig. 15.1A. Scleral pocket is created and 26 G needle is passed and kept under the edge of the dialysed peripheral iris. Prolene needle comes from the top of the iris and perforates it and enters the 26 G needle and then comes out of the eye. Procedure is repeated with second needle. Both these threads are tied which pull the dialysed iris up.

CAPSULAR COMPLICATIONS

Zonulodialysis

Pre-existing zonulodialysis should be picked up pre-operatively especially in cases with a predisposition to zonular weakness such as pseudoexfoliation syndrome, high myopia, and trauma. In such predisposed cases, zonulodialysis may be extended while trying to rotate the nucleus or at the time of insertion or dialing of the IOL. If zonulodialysis is upto 2 clock hours, CTR is good enough but if it is more than that then Cionni's ring with scleral fixation is a better choice.

Cionni's ring fixation in cases of zonulodialysis

Scleral wall fixation of capsule with the help of prolene sutures can be done. Scleral flaps/pockets can be made as explained during scleral fixated IOL.

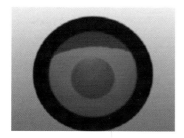

Superior zonular dialysis can be appreciated.

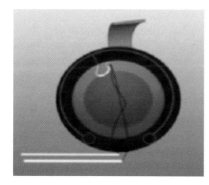

Cionni's ring needs fixation at only one point most of the time, so we need only one scleral flap at the site of maximum zonular dialysis. Prolene threads are fixed to the eyelet of Cionni's before inserting the Cionni's into the capsular fornices. The loop of Cionni's, which fixates it to the sclera, comes out of the rhexis margin and lies outside the capsule and underneath the iris along with prolene traction sutures.

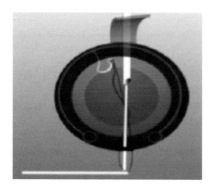

Needle is brought out through the scleral pocket, using the same technique as in scleral fixated IOL.

Fig. 15.1B.

POSTERIOR CAPSULAR TEAR

PREDISPOSING FACTORS

PCT can be defined as an iatrogenic breach in the continuity of posterior capsule. The incidence of PCT in various studies varies between 1–4%. This largely depends upon the equipment, setup and surgeon's experience and skill. The incidence of PCT goes down as the surgeon develops a better understanding of the equipment and his surgical skill improves. If beginners are able to understand the causes and factors responsible for PCT, they can take essential steps to prevent its occurrence.

Our aim is to analyze how and why PCT takes place and, in case it occurs, how can we have a surgical outcome comparable to an uncomplicated surgery, in terms of good visual outcome, early visual rehabilitation and prevention of secondary consequences of PCT like Glaucoma, Nucleus drop, IOL drop, Distorted pupil, Decentred IOL, Corneal decompensation, Cystoid macular edema, Prolonged inflammation, Retinal detachment, etc. To have a satisfactory outcome, when there is an IOL or nuclear drop, it has to be managed by a posterior segment surgeon.

Prevention is the best form of management. Prevention is possible only if we know what causes PCT. The predisposing factors can be classified as follows:

1. Equipment related
   (a) Operating microscope
   (b) Phacomachine
2. Extraocular – Ergonomics
   (a) Prominent eyebrows
   (b) Deep set eyes
   (c) Narrow palpebral fissure
   (d) Disorders of spine
3. Ocular
   (a) Corneal causes
   (b) Anterior chamber depth
   (c) Iris and pupillary factors
   (d) Capsule, lens and zonules
4. Surgeon's factor

1. Equipment related

(a) Operating microscope

Focussing of the oculus, proper interpupillary distance (IPD) selection, well positioned microscope, and comfortable seating are essential prior to surgery.

- **Adjusting the oculus:** If there is no anisometropia, the surgeon can keep the oculus at 0, in both eyes. In case of anisometropia, the surgeon keeps one oculus at 0 and focusses with the other eye closed; now the surgeon closes the focussed eye and adjusts the oculus of the other eye. Maximum plus which provides a clear view should be chosen in the oculus, so as to relax the accommodation.

- **IPD:** Maximum IPD which does not cause diplopia should be selected.

(b) Phacomachine

Proper understanding of phacodynamics and the machine is an essential prerequisite for a successful surgery.

2. Extraocular – Ergonomics

For the ease of surgery it is important to have the eye horizontally placed. Any angulation may lead to an oblique plane causing rotation and distortion of the globe, leading to unfocussed surgical field and difficulty in depth perception. Optimum exposure of the surgical field and unhindered access to anterior chamber are prerequisites for a good surgical outcome. Attaining a horizontal position of the eye during surgery by either adjusting the table, sutures, block or extra support under the head or the shoulders is essential.

(a) Prominent eyebrows

Chin can be raised and extra support if needed can be given below the shoulders to position and stabilize the head.

(b) Deep set eyes

Temporal incision is better as eyebrows can be avoided. If needed, superior and inferior rectus bridle sutures can be passed to elevate and stabilize the eyeball.

(c) Narrow palpebral fissure

If it is felt that the speculum is pressing on the globe and the exposure is not adequate then lid traction or bridle sutures can be passed. If the exposure is still not adequate, cantholysis (crushing and cutting of lateral canthus can be done, which can be sutured after phacoemulsification) is a good option.

(d) Disorders of the spine

Extra support may be needed behind the shoulders or the spine to make the patient comfortable. This may lead to elevation of the patient's head. To compensate this we can elevate the foot end of the table to make the head horizontal. Being a closed chamber technique, elevating the foot end of the table will not alter the surgery as it used to do in open chamber surgeries due to increased orbital pressure and vitreous thrust.

> *Never hesitate to give blocks in patients in whom you consider eye positioning may be suboptimal.*

Certain modifications in the surgical practice can help in overcoming the problems posed by the ergonomic factors, such as:

- If doing superior phacoemulsification, shift to a temporal incision.
- Side port incision can be made more central i.e. corneal instead of limbal, if there is obstruction due to prominent eyebrows or cheek bones.
- If there is excessive pooling at the medial side, causing annoying reflexes, then slight temporal tilting of the head can be done or drainage through merosel sponges/gauze, placed at the lower fornix and draining out can be done.

3. Ocular factors

Assessing ocular risk involves evaluation of the corneal clarity, anterior chamber depth, extent of pupil dilation, iris, capsular status, cataract density and extent of zonular weakness, if any.

(a) Corneal problems leading to poor visibility

Scarring from any corneal pathology can cause irregular corneal haze, increasing light scatter and reducing contrast during surgery. The use of trypan blue to stain the anterior capsule during capsulorhexis is a must.

The annoying reflexes by the microscope light in presence of corneal pathology during Continuous Curvilinear Capsulorhexis (CCC) can largely be overcome by the use of an endoilluminator (used by retinal surgeons). It can be placed on the limbus or inside the AC with the microscope light off, which enhances the visibility and facilitates the CCC.

(b) Anterior chamber depth (ACD)

Proper evaluation of ACD is essential prior to surgery, as ACD can be shallow in high hypermetropes, intumescent and hypermature cataracts with secondary glaucoma which decreases the safety margin, as there is a reduction in the central safe zone (CSZ). We will discuss the concept of CSZ later.

ACD is deep in high myopes, vitrectomized eyes and zonulopia (stretched weak zonules) which makes the lens lie deep. So when we access the lens during phacoemulsification, the direction of the phaco tip is more posterior. This leads to corneal striae and folds along with a posterior direction force, which increases the chances of PCT. To prevent this, bottle height should be low; a small corneal tunnel is warranted with no undue pressure on the nucleus.

(c) Iris and pupillary factors

Small pupil and floppy iris increase the risk of PCT. If pupil is smaller than 5 mm then appropriate measures have to be taken for sustained dilation of pupil.

- **Sclerosed pupil:** Easier to handle as compared to floppy iris. Stretching of pupil or multiple sphincterotomies (8–12) of about 400–500 μ each can be done.
- **Floppy iris:** More dangerous than the above. Prolapse of the iris from the wounds and progressive miosis being a major problem. Hence careful evaluation of a floppy iris should be made and iris hooks or expanders (Malyugin rings) should be kept ready and used whenever required.

Even if during surgery the pupils get miosed, there should be no reluctance in usage of hooks and expanders.

(d) Capsule, zonules and lens

Thin friable PC in certain situations, such as posterior polar cataract, pseudoexfoliation, vitrectomized eye, high myopia and **floppy and lax PC**, as in hard cataract, zonulopia, zonular dehiscence, poses increased threat of posterior capsule tear.

Hard cataract is one of the most important risk factors for PCT. The capsule is generally thin and friable in such cases (Fig. 15.2). Overstretching of the capsule because of the large volume of the nucleus increases the tendency of the PC to keep coming forward. Also, it is difficult to separate and chop the leathery fibres.

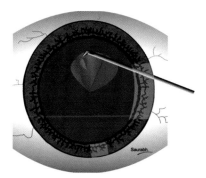

Fig. 15.2. Friable capsule. Note: Not only turned capsular flap but the capsule underneath gets torn inadvertently.

4. Surgeon's factor

As the surgeon keeps on gaining experience, the incidence of complication goes down, but any complication due to lack of understanding of the basics is unacceptable. Every surgeon should be aware of the mechanism of surge and should know how to prevent or control surge during the surgery. Before going to various stages and how PCT happens, let us understand the mechanism of surge.

For that we first need to understand the concepts of:

- (a) Central safe zone,
- (b) Peripheral unsafe zone,
- (c) Compliance,
- (d) Flow rate, vacuum and their relationships.

(a) Central safe zone (Fig. 15.3)

The **central safe zone** is not an anatomical area but a concept that needs to be understood for performing safe aspiration. This is an area within the CCC margin which is bounded vertically by the cornea on the top and the posterior capsule in opposite direction. This is the area with maximum space in the AC. All aspiration—nuclear, epinuclear or cortical—should be done here as there is maximum safety here. Even if there is AC flutter, the probe will not damage any vital structures. The nuclear pieces and cortical matter can be held in the periphery and then brought to the CSZ for aspiration. This is a dynamic area – as more of the nuclear pieces are removed, the space and thus the safety margin keeps on increasing. **In myopes, zonular stress syndromes and vitrectomized eyes the CSZ is further increased whereas in hypermetropes, small pupil and small CCC the CSZ is smaller.**

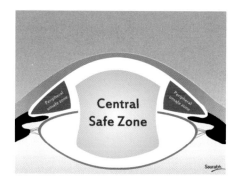

Fig. 15.3. Central safe zone (CSZ).

(b) Peripheral unsafe zone (Fig. 15.3)

Due to the corneal curvature, as one proceeds towards the periphery, one enters an unsafe zone as there is less space for manoeuvering. The capsular fornices and the angle region are thus areas where it is dangerous to do phacoaspiration since the vital structures are extremely close. This constitutes the **Peripheral unsafe zone** (PUSZ).

(c) Compliance

A silicon tube connects the aspiration system with the handpiece in both types of pumps. Additionally thick wide bore tubing is required for the rollers to be effective in a peristaltic pump. While the rollers are rotating, there is no occlusion and no collapse of tubing. When occlusion occurs, vacuum builds up, the rollers stop and negative pressure is generated within the whole system. This causes the tubing to collapse.

Property of the tubing to collapse (deform under pressure) is the compliance of the tubing. Once the occlusion breaks, there is a release of negative pressure and the tubing re-expands to the original size. Fluid is drawn from the AC to fill up this extra volume (this is what causes surge). Though this volume is not much, it is this instantaneous withdrawal of fluid over an extremely short period of time which causes the surge (Fig. 15.4A).

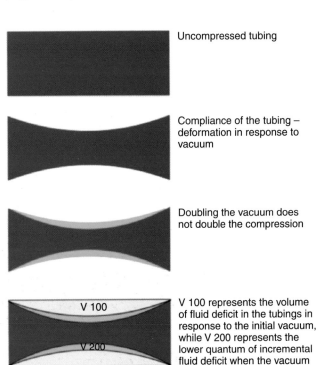

Uncompressed tubing

Compliance of the tubing – deformation in response to vacuum

Doubling the vacuum does not double the compression

V 100 represents the volume of fluid deficit in the tubings in response to the initial vacuum, while V 200 represents the lower quantum of incremental fluid deficit when the vacuum is doubled.

Fig. 15.4A. Compliance.

This extent of collapse of the tubing will depend on the lumen size, the level of vacuum generated and the thickness of the tube. The collapse is more at higher vacuum levels and less if the lumen is smaller and the walls are thicker (less compliant tubing). Tubings of these characteristics are known as 'High Vacuum' tubing.

SURGE

Sudden withdrawal of fluid from AC after occlusion breaks is called surge. Beyond a certain limit it may cause collapse of chamber, jeopardizing the vital structures of eyes and making the surgery filled with complications. In fact modifications introduced over a period of time have taken place to manage this surge and thus make phaco surgery free from complications. If there was no surge, any one could have mastered phacoemulsification. To maintain a constant volume and IOP of the AC, inflow, i.e. infusion has to be equal to outflow, which is the sum of aspiration by pump and the wound leakage. For a given bottle height inflow is constant and so is the leakage. The only variable parameters left in the above equation are the aspiration flow rate and the vacuum, i.e. the outflow by aspiration (Fig. 15.4B).

THE GENESIS OF SURGE

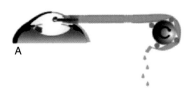

A. The tip is not occluded and fluid is passing through the system.

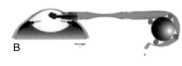

B. A nuclear fragment occludes the tip while the aspiration continues to draw fluid away from the tubings. This creates a negative pressure inside the tubings.

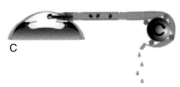

C. As the fragment is emulsified, occlusion breaks, and the accumulated negative pressure causes a sudden withdrawl of fluid from the anterior chamber, resulting in **SURGE**.

Fig. 15.4B. Surge.

(d) Relationship between vacuum, surge and flow rate

Suppose there is surge beyond acceptable limits. Now there are two options—either reduce the flow rate or the vacuum. Decreasing the AFR has a direct and linear effect but increases the rise time and makes the procedure slower, which may not be such a disadvantage to a beginner. On the other hand decreasing the vacuum will decrease the holding power which is not desirable in steps like chopping/phacoaspiration of a hard cataract. So, it is better to lower the FR in such a situation to decrease the surge, while maintaining high vacuum. On the other hand, in situations where a firm hold is not so important, like divide and conquer technique, soft cataracts or epinuclear plate removal, one can lower the vacuum settings to decrease the surge while maintaining the AFR.

Control of surge

There are various methods of controlling the surge. Some are incorporated into the newer machines and there are some measures that the surgeon can apply.

Surge prevention by the machine

Venting, high vacuum tubings, use of cassettes, delay in start of motor after breaking of occlusion, differential settings for flow rate and vacuum at different stages of surgery, dual/linear foot pedals, microtips and above all highly responsive sensors and computing have been successful in decreasing the surge.

Surgeon's control of surge

1. **Decreasing the effective flow rate:** Without changing the actual setting on the machine, the surgeon can decrease the effective FR by using a smaller bore aspiration port, e.g. Microflow tip.
2. **Increasing the infusion** by raising the bottle height or using a TUR (Transurethral resection) set may be useful in some cases.
3. The use of an **ACM** is useful for decreasing surge (especially for beginners).
4. **Proper wound construction:** A leaking wound will disturb the equilibrium of the chamber so that even a very small amount of fluid withdrawn can cause it to collapse. This highlights the importance of making a good main wound and side port. The wound construction should be such that it conforms to the tip that you are using. Premature entry also results in a leaking wound. Distortion of the wound, with the co-axial IA handpiece may cause a leaky wound. Too tight a wound or too long a tunnel can also cause a problem by reducing the inflow. Thus both a leaky and too tight a wound can increase the surge.
5. **Increased viscosity of the AC contents:** The flow rate settings are for clear fluids like BSS/Ringers. A thicker fluid increases the resistance and does not flow out easily. The use of viscoelastic substance (VES) can cause a decrease in the effective FR and thus decrease the surge. This is particularly useful in hard cataracts where the settings are usually high and whilst aspirating the last nuclear fragment.

6. **Partial occlusion of the tip:** Partially occluding the tip with another piece before the occlusion breaks and the occluding fragment gets aspirated ensures that any surge that occurs will be used to draw in the next piece to occlude the tip. This will maintain occlusion and prevent fluid from the AC being aspirated.

7. **Foot control:** Above all, good foot pedal control is of paramount importance in controlling surge and utilizing it to your own advantage. If one can anticipate the events then surge control is not a problem. That is why experienced surgeons can operate on any settings and any machine. As soon as the occlusion is about to break (i.e. the piece is about to be aspirated into the tip), the surgeon lifts the FP to IA_0 (position 1 of foot pedal or completely in the Continuous Infusion Mode), the piece will go in on its own momentum and without any of surge as the FR will decrease. Thus fluid withdrawn from the AC will be very little to overcome the compliance of the system. However, if the FP is withdrawn too early and there is not enough momentum then it will take more time to build up vacuum again. This balancing between the AFR, vacuum and the momentum of the pieces needs to be done very carefully.

MECHANISM OF PCT

It is indeed surprising that just a 4 μ thin posterior capsule can withstand so much stress and pressure, arising because of the various forces during phaco surgery. Why then, under certain situations, does its tenacity give way? To understand this we have to assess each and every step of the surgery, understand what predisposes to PCT and what remedial measures can be taken.

1. Wound construction

Though wound construction may not be directly responsible for PCT, but leaky wounds are the most important factor for unstable AC. A sharp keratome, according to the size of the phaco tip is a must for a good wound construction. Trying to create a 2.75 mm incision with a 3.2 mm keratome will always result in a leaky wound. Even a tight wound will lead to increase in surge by reducing the inflow.

Side port incisions are even more important. The chopper is much thinner than the aspiration cannula used in bimanual I/A system. We generally create the side port incisions to the size of the I/A cannula and when we are at the highest parameter setting of phacomachine, i.e. during chopping and phacoaspiration this wound keeps on leaking. Due to the same reason beginner can make initially small incision corresponding to the size of chopper and then enlarge it afterwards for I/A.

2. Anterior continuous curvilinear capsulorhexis (CCC)

The CCC can withstand turbulence, pressure and mechanical stress created by the fluid, nucleus, chopper, IOL, etc., during phacoemulsification. If CCC is not intact, or there is cone formation in the CCC, then these forces may cause the anterior rhexis margin to extend posteriorly leading to a PCT. Rhexis margin tear (RMT) could be primary, occurring at the stage of performing anterior CCC or secondary, i.e., happening at any other stage of the surgery.

Primary RMT

There are certain situations which are more prone to RMT, such as:

1. Intumescent or hypermature cataract
2. Pediatric cataract
3. Hard cataract
4. Fibrosed capsule

1. Intumescent or hypermature cataract

Due to the high intralenticular pressure, many a time as soon as a nick is made on the anterior capsule, the rhexis tends to run away, or one is able to start the rhexis, but it tends to run to the periphery midway. In such a scenario use of **Healon 5 or Healon GV** to flatten the anterior capsule may prevent it.

To prevent this, one may try to reduce the intra-lenticular pressure by doing multiple **YAG capsulo-tomies**, few hours before the surgery. This is the best method as holes created by YAG are round and don't have the tendency to run away. Same can also be achieved by **multiple small punctures** at the centre instead of one linear cut to relieve the intralenticular pressure. Fluid is allowed to escape slowly, but these punctures are not round, and will have a tendency to run away.

After making the punctures, some of the released fluid can be manually **sucked by a syringe** by putting the cannula at various locations underneath the anterior capsule or viscoexpressed. **Viscoexpression** is better as it maintains the pressure from the top and thus prevents the rhexis from running away.

Another, very good option is to make a **small rhexis** initially and enlarge it before or after phacoemulsi-fication, depending upon the size of the rhexis and hardness of the cataract. If the CCC is less than 3.5 mm and the nucleus is large and hard, it's better to enlarge it before doing phacoemulsification.

Many surgeons prefer to make a **sinusoidal CCC**, i.e. start as small CCC and after completing 120–180° start enlarging it and instead of finishing it at the site of origin go beyond and get an adequate CCC.

2. Pediatric cataract

Younger the patient, more are the chances of RMT. To perform CCC in such cases requires special surgical skill. Capsule has to be stained, high viscosity viscoelastics are a must and CCC has to be done with a forceps.

Small CCC is attempted and instead of applying tangential force, the cut end is **pulled in towards the centre**. AC has to be maintained at all times, as even a slight collapse of the AC will make the CCC run away.

3. Hard cataract

Hard cataracts in older patients usually have a very thin and friable capsule. Trying to do an anterior CCC by cystitome, many times leads to tears in the anterior capsule underneath the turned flap, making it difficult to get a round CCC. If such tears go unnoticed, these lead to RMT (Fig. 15.5).

Use of **forceps and trypan blue** stained capsule is a better choice.

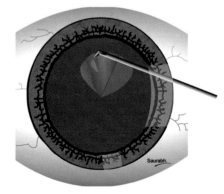

Fig. 15.5. Friable capsule – hard cataract.

4. Fibrosed capsule

Sometimes in long standing traumatic and hypermature cataract, the cataract gets partially absorbed and the patient develops plaque, fibrosis of the capsule and wrinkling of the anterior capsule. In such situations CCC is difficult and one may land up in incomplete and irregular CCC.

Secondary RMT

This occurs because of inadvertent injury to the anterior CCC, which can be due to the chopper, phaco tip, IOL or the hard nucleus. The most common culprit is the sharp chopper.

Types of RMT

There are two types of RMT:
1. Curved or tangential
2. Radial or coned

1. Curved

When trying to do a CCC, it goes to the periphery in curvilinear fashion and you are not able to retrieve it. This retrieval is difficult in younger patients due to high elasticity of the zonules. When the rhexis is pulled in, zonules get stretched and prevent this force to be applied on to the cut end of the rhexis margins in proper direction (Fig. 15.6).

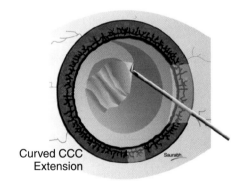

Curved CCC
Extension

Fig. 15.6. Rhexis margin tear.

2. Radial

This happens in morgagnian or intumescent cataract when rhexis runs away to the periphery or due to injury to the rhexis margin by chopper or phaco tip during surgery, which leads to the formation of a cone (Fig. 15.7).

In presence of RMT, excessive pressure by nuclear fragment, while dialing or during chopping may cause RMT to extend posteriorly. Collapse of the chamber during any phase of the surgery will cause vitreous to

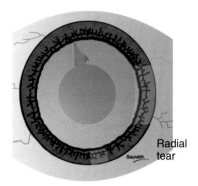

Radial tear

Fig. 15.7. Rhexis margin tear.

bulge forward and cause RMT to run posteriorly. This happens more when the last nuclear fragment is being removed. As long as some nuclear fragment is present in the capsular fornices, it prevents PC to come forward.

> **Curved RMT is not as dangerous, as its chance to run to the posterior capsule is much less as compared to the radial RMT.**

The most important strategy to prevent PCT is to **maintain AC depth at all times**. For this reason do not lower the bottle height, but lower the fluidics parameter by 20%, so as to avoid any chamber fluctuation.

Viscoelastics have to be injected before removal of the probe, at every step of the surgery, even after cortical aspiration before removing the infusion cannula inject viscoelastics from the side port.

Alternatively nucleus can be prolapsed into the AC and supracapsular phacoemulsification can be performed, but still ACD should be maintained during every step of the surgery.

3. During hydrodissection

There are 3 main reasons for posterior capsular rupture during hydro procedures:

1. Block to outflow

The outflow may be blocked due to increased resistance offered by viscoelastic in the chamber or a small CCC/ small pupil. Also injecting from the side port when main wound is sealed can lead to a PCT due to increased pressure (Fig. 15.8).

2. Injection of too much fluid

Injection of too much fluid with too much force or using a faulty technique/wrong syringes and cannula can lead to PCT.

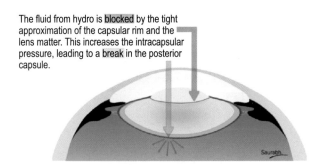

The fluid from hydro is blocked by the tight approximation of the capsular rim and the lens matter. This increases the intracapsular pressure, leading to a break in the posterior capsule.

Fig. 15.8. Hydrodissection.

3. Inherent weakness

Weak capsule may be seen in case of posterior polar cataract, high myopes, post-vitrectomy, traumatic cataracts, pseudoexfoliative syndromes and some cases of posterior subcapsular cataract. In these cases one can avoid hydrodissection (since this step can lead to a nuclear drop) and perform a careful hydrodelineation.

If the PCT goes unnoticed and if the phaco probe is placed in the anterior chamber, the nucleus will be dislodged in the vitreous cavity. So, early recognition of the PCT is of utmost importance at this step. Few signs that help in the recognition of PCT are as follows.

Signs of a PC rupture during hydrodissection
These are:
- **Sudden deepening of the chamber**
- **Abnormal tilt in the nucleus**
- **Inability to rotate the nucleus**
- **Sudden dilation of the pupil – Snap sign**
- **Bright red reflex.**

4. During nucleotomy

Nucleotomy comprises of Trenching, Splitting, Chopping and Aspiration. Any of these steps if not performed properly can lead to a PCT.

1. Trenching

In case of a **soft cataract**, while trenching if the power has not been adequately lowered, one can go through and through, which can lead to a PCT in the periphery. On the other hand, in case of a **hard cataract** if the power has not been adequately increased, surgeon tends to apply excessive force on the nucleus pushing it down, which can lead to PCT or zonular dehiscence.

2. Splitting

If trenching depth is not adequate, excessive force applied during splitting can lead to damage to the capsule. If the fibres are very leathery, on attempted splitting we tend to dip the periphery of the nucleus which may lead to development of zonular dehiscence or a peripheral PCT. In such cases make sure, not to push the nucleus too far away, and keep on moving your instruments closer to the area of the split, so that the fragments do not move very far apart.

3. Chopping and aspiration

At this stage of surgery fluidic parameters are highest and surge is the most important causative factor. Sudden surge or collapse of anterior chamber can lead to a direct injury to the posterior capsule by the chopper. When chopping in a soft cataract, the soft part tends to be sucked in, and the probe may damage the posterior capsule (PC) more so in the periphery.

Epinuclear plate, the cortical matter and nuclear pieces in capsular fornices keep the PC away from the probe, while emulsifying the last nuclear piece the capsular fornices are empty and a slight surge moves PC towards the probe, causing PCT. This is more common in conditions where the capsule is lax and floppy as in hypermature, brown hard cataracts. In such cases the nucleus size is very large, which stretches the capsule and the capsule becomes large and floppy. This also occurs in cases of zonular dehiscence and weakness wherein the PC is lax again.

In such cases various steps can be taken to prevent a PCT, such as:

- **Lowering the aspiration parameters.**
- **Increasing the bottle height.**
- **Using an AC maintainer (another port for fluid to go in).**
- **Removal of last piece under viscoelastic.**
- **Extreme cases – assistant can keep on injecting viscoelastic from the side port, to keep the PC away.**
- **Use of micro tip instead of kelman.**
- **Phacoaspiration to be done in Central Safe Zone.**

Partial occlusion of tip

Sometimes the aspiration tubing or the phaco tip may get blocked, particularly in hard cataracts, and on sudden release of this blockade there will be increased surge and increased chances of chamber collapse and PCT. In such cases when a tube blockade is expected (poor followability and poor hold on the nucleus) one should take out the probe from AC and flush it. The probe should be tested in a test chamber, before use.

5. During epinuclear plate removal

Many a time one is left with a posterior epinuclear plate with no anterior extension. In such cases turning the bevel of the phaco tip down to lift the EPN may lead to PCT. Any attempt to lift the posterior EPN with iris repositor may lead to PCT if the eye is not adequately visco-compressed.

While doing cortical aspiration with the bimanual I/A system, EPN gets automatically prolapsed and suck out along with the cortex.

6. During cortical aspiration

High incidence of PCT occurs during cortical aspiration, especially in the sub-incisional area. This is because of poor access and decreased visibility, problem being exaggerated by small capsulorhexis. A coaxial handpiece leads to further distortion of the wound, causing the PC to come anteriorly.

GOLDEN RULE

When the PC is caught in the suction port a star-shaped tented area appears. Immediately, **without moving the handpiece/cannula**, release the foot pedal to stop suction (Fig. 15.9).

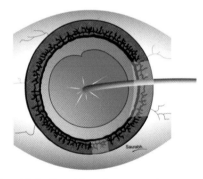

Fig. 15.9. Catching the posterior capsule.

In some cases, reflux may be required. Catching does not tear the posterior capsule but pulling does. Use of bimanual technique reduces the incidence of PCT.

PCT does not occur if the PC is only caught in the probe; sudden movement after holding with the probe/cannula is what causes it to tear.

7. During capsular polishing

During polishing, a well-focused PC in retro-illumination view under high magnification and a bag filled with VES is a must to prevent PCT (Fig. 15.10). The bag must always be concave and viscocompressed so as to provide

easy sliding of the instruments. If the bag is lax and some wrinkling appears on the capsule during the movement of rounded repositor/polisher, the chances of creating a PCT are high (Fig. 15.11).

Patients with thin PC (as discussed during hydro procedures) are particularly prone to PCT.

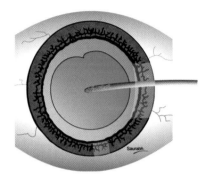

Fig. 15.10. Well filled bag – no striae.

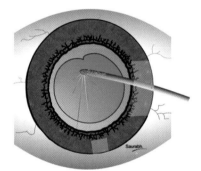

Fig. 15.11. Poor filled bag – capsular striae.

8. During IOL implantation

IOL implantation should be done under a well pressurized globe. The bag should be filled with viscoelastics. If the viscoelastic leaks or the capsule is not taut, then chances of capsule getting entangled in the leading loop are very high. While using an injector system, the leading loop has to be kept horizontal all the time, for that one has to observe the leading loop carefully and keep on rotating the nozzle of the cartridge as and when required.

In this era of micro-incision surgeries with reducing incision size, there may be leakage of viscoelastic from the wounds, particularly in wound-assisted insertion of the IOL. In such cases one can re-inject the viscoelastic or release the IOL in the sulcus rather than the bag. The IOL is positioned in the bag, after re-injection of viscoelastics.

All the companies provide same cartridge size for all IOL powers. High power IOLs are much thicker and excessive force is required to inject these IOLs. This at times causes sudden and jerky release inside the bag causing PCT.

DIAGNOSIS AND GOALS

GOLDEN RULE

Once PCT is noted, or one is in doubt about the status of the posterior capsule, be calm and maintain the phaco probe in the AC, keep the infusion on and inject visco-elastics from the side port. After ensuring that the AC is well pressurized, the phaco probe is withdrawn (Fig. 15.12).

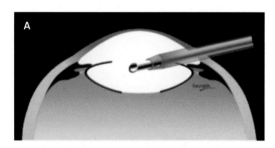
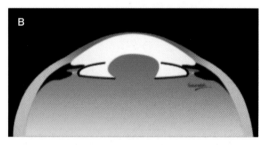
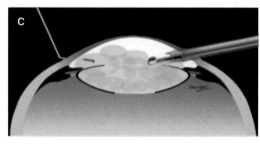
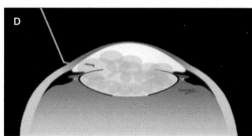

Fig. 15.12. A. Posterior capsular tear. **B.** Removal of probe – vitreous prolapse in AC. **C.** Pressurizing the AC from the side port. **D.** Removal of probe – no prolapse of vitreous into AC.

If one withdraws the phaco probe suddenly, then the anterior chamber collapses, causing the PCT to enlarge and the hyaloid face may get disrupted, leading to prolapse of the vitreous in the AC and prolapse of the nuclear fragments into the vitreous cavity.

Converting tear to PCC

Converting a PCT into a PCC is ideal, but most of the times impractical. Conversion to PCC is possible only if PCT is small and central and the hyaloid faces nearly intact. Also, if the hyaloid face is intact, risk of disrupting it while attempting PCC is very high.

One should attempt conversion to PCC only when one has small central/paracentral PCT (not more than 3 mm), good viscoelastics, excellent capsulorhexis forceps and a good operating microscope. However, the failure rate is still very high.

Diagnosis

Confirmation of PCT and hyaloid face rupture (HFR)

The next step is to confirm the presence and extent of PCT, and even more important is to ascertain whether hyaloid face is intact or not. Majority of the cases of PCT will have a disrupted hyaloid face, but an intact hyaloid face can be encountered if PCT occurs at the stage of capsular polishing, IOL insertion or cortical aspiration.

Signs of HFR

- Torn edge
  - Shiny/golden
  - Rolled up
- Anterior chamber
  - Irregular depth   Indicate disruption
- Nucleus   of hyaloid face
  - Restricted movements of the fragments

Tests

One can do the following tests:
- **Sponge test** (Fig. 15.13): One can sweep a sponge along the incision to detect the presence of vitreous.
- **Sweep test:** One may also try to sweep the spatula from the anterior chamber angle under the incision towards the PCT. Vitreous, if present, will be seen dragging in (due to tendency of the vitreous to come towards the wound).

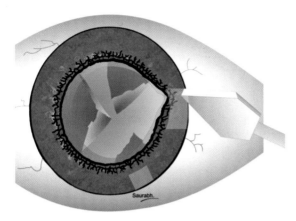

Fig. 15.13. Sponge test.

• **Halo test** (Fig. 15.14): Put viscoelastic in the bag, to flatten it or keep it slightly convex to elicit the halo test. Try to look for the ring reflex by applying the pressure in the centre of the capsule with the help of a rounded repositor. If the hyaloid face is intact, a halo will be seen which will vary in size depending upon the amount of pressure applied. This ring reflex will be broken at the site of PCT.

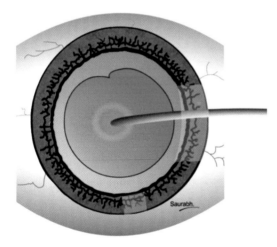

Fig. 15.14. Halo test.

• **Stain test:** One can also inject Triamcinolone into the anterior chamber just adjacent to the PCT (not above it as it will fall back into the vitreous cavity), to stain the vitreous. However, *when one is in doubt consider the hyaloid face as disrupted*.

Goals of management

The goal of every complication created during surgery is to minimize the short term and long term damage to the eye. For this purpose we can divide the goals of management into major goals and important goals.

Major goals

1. To avoid posterior dislocation of nucleus, nuclear fragments, epinucleus or cortical matter into the vitreous cavity.
2. Prevent any damage to the corneal endothelial surface.

Important goals

These goals are very important to achieve so that the end result of the surgery is as good as if nothing had happened. Surgery remains sutureless, astigmatically neutral with well-centred IOL and without any secondary complications.

1. Prevent enlargement of tear.
2. Prevent damage to capsulorhexis.
3. Minimize size of vitrectomy, avoiding traction.
4. Removal of left over cortex.
5. Maintain the wound size.
6. Proper positioning of the IOL.

Management by Anterior Segment Surgeon

GOLDEN RULE

DO NO HARM TO THE PATIENT

If the primary surgeon is ill-equipped or inadequately trained, secondary management by a senior or trained surgeon should be done. If nucleus is not retrievable from the anterior route, then leave it for the posterior segment surgeon to do the needful. Be truthful to yourself and the patient, inform the patient about the scenario. Your ego might get hurt, but you will have better peace of mind, with the shared responsibility.

Factors in decision making

Management will depend on various factors, such as:

• Extent of PCT
• Hyaloid face intact or not
• Location of the nucleus – whether dislodged into the vitreous cavity
• Availability of equipment – vitreous cutter, vitrectomy machine
• Availability of alternative IOLs
• Availability of specialized instruments

- Knowledge about anterior vitrectomy and confidence of the surgeon
- Availability of VR surgeon.

Above factors help in deciding the plan of management:

- Management by Anterior Segment Surgeon
  - Primary
  - Secondary
- Management by Posterior Segment Surgeon
  - Primary
  - Secondary

PRIMARY MANAGEMENT STRATEGIES

Primary management is the best approach, as it causes least stress to the patient and harm to the reputation of the surgeon. It causes a lesser amount of inflammation and provides an early rehabilitation as promised to the patient. We need to have strategies to manage:

1. Nucleus/nuclear fragments
2. Epinucleus
3. The cortex
4. IOL implantation
5. Final vitrectomy and closure

1. NUCLEUS / NUCLEAR FRAGMENTS

Managing of nucleus/nuclear fragments is the most important step in a case of PCT. The main goal is to prevent any dislocation of the nucleus/nuclear fragment into the vitreous cavity. There are two main steps but many techniques for the same.

1. **Supracapsular relocation**
   - Dislodging
   - Tumbling
   - Chopstick technique
2. **Extraction from eye**
   - Manual
     (i) Viscoexpression
     (ii) Chopstick technique
   - Automated
     (i) Vitrectomy cutter
     (ii) Phacoemulsification
       (a) Without scaffold

       (b) With scaffold
         1. HEMA Contact lens
         2. Lens glide
         3. IOL
   - Conversion to ECCE/SICS

1. Supracapsular relocation

In a viscopressurized eye, nuclear fragments are relocated anteriorly infront of the CCC and iris, preferably at the angle of the AC to prevent these from dropping into the vitreous cavity by any of the following techniques:

Dislodging

Small fragments of the nucleus are moved just sideways into the capsular fornices and then brought gently upwards towards the iris plane and then pushed towards the angle of AC.

Tumbling

This is a very good technique for small fragments. It can also be used for soft cataracts and epinuclear plate. In this technique the repositor pushes the nucleus to the periphery initially (Fig. 15.15), and then upwards, maintaining a constant counter-pressure from the anterior capsule, the nucleus can be easily brought out from anterior CCC (Fig. 15.16).

Even, if the pupil is small, which is obscuring the peripheral view, this technique comes in handy.

Chopstick technique
Chopstick technique in PCT

As the name suggests, two instruments are used in this technique, through which the nucleus/nuclear fragments can be held and repositioned to a desired site. The instruments that could be used are the Sinskey hook, chopper, rounded repositor or dumbbell dialer. Sinskey hook is particularly good as it gets buried into the nucleus and provides a good grip. Both the instruments can be introduced from the main port or one from the main port and another from side port. One is put below and the other above, or alternatively one on each side of the fragment, so that the fragment is sandwiched. The fragment is gripped firmly between the two instruments and is now moved into the supracapsular area away from the site of tear (Fig. 15.17).

Chopstick technique in impending nuclear drop

In case the nucleus is hanging down in the anterior vitreous cavity, never try to fish it out through the anterior

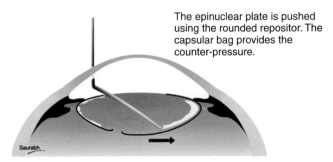

Fig. 15.15. Rounded repositor pushes the nucleus to the periphery initially.

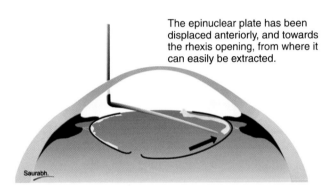

Fig. 15.16. Upward pressure is maintained and a constant counter pressure from the anterior capsule facilitates easy removal of the nucleus from the anterior CCC.

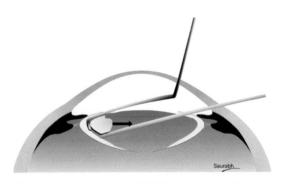

Fig. 15.17. In case of a PCT if a nuclear fragment is remaining in the bag then two instruments can be used to grip the fragment. It is now moved into the supracapsular area away from the site of tear.

route. Such an impending nucleus drop is best managed by either the 'Chopstick technique' as described by Dr. Harbansh Lal or the "Posterior assisted levitation" as described by Dr. Kelman. In both these techniques, one port is made through the pars plana by giving a stab incision with 15 degree blade or V-lance knife, 3.5 mm away from the limbus.

Through the pars plana incision, in PAL technique Viscoat is injected behind the nucleus and the thin cannula

of Viscoat or iris repositor is used to push the nucleus forward. In chopstick technique an instrument (Sinskey hook) is passed through the pars plana incision and buried into the undersurface of the nucleus, which helps to support the nucleus and prevents it from sinking into the vitreous. The nucleus is sandwiched and stabilized with the second instrument from above which may pass through the side port or the main port. The nucleus is then brought into the supracapsular area after having been stabilized (Fig. 15.18).

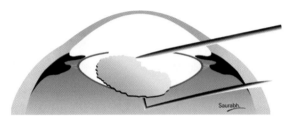

Fig. 15.18. In case of an impending nuclear drop an instrument (Sinskey hook) is passed through the pars plana incision and buried into the undersurface of the nucleus, which helps to support the nucleus and prevents it from sinking into the vitreous. The nucleus is sandwiched and stabilized with the second instrument from above which may pass through the side port or the main port. The nucleus is then brought into the supracapsular area after having been stabilized.

Chopstick technique without PCT

Chopstick technique is not only helpful in case of PCT, but also in any case where we want to reposition the nuclear fragment to prevent the PCT. In case of a miosed pupil, the visibility of the surgeon particularly in the area of capsular fornices is hampered. If a small nuclear fragment has gone in the capsular fornices or between the iris and the anterior capsule or as in a case of resistant sub-incisional nuclear fragment, which fails to rotate, the surgeon can use two instruments to hold and reposition the nuclear piece in the central safe zone (Figs. 15.19 and 15.20). In case of failure of the phacomachine, this method can be used to bring the nucleus/nuclear fragments not only into the anterior chamber but also for removal from the eye.

2. Removal from eye

Manual

(i) Viscoexpression

Soft nuclear fragments are crushed between two instruments, such as chopper, Sinskey hook or a repositor. Thick cannula of viscoelastic is passed underneath and

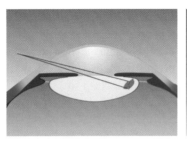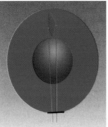

Figs. 15.19 & 15.20. If a small nuclear fragment has gone in the capsular fornices or between the iris and the anterior capsule, two instruments can be used to hold and reposition the nuclear piece in the central safe zone.

well beyond the nuclear fragments (Fig. 15.21). Now viscoelastic is injected with simultaneously minimal pressure at the posterior lip of the wound with the cannula, causing the viscoelastic to flow out along with the nuclear material (Fig. 15.22). Care is taken to maintain AC depth at all times.

(ii) Chopstick technique

As already discussed in the relocation of nucleus, the chopstick technique can also be used for removal of the fragments from the eye. The incision size will depend upon the size of the nucleus. If half of the nucleus is remaining then 5 mm incision is adequate, and if less than that a 4 mm incision would be sufficient.

Long axis of the nuclear fragment is positioned perpendicular to the long axis of the wound. The eye is now viscopressurized, and any two instruments, as discussed earlier, are inserted through the main port. These instruments are buried one on each side of the long axis of the fragment. Now both instruments along with the nuclear fragment are pulled out through the wound.

Advantages of the chopstick technique:

- Non-bulky instruments.
- Small incisions are needed.
- Any number of side ports can be made.
- Better than other techniques, such as wire vectis which relies on counter pressure, leading to damage to the cornea.
- Least traction on the vitreous, as instruments are even thinner than vitreous cutter.
- AC is maintained at all times.
- Better than PAL as counter pressure provides more controlled elevation of the nucleus with no risk of viscoelastic going into the vitreous cavity. No risk of increased IOP.

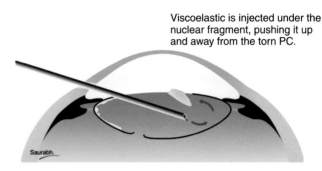

Viscoelastic is injected under the nuclear fragment, pushing it up and away from the torn PC.

Fig. 15.21. Thick cannula of viscoelastic is passed underneath the nuclear fragments.

Depress the posterior lip of the main wound while slowly injecting the viscoelastic. This creates a directional flow that forces the nuclear fragment out of the main incision.

Fig. 15.22. Viscoelastic is injected with simultaneously minimal pressure at the posterior lip of the wound with the cannula, causing the viscoelastic to flow out along with the nuclear material.

Disadvantage:

- Not suitable for soft cataracts or epinuclear plate as it will cheese wire through.

If the posterior capsular tear occurs early in the surgery with almost the entire nucleus remaining in the bag, it is of utmost importance to secure the nucleus by bringing it out of the bag and positioning it above the anterior rhexis margin. If CCC is small, release it by giving appropriate number of small relaxing cuts in the CCC margin, according to the size of the nucleus.

Automated

(i) Vitrectomy cutter

Using automated vitreous cutter is a very good option for soft cataracts and epinuclear plate. For using the cutter an infusion cannula is needed, which can be placed through the corneal side port, through the pars plicata (i.e. 1.5 mm from the limbus) or via the pars plana route (i.e. 3.5 mm from the limbus). Self-retaining infusion cannula from the pars plana route would be ideal as it causes the least disturbance of vitreous, with lesser chances of enlargement of the PCT and diminishes the chances of epinuclear plate or the nucleus fragment falling into the vitreous cavity.

A 20 G cutter system would be ideal, because of its larger port size, but 23 G system is equally effective if the cataract is soft and there are minimal nuclear fragments. Limbal, pars plicata or pars plana routes can be used for the cutter (Fig. 15.23). If most of the nuclear fragment has been relocated to the supracapsular area, then the limbal route is preferred. If the nuclear material is still in the capsular fornices, either a pars plicata or pars plana route would be preferable.

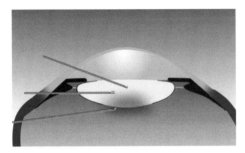

Fig. 15.23. Automated vitreous cutter can be placed through the corneal side port through the pars plicata (i.e. 1.5 mm from the limbus) or via the pars plana route (i.e. 3.5 mm from the limbus). Self-retaining infusion cannula from the pars plana route would be ideal as it causes the least disturbance of vitreous, with lesser chances of enlargement of the PCT and diminishes the chances of epinuclear plate or the nucleus fragment falling into the vitreous cavity.

For pars plicata vitrectomy, stab incisions are given at about 1.5 mm from the limbus, through which the cutter enters the AC, behind the iris. The advantage being that there is no disturbance to the vitreous base, whereas the disadvantage would be a risk of bleeding and inadvertent damage to the iris.

Cut rate for nuclear removal should ideally be in the medium range, at a very high cut rate the suction port of the cutter gets occluded leading to a loss of vacuum and grip on the nucleus. The rate of 800/cuts per minute should be ideal for the nucleus. A vacuum of 300–400 is preferred for the nucleus removal AC depth should be maintained at all times with no fluctuation.

For vitrectomy, the cut rate is kept at maximum and an aspiration rate of 150–200 is preferred so as to avoid any traction on the vitreous.

(ii) Phacoemulsification

(a) **Without scaffold:** This is a safe technique if PCT is small and vitreous face has not been disturbed. If the capsular support is good and there is no vitreous in the anterior chamber, the most important step is to secure the nucleus by bringing it away from the site of PC defect.

Viscoat is placed below the nuclear fragment and infusion bottle is kept at approx. 3 feet. All other fluidic parameters are lowered. The tip is then placed close to the nuclear fragment so as to achieve a full occlusion of the aspiration port and minimal phaco energy is used to emulsify the nucleus. This will reduce the risk of further damage to the capsule and aspiration of vitreous.

The main aim in such a case is to avoid any fluctuation in the anterior chamber, either by lowering the parameters or by the use of viscoelastics.

If vitreous face has been disrupted a limited anterior vitrectomy is done before coating and pushing back the hyaloid face with chondroitin sulphate (Viscoat). Viscoat being a viscodispersive material stays longest in the eye, the next best choice would be methyl cellulose. Hyaluronic acid is not preferable as it disappears at the earliest during phacoemulsification.

(b) **Use of scaffold:** Use of scaffold is generally advocated when there has been a disturbance to the hyaloid face. Various scaffolding techniques have been described. These are:

1. **HEMA boat** as described by Dr. Keiki Mehta, which utilizes a HEMA contact lens as a scaffold. Ideally any soft contact lens can be punched with the help of a corneal trephine of 8–9 mm in size.

   The C.L. is rolled and injected by the IOL injector beneath the fragment after the fragment has been relocated to the supracapsular area. Before injecting the C.L. limited anterior vitrectomy should be done. After the C.L. has been injected it should be made sure that there is no vitreous above the C.L., before starting phacoemulsification. If need be vitrectomy can be repeated after staining the vitreous with diluted tricort (1 : 2, 1 : 4).

2. **Lens glide:** Lens glide is a thin long plate which is passed underneath the nuclear fragment, supporting the leading end at the iris angle and second end is kept outside the wound. After proper vitrectomy, phacoemulsification is performed on top of the glide.

3. **IOL scaffolding:** IOL scaffold is one of the very good techniques for removal of nucleus, nuclear fragment and epinuclear plate, which has been popularized by Dr. Amar Agarwal.

This procedure is intended for use in cases where PCT occurs with a non-emulsified, moderately hard to soft nucleus. After anterior vitrectomy the nucleus/nuclear fragments have to be prolapsed into the AC by the techniques described earlier.

Combining the 'Chopstick technique' and the IOL scaffolding would be the ideal method of managing cases of PCT with soft to moderate cataracts. The chopstick technique would be used to reposition all of the nuclear fragments above the rhexis margin, followed by insertion of a three-piece foldable IOL, which would act as a scaffold.

TECHNIQUE

(a) Thorough anterior vitrectomy.
(b) Prolapsing nucleus, Nuclear fragment or Epinucleus plate in the AC.
(c) IOL positioning: 3-piece foldable IOL is injected into the AC above the iris plane, keeping the trailing loop out of the wound to prevent IOL drop, and allow for easy manoeuvering of IOL afterwards (Fig. 15.24). Use of the second hand sometimes becomes necessary to stabilize the IOL and keep it in the centre, by holding it at the optic-haptic junction.

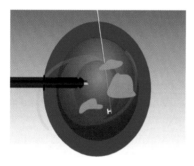

Fig. 15.24. One haptic is kept out, and another instrument supports the IOL.

Alternatively – We can place both the loops above the iris (Fig. 15.25), or else the IOL can be directly placed in the sulcus (Fig. 15.26).

(d) Check for vitreous again and make sure there is no vitreous in AC.
(e) Phacoemulsification: Phaco energy is used to emulsify the nucleus/nuclear fragments.

Advantages of the IOL scaffold technique are as follows:

1. The three-piece foldable IOL as a **scaffold or barrier to compartmentalize the anterior and posterior chamber**, thereby preventing

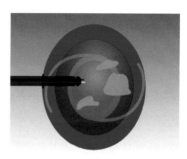

Fig. 15.25. Both the loops are placed above the iris.

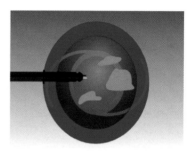

Fig. 15.26. IOL is placed in the sulcus after repositioning the remaining nuclear fragments in the supracapsular area. Phacoemulsification can be done after confirming the absence of vitreous.

(a) vitreous prolapse,
(b) vitreous hydration, and
(c) nucleus drop.

2. IOL is **inserted through the existing corneal incision**.
   (a) Hence maintenance of anterior chamber stability and IOP.
   (b) Preserving the astigmatic benefits of sutureless, small incision surgery.

3. Same IOL can be used for sulcus or bag fixation, or in cases with absence of adequate capsular support can be used for glued IOL, which will be discussed later.

In cases of hard cataract, the damage to the cornea during phacoemulsification can be there; hence this technique is not advised in such cases.

Conversion to ECCE/SICS

The supracapsular phacoemulsification of nearly complete and comparatively hard nucleus may damage the corneal endothelium permanently. In such case it is better to convert to SICS/ECCE. Viscopress the eye, give peribulbar or subtenons block, do gentle compression decompression of the orbit by fingers between the globe and inferior orbital margin without applying much force on the globe.

If the **initial incision was temporal**, leave it undisturbed and move superiorly to create a pocket for SICS or a limbal incision for ECCE, according to the size of the nucleus. If the **initial incision was superior**, enlarge the pocket for SICS, whereas for ECCE the scleral pocket is released and incision is enlarged at the limbus. Now the wound configuration will be like the incision which we make for combined ECCE and Trabeculectomy.

Nucleus delivery
- SICS – Bluementhal technique, irrigating wire vectis or surgeon's preferred technique
- ECCE – Chopstick technique

2. EPINUCLEUS

A remaining epinuclear plate in cases of PCT has to be managed very carefully, and should never be taken lightly, as an epinuclear plate falling into the vitreous cavity is much more common than a nucleus falling into the vitreous cavity. Even a small epinuclear plate can lead to intense inflammation, as it takes longer time to absorb, and can lead to various complications such as CME, increased IOP, iris neovascularization, neovascular glaucoma.

Before any manoeuvre, at this stage a proper assessment should be made about the presence or absence of vitreous. It is important to clear the chamber of any vitreous by doing a *good vitrectomy* **with an automatic cutter**. After clearing most of the vitreous, fill the capsular bag with viscoelastics to open the capsular fornix. The epinuclear plate is tough to remove because it is difficult to hold it with anything.

Relocation of epinuclear plate
1. Use of rounded repositor
2. Use of suction

Use of rounded repositor
The EPN is mobilized using a rounded repositor, taking counter pressure from the capsular fornices or anterior capsule. Rotating the epinucleus helps to dislodge it from the fornix and prolapse into the anterior chamber (Figs. 15.15 and 15.16).

Use of suction
With the help of I/A cannula, under low bottle height

and low aspiration parameters, the cortical fibres can be held at various places and can be pulled gently to the centre. This leads to the dislodgement of the epinuclear plate, which lies in front of the cortical fibres.

Extraction from eye
1. IOL scaffold technique
2. Viscoexpression
3. Automated vitreous cutter

1. IOL scaffold technique
This technique has already been described in the text.

2. Viscoexpression
Once the EPN has been prolapsed, the technique is same as described for soft cataracts.

3. Automated vitreous cutter
Anterior relocation of the EPN particularly of the sub-incisional area is difficult. While doing removal by vitrectomy cutter, if the fluid is coming from the top, i.e. from the limbus, it may push the EPN into the vitreous cavity. In case of failed relocation of EPN, infusion from the pars plana is recommended, as it will push the EPN forward. Rest of the technique is same as for soft nucleus.

3. CORTEX

Cortex removal can be broadly divided into the following categories:
- Manual
  - Dry – Suck and spit
  - Semi-dry – Simcoe cannula
- Automated
  - Vitrectomy cutter

Dry – Suck and spit
Mechanical suck and spit is a better controlled system than irrigation and aspiration. In a viscopressed chamber, with a 27 gauge cannula mounted on a viscoelastic syringe go underneath the capsulorhexis margin, hold the cortical fibres and do not try to aspirate there, instead hold and pull them out of the incision and then spit (Fig. 15.27). Take the cannula back, and repeat the same process. Sometimes the spitting can be done in the AC and can be removed later. While sucking if the vitreous is caught, spit the cortical matter within the eye, which can be washed afterwards. Sometimes, cortical matter may be removed after insertion of IOL.

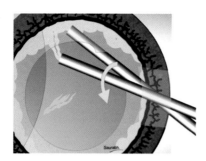

Fig. 15.27. Cortex removal: dry – suck and spit.

Semi-dry – Simcoe cannula (Fig. 15.28)

The chamber is formed with VES and aspiration is done using Simcoe cannula. Always aspirate at the site where there is no vitreous. If need be, another side port may be constructed. A little infusion is required to release the cortical matter. For this purpose, enter with irrigation tube of Simcoe cannula pinched between thumb and forefinger and as and when required, allow the irrigating fluid through. Continuous irrigation should be avoided.

Cortex should be removed by dry aspiration after ensuring that no vitreous is in the chamber.

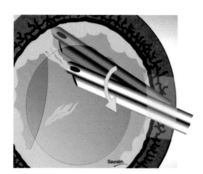

Fig. 15.28. Cortex removal – Simcoe cannula.

Automated – Vitrectomy cutter

Best method for handling the cortex in presence of PCT is with a bimanual vitrectomy cutter. The best part of the system is that, on pressing the foot pedal you can change the system into vitrectomy mode or bimanual irrigation and aspiration system. Once inside do vitrectomy and switch to I/A system for cortical aspiration. During this if at any time one feels the vitreous is being held, the surgeon can shift back to vitrectomy mode to cut the vitreous. This causes least traction and best possible cleanup of the cortical fibres.

4. IOL IMPLANTATION

1. No IOL
2. IOL in bag

3. IOL in sulcus
4. Anterior chamber IOL
5. Scleral fixated IOL
6. Iris fixated IOL
7. Glued IOL

1. No IOL

Indications

- Lenticular matter is not cleared adequately.
- Not sure about the capsular support.
- Status of vitreous in AC can't be assessed.
- Nonavailability of instruments or IOLs.

After 2–3 days the cortex becomes fluffy, and vitreous gets organized. So, at this point of time, secondary anterior vitrectomy and removal of lenticulate material becomes easier. In majority of the cases secondary PCIOL insertion is possible as fibrosed capsule is taut and able to support the IOL well, particularly if surgery is delayed for 2–3 weeks or more.

2. IOL in the bag

Indications

- If *hyaloid face is intact*, in the bag fixation of IOL is ideal.
- In case of a *small capsular tear with a good capsular support* where the *hyaloid face has been disturbed* – adequate anterior vitrectomy may make in the bag fixation possible.

Many a time it is difficult to ascertain whether all the vitreous has been cleared or not. In such a situation there are certain techniques which have to be followed for IOL implantation.

- **Inflate the bag with viscoelastics:** Viscoelastics serve as essential adjuncts in such cases. Viscoelastic of choice for this step would be hyaluronic acid (Healon GV). Firstly, they help in maintaining the AC and prevent further prolapse of vitreous. Secondly, they push the already prolapsed vitreous back into the cavity. Finally, due to the inflated capsular fornices it is easier to place the IOL in the bag.
- **Do not dial the IOL:** Dialing the IOL may entangle the vitreous, which may cause traction on the retina and can even enlarge the tear. We will be describing techniques of haptic placement into the bag without dialing the IOL, for PMMA as well as foldable IOL.

A. PMMA IOL

We will be describing 2 techniques here, depending upon the remaining area of capsular support.

1. Pronate and Release
2. Hook and Release

1. Pronate and Release

In cases where there is adequate capsular support in the **cross-incisional area**, place the leading haptic in the bag. Hold the tip of the trailing haptic with a Mcpherson forceps. The IOL is pushed down till the loop of the trailing haptic is well beyond the CCC margin. Pronate your hand so that the tip is lifted up and the loop of the haptic dips down. This brings the loop of the haptic underneath the CCC and then the haptic is released.

2. Hook and Release

The IOL is placed over the anterior capsule or iris and positioned in such a way that the haptics come to rest at the site of maximum posterior capsular support (Fig. 15.29). Once the IOL has been positioned, the haptics are guided one by one underneath the CCC. Dumbbell-dialer, Sinskey hook or chopper can be used for this purpose.

In this technique, the dumbbell-dialer is used to hold the haptic close to its apex and is pulled beyond the CCC margin. Now, the dumbbell-dialer along with the haptic is taken underneath the CCC margin. The dialer is disengaged by sliding it sideward (Fig. 15.30), thus positioning the haptic in the bag (Fig. 15.31).

If the visibility is poor, or the rhexis margin is too large or small, another instrument, preferably a Rounded Repositor (RR) can be used to guide the haptic underneath the CCC. In this technique the haptic is hooked with the dumbbell-dialer as described previously, the second instrument lifts the CCC, ensuring that the haptic is released into the bag.

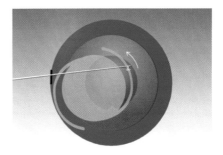

Fig. 15.30. The dumbbell-dialer is used to hold the haptic close to its apex and is pulled beyond the CCC margin. Now, the dumbbell-dialer along with the haptic is taken underneath the CCC margin. The dialer is disengaged by sliding it sideward, thus positioning the haptic in the capsular bag.

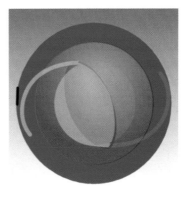

Fig. 15.31. One haptic is inside the capsular bag and other is still outside the bag.

Same procedure is repeated for the second haptic (Fig. 15.32). It is ideal to have the entry point of the dialer diagonally opposite to the position of the haptic. Now, if the surgeon feels that he can't access the second haptic from the existing incisions, he can create a new side port incision for this purpose.

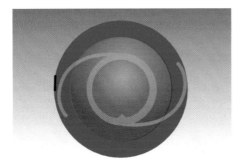

Fig. 15.29. The IOL is placed over the anterior capsule or iris.

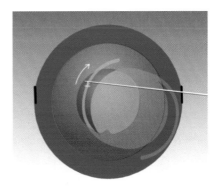

Fig. 15.32. Same procedure is repeated for the second haptic to place it inside the capsular bag.

GOLDEN RULE

If there is doubt about the stability and centration of the IOL, a 10-0 silk suture can be tied to the trailing haptic for retrieval if needed, which can be cut if IOL is well positioned.

B. Foldable IOL

Three-piece hydrophobic acrylic IOLs are ideal, to be used for bag fixation in cases of a PCT. However, if the hyaloid face is intact any IOL can be used. Holder-folder technique is safer as compared to the injector system, as it ensures a more controlled opening of the IOL.

Fill the anterior chamber and the bag with cohesive viscoelastic (Healon GV), which maintains the AC depth and prevents a jerky opening of the IOL. Using the insertion forceps the IOL is released inside the AC on top of anterior capsule or iris.

In case using the injector system, make sure that the leading loop remains horizontal inside the eye. This can be achieved by constantly positioning the cartridge by rotation of the injector system. Release the IOL on top of the anterior capsule.

Now, the haptics are positioned into the bag, as described for the PMMA IOLs.

Another technique which should be mentioned here is the technique of optic capture.

OPTIC CAPTURE

The chances of decentration of IOL are high in cases of PCT because of uneven contraction of the capsule. Incomplete anterior vitrectomy increases the incidence of decentration drastically.

To prevent decentration of IOL, optic capture can be done, wherein if the haptics are in the bag, optic is outside the bag (Figs. 15.33 and 15.34) i.e., anterior to CCC and

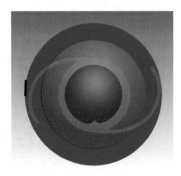

Fig. 15.33. IOL in the bag.

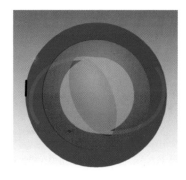

Fig. 15.34. Optics is prolapsed out of CCC into the AC while haptics remain in bag.

if the haptics are in the sulcus then the optics is posterior to the CCC, i.e., in the bag (Figs. 15.35 and 15.36).

This enables centration and stability of the IOL. There are certain pre-requisites for doing an optic capture; the anterior CCC should be uniform, central and 4–5.5 mm in size.

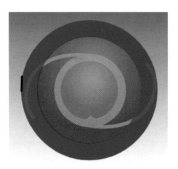

Fig. 15.35. IOL placed in the sulcus.

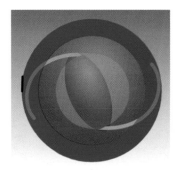

Fig. 15.36. Optic is pushed in the bag and haptic remains in the sulcus.

3. Sulcus fixated IOL

In case of a large PCT with or without a damaged CCC it is better to place the IOL in the sulcus.

• **CCC is not intact:** Best is to choose a large optic PMMA IOL (6.5 mm with an overall diameter of 13 mm).

• **CCC is intact:** If the anterior rhexis is intact and a large posterior capsular tear lies underneath, foldable IOL can be placed in the sulcus with or without a reverse optic capture. After releasing the IOL in the sulcus the optic is gently pressed underneath the anterior rhexis margin (Figs. 15.35 and 15.36).

Single-piece foldable IOLs should be avoided when sulcus fixation is planned, as rubbing of the large area of the haptic will lead to increased inflammation and iris chaffing.

4. Anterior chamber IOL (ACIOL)

In case of excessive damage to capsule and zonules, the stability of in the bag or sulcus fixated IOL becomes doubtful. In such cases ACIOL implantation is the easiest and most often performed procedure. Though ACIOL appears to be an inferior technique, in comparison to iris fixated, scleral fixated or glued IOLs, there is no conclusive evidence for the same.

Do not place PCIOL in the AC. PCIOL in the AC can cause fibrosis of the angle structures leading to glaucoma. The angulation of the PCIOL is unsuitable for the angle. The forward angulation leads to corneal problems and if placed the other way, the backward angulation may lead to pupillary block. ACIOL may cause ciliary tenderness, inflammation, glaucoma, CME and corneal complications such as decompensation; hence regular follow-up is a must.

TECHNIQUE

1. Choose the correct powered ACIOL, which is less than that of PCIOL by 4–5 D, depending upon the A constant.
2. Anterior vitrectomy: Constrict the pupil using 0.5% pilocarpine, inject diluted triamcinolone acetonide (tricort; 1 : 4 dilution) into the AC, so as to stain the vitreous. Anterior vitrectomy is performed to take care of any remaining vitreous.
3. Enlarging the incision: Inflate the AC with viscoelastics and enlarge the incision to 5.5 mm, or to the width of the IOL.
4. Inserting the IOL: The IOL is held with a McPherson forceps, and the leading loop is advanced in the AC. While advancing the leading loop of the ACIOL towards the opposite angle, make sure it does not touch the iris (Fig. 15.37). **In fact the IOL should be kept closer to the cornea, till the loop is about to reach the angle** (Fig. 15.38). This will prevent any distortion or ovalization of the pupil post-operatively.

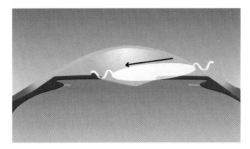

Fig. 15.37. Wrong placement of an ACIOL – If an ACIOL is inserted with a downward direction, its haptic will get stuck in the iris which can lead to an irregular pupil.

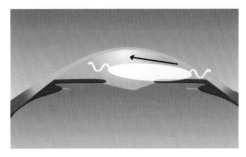

Fig. 15.38. Correct placement of an ACIOL – An ACIOL should be inserted with an upward direction, so that the haptic does not interfere with the iris, and on reaching just before the angle the direction of the IOL is changed.

The convexity of the IOL should always be away from the pupil, to avoid pupillary block. Now the trailing IOL is pushed below the incision.

5. Iridectomy: One or two iridectomies, at the site where there is no vitreous, should be done, preferably with the help of vitreous cutter. This prevents the chances of pupillary block glaucoma.
6. Wound closure: Suturing of the wound is essential, as a shallow AC in presence of an ACIOL can lead to damage to the cornea. When using ACIOLs certain points have to be taken care of:
    (i)   "A constant" of the IOL – lesser power required as compared to a PCIOL
    (ii) Proper positioning of ACIOL – maintaining forward convexity of the IOL
    (iii) Need for peripheral iridectomy – should be at a site where there is no vitreous

We usually prefer to wait and insert a secondary PCIOL later, as compared to ACIOL.

5. Scleral fixated IOL (SFIOL) (Figs. 15.39–15.45)

Scleral fixation of IOL is a good option if there is inadequate capsular support for bag or sulcus fixation of

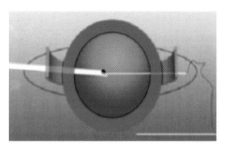

Fig. 15.39. 2 points are marked 180º apart, fornix based conjunctival flaps are raised and light cautery is applied. Limbus based partial thickness scleral flaps are raised, 2.5 ´ 3 mm and 500 µ in depth. At 1.5 mm from the limbus, through the scleral bed a 26 G needle is passed from one side and a straight 9-0 needle from the other side, which is loaded into the barrel of the 26 G needle in the centre of the eye.

IOL. Usually specialized IOLs are available for scleral fixation, which have extra eyelets. We need SFIOL and double armed straight needle prolene sutures (9-0/ 10-0).

If SFIOL is not available, foldable or non-foldable IOL can be used for scleral fixation.

TECHNIQUE
1. 2 points are marked 180º apart, either by RK marker or toric marker (Fig. 15.39).
2. Fornix based conjunctival flaps are raised and light cautery is applied (Fig. 15.39).
3. Creation of scleral flaps (Fig. 15.39): Two partial thickness quadrangular scleral flaps are created 180º apart at limbus, 3 × 2.5 mm in dimension, as for trabeculectomy.

ALTERNATIVES TO SCLERAL FLAP CREATION

Scleral pockets may be created which may be limbus- or fornix-based.

Alternative 1 – Limbus-based scleral pocket: Instead of making flaps we can make scleral pockets (limbal based pocket), of the same size as we make for phacoemulsification. The advantage of this technique is that scleral flap closure is not required at the end of surgery.

Alternative 2 – Fornix-based scleral pocket:
• Straight 3 mm incisions are given 180º apart at the limbus without removing the conjunctiva.
• 2.5 mm deep pocket is made towards the sclera, making fornix based scleral pocket.

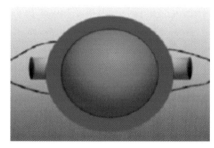

Fig. 15.39A. Limbus based scleral pocket.

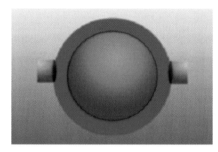

Fig. 15.39B. Fornix based scleral pocket.

• As the direction of the pocket is opposite to the direction of the needle, it is not possible to insert the needle directly at the base underneath the flap. The needle perforates the conjunctivoscleral upper flap and scleral base to enter the eye.
• The threads are passed and tied into the IOL. Then these threads are pulled out from the scleral pocket by Sinskey hook for tying and burying the knot in the pocket.

This is a little more complicated, with more chances of bleeding, but still a great technique to master as it is faster and requires no cautery and suturing of conjunctiva or scleral flap.
4. Rail road technique (Fig. 15.39):
• 26 G needle is mounted on the back of a repositor or a chopper.
• The needle is bent at an angle of 45–60° from its hub.
• At the junction of the lower 1/3rd and upper 2/3rd of the scleral bed, about 1.5 mm away from limbus, the needle is passed.
• First we go perpendicular to the globe and then turn the needle in such a way that it comes to lie parallel and just behind the iris. If it tucks the iris, or comes anterior to the iris, the needle can be withdrawn and passed again slightly posterior to the original site.

- Straight needle of prolene suture is passed through the opposite scleral pocket at the same location.
- In the centre of the eye, the straight needle is threaded into the barrel of 26 G needle, and both are withdrawn from the side of 26 G needle.
- Now, similar procedure is repeated, at the junction of upper 1/3rd and lower 2/3rd of the scleral bed (Fig. 15.40).
- Hence now we have 2 prolene threads in the eye (Fig. 15.40).

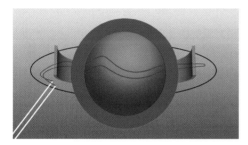

Fig. 15.40. The prolene needle is brought out along with the 26 G needle. Similarly the second arm of the needle is also brought out through the opposite scleral bed. Hence, we have now two threads in the eye.

5. Placing sutures on the IOL:
   - The 2 prolene threads are brought out through the corneal/limbal incision, which is created for the insertion of IOL, and are cut in the centre (Fig. 15.41).

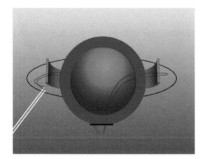

Fig. 15.41. The two threads are brought out through the main wound and cut in between.

- Now, we have two threads on each side of the incision, which have to be tied to respective haptics.
- For tying, one thread is passed 2–3 times in the eyelet and the other thread is passed from the opposite direction before tying (Fig. 15.42).

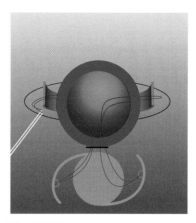

Fig. 15.42. The SFIOL is positioned and the cut ends of threads are tied at the eyelets of the SFIOL on both sides.

- After securing both the haptics, the leading haptic i.e., the haptic fixed on the right side suture is gently introduced inside the AC, maintaining a slight pull on the prolene sutures. A gentle pull is maintained by the assistant on this while inserting the leading haptic as well (Fig. 15.43).

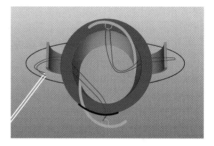

Fig. 15.43. The SFIOL is introduced in the AC.

6. Securing the sutures: Once the IOL is inserted, slight traction is given to the prolene sutures, which are secured onto the sclera after proper centration of the IOL (Fig. 15.44).
7. Suturing the flaps: The partial thickness scleral flaps and the conjunctiva are sutured back to the scleral bed with 10-silk suture (Fig. 15.45).

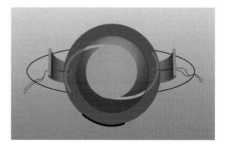

Fig. 15.44. The SFIOL is positioned with slight traction on the threads.

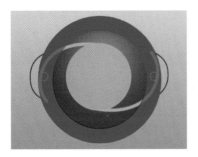

Fig. 15.45. The sutures are tied to the scleral bed. The scleral flaps are sutured, one by one on both the sides. Conjunctiva above is sutured.

8. Main incision is closed. Pupil is constricted and diluted tricort is injected in the AC to look for any vitreous. Anterior vitrectomy has to be done if vitreous is present.

9. Corneal wounds are hydrated if foldable IOL is used, or sutured if non-foldable IOL is used.

If especially designed SFIOLs are not available, same procedure can be done with single or 3-piece PMMA IOLs. It is advisable to use ECCE IOL, as compared to the phacoemulsification profile IOL, due to its bigger optics and overall size, though it's not a must.

In case using a foldable IOL, it's possible to do the same procedure with a 3-piece foldable IOLs. The only modification being that, one set of sutures have to be passed through the barrel of the cartridge before securing it on the leading haptic of the IOL. Once the leading haptic is secured, the IOL is injected inside the eye. Trailing haptic is left outside and second set of prolene threads are tied. Now, the trailing haptic is dialed inside the AC. Alternatively the holder folder method of IOL insertion can be used.

6. Iris fixated IOL

Iris fixation of PCIOL

Technique 1 (Figs. 15.46–15.52)

1. Two side port clear corneal incisions, nearly 3'o clock away from the site of the haptic fixation on either side, directing towards each other are made.

2. After releasing the IOL in the AC, both the haptics are placed behind the iris and the optic is kept above the iris.

3. Now pilocarpine is injected into the AC to constrict the pupil.

4. The IOL is lifted up with the forceps (lens holding forceps), to identify the position of the haptics.

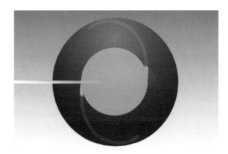

Fig. 15.46. The IOL is positioned such as the optic is above the iris plane and the haptics are behind the iris. Lens holding forceps or a rounded repositor is used to elevate the optic so that the haptics can be appreciated better behind the iris.

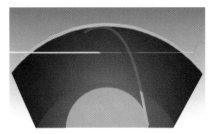

Fig. 15.47. Railroad technique – 9-0 straight needle is passed from the corneal incision going beneath the iris and haptic elevation and re-emerging from the iris soon after. 26 G needle is inserted from the opposite site, and the prolene needle is loaded into its barrel and is brought out of the eye.

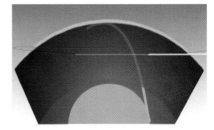

Fig. 15.48. Now the prolene needle is reinserted through the same wound from which it was externalized. 26 G needle is now inserted from the opposite site and again the prolene is loaded into its barrel. This complex is above the iris haptic elevation.

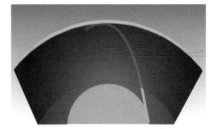

Fig. 15.49. Both threads are externalized from the same wound.

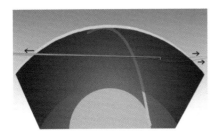

Fig. 15.50. A knot is given and an instrument is introduced from the opposite side, so as to slide the knot to the appropriate position.

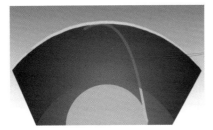

Fig. 15.51. The knot is finalized and the threads cut. Similar procedure is repeated on the opposite haptic.

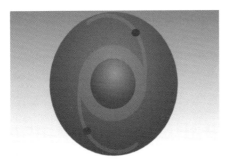

Fig. 15.52. Final position.

5. Now prolene 10-0 is passed through the clear corneal incision behind the iris and haptics and then taken out in front of the iris from the other side. 26 G needle is introduced and by rail road technique needle of prolene thread is brought out.

6. Now hands are changed and 26 G needle comes from the opposite CCI and prolene needle is brought out from the other side by rail road technique passing in front of the iris. Thus we have both the threads on one side of the wound one behind and one on top of the iris and lens haptics.

7. Now tie the triple knot outside the wound. Push the tied knot into the AC. Sinskey hook or double dialer is introduced from the opposite incision to pull the knot on the iris while maintaining gentle traction in the opposite direction on both the threads outside the eye.

8. Second and third knots are given the same way to firmly anchor the haptic behind the iris.

9. Suture is cut by Vannas just above the iris.

10. Same technique is repeated on the other side.

Technique 2 (Figs. 15.53–15.57)

In this technique only one side port incision is required but it needs 9-0 or 10-0 curved prolene needle. If curved needle is not available surgeon can make straight needle curved by himself. In this technique instead of using rail road technoique surgeon takes out the needle by perforating the cornea from the other side. If the needle is not sharp it becomes difficult. Then threads are brought out as demonstrated in the picture and tied.

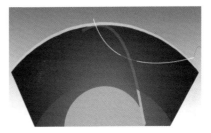

Fig. 15.53. Alternative. A curved 9-0 needle is passed from the corneal incision and behind the iris haptic elevation, and re-emerges soon after. The curved 9-0 needle now re-emerges from the cornea at a different site.

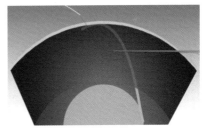

Fig. 15.54. An instrument is used to hook the thread (Siepser's technique).

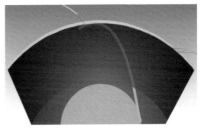

Fig. 15.55. Now the thread is brought out from the initial wound.

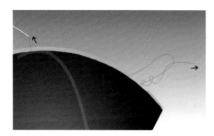

Fig. 15.56. The threads are externalized and a double knot as shown is placed.

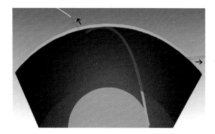

Fig. 15.57. The threads are pulled so as to position the knot. A similar knot is placed again by repeating the above steps. The opposite haptic is similarly fixated.

Iris fixation of iris fixated IOL

These IOLs are very easy to fix.

- IOL is placed in the AC over the iris.
- IOL is gripped at the centre, and one end of the IOL is placed behind the iris and lifted up to identify the site of enclavation.
- Having a firm grip at the optics and ensuring the centration of IOL, a fine enclavation rod or an iris repositor pushes the iris tissue down to have a pincer like grasp of the IOL, on the iris.
- Same procedure is repeated on the other side.

7. Glued IOL

The glued IOL technique is a relatively new method for fixing a posterior chamber IOL in an eye without a capsule, which has been popularized by Dr. Amar Agarwal.

TECHNIQUE

1. 2 points are marked 180° apart, fornix based conjunctival flaps are raised and light cautery is applied (Fig. 15.58). It is essential to mark, as improper placement of haptics can lead to a decentred IOL.
2. After light cautery, limbus based partial thickness scleral flaps are raised, 2.5 × 3 mm and 500 μ in depth (Fig. 15.58).

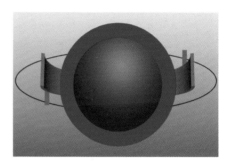

Fig. 15.58. 2 points are marked 180º apart, fornix based conjunctival flaps are raised and light cautery is applied. Limbus based partial thickness scleral flaps are raised, 2.5 ´ 3 mm and 500 μ in depth. 26 G needle or V-lance is used to create a scleral pocket, on both sides, in which the loop can be guided in later.

3. Main port is made for insertion of IOL, which depends upon the type of IOL we will be placing. Foldable IOLs are preferred over non-foldable IOLs, as a sutureless surgery with a limbal or clear corneal incision is possible.
4. Choice of IOL: Any 3-piece IOL would be preferable. AMO Sensar IOL is a very good option, because of the slow release of the IOL through the cartridge.
5. Formation of AC: When we are going to place the IOL the eyeball has to be reasonably pressurized either by:
   (a) Viscoelastics
   (b) Anterior chamber maintainer – through limbus
   (c) Infusion via pars plana route – if pars plana vitrectomy is done, for removal of dislocated nucleus, the infusion port can be used for the IOL implantation.
6. IOL insertion and externalization of haptic: V-Lance knife is introduced at the base of the bed of the scleral flap 1.5 mm from the limbus (Fig. 15.59). The V-lance should be just behind the iris, and if by any chance it is in front of the iris it can be positioned again so that it enters the eye behind the iris. Same procedure is repeated on the other side. This wound is used both to introduce the vitrectomy pick or MST forceps in the eye as well as to externalize the haptic.

   Foldable IOL is loaded and advanced to an extent that a small tip of the haptic is outside the cartridge. Cartridge is passed into the AC by the surgeon; the assistant holds the exposed tip by MST forceps. Surgeon injects the IOL and assistant externalizes the leading haptic and holds it there (Figs. 15.59 and 15.60).

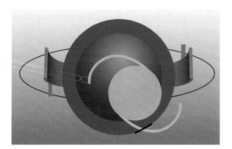

Fig. 15.59. V-Lance knife is introduced at the base of the bed of the scleral flap 1.5 mm from the limbus. This wound is used both to introduce the MST forceps in the eye as well as to externalize the haptic. Surgeon injects the IOL and the assistant holds the leading haptic with MST forceps.

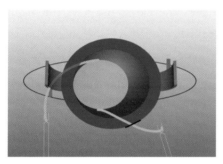

Fig. 15.60. Now the assistant externalizes the leading haptic and holds it there.

The commonest mistake that occurs here is breakage, damage or distortion of the haptic, if the forceps is not holding the tip of the haptic or there is loosening of the grip due to poor quality of the forceps.

A firm grasp is maintained by the assistant on the externalized haptic so that it does not become internalized due to traction on the trailing haptic (Fig. 15.61). Now, a MST forceps is placed inside the AC, and another MST forceps holds the trailing haptic of the IOL, close to the tip and brings it into the AC (Fig. 15.62). Now, another forceps holds the tip of the haptic and externalizes it (Fig. 15.63).

7. Haptic fixation: The haptic needs to be placed into a pocket made at the same level as the base of the flap, in the direction of the natural direction of the haptic (Fig. 15.58). 26 G needle or V-lance can be used to create a scleral pocket, on both sides, in which the loop can be guided in (Fig. 15.64). Because of good IOP, it's easier to create these pockets before entering the AC.

IOL centration is checked; a little pull on the haptic to readjust the IOL may be required.

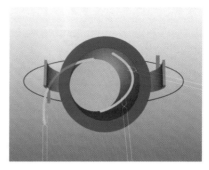

Fig. 15.61. One MST forceps is placed inside the AC, and another MST forceps holds the trailing haptic of the IOL, and brings it into the AC.

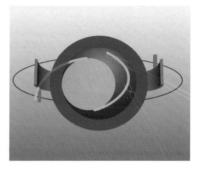

Fig. 15.62. Now the MST forceps are relocated to the tip of the haptic after pulling the haptic with another MST forceps.

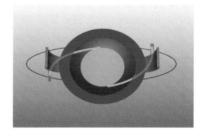

Fig. 15.63. The loop is externalized.

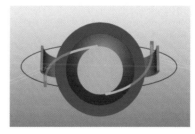

Fig. 15.64. Both the loops are guided into the scleral pockets with the help of MST forceps.

8. Glue fixation: Once the IOL is in centre, glue is applied at the base of the flap and scleral flaps are pressed and stuck over it, one by one on both the sides (Fig. 15.65). Glue provides strong closure over

the area and also closes the V-lance opening. Conjunctiva above can be sutured or can be fixed with glue.

9. After the IOL has been positioned, pupil is constricted and any vitreous is looked for. Tricort can be used to stain the vitreous. If present a thorough vitrectomy is done.

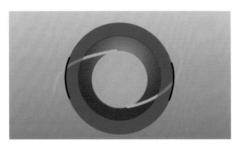

Fig. 15.65. Glue is applied at the base of the flap and scleral flaps are pressed and stuck over it, one by one on both the sides. Conjunctiva above can be sutured or can be fixed with glue.

SPECIAL POINTS

1. 3-Piece IOL with prolene haptic preferred.
2. Single-piece PMMA IOLs can also be used – though more chances of breakage.
3. Large optic PMMA IOLs preferred.
4. In case of a dropped IOL: The IOL can be brought into the AC after thorough pars plana vitrectomy. The haptics are held and externalized as described earlier.

Advantages of glued IOL

- Better fixation
- Better centration
- Pseudo tilting
- No phacodonesis
- Faster technique.

Disadvantages of glued IOL

- Special forceps needed
- Glue needed
- Higher cost due to glue and special forceps.

Summary

Choice of IOL depends upon the extent of the capsular damage, the availability of IOLs, instruments and the expertise of the surgeon. If reasonable centration of the IOL can be ensured, then in the bag fixation or sulcus fixated IOL, with or without optic capture would be ideal.

If there is extensive capsular damage, then we have no choice but to go for ACIOL, SFIOL, Glued or Iris fixated IOL. ACIOL is the fastest, easiest and can be done even without proper vitrectomy, as insertion of ACIOL causes least pull on the vitreous. Secondary vitrectomy can be performed if there is increased IOP, inflammation, distortion of the pupil, CME etc. Specifically designed Iris fixated IOL are also a good option, because the time taken is same as for ACIOL.

Ideal technique in such cases, as of now, looks to be the glued IOL, which provides excellent centration and fixation, with no pseudophacodonesis. This technique needs special instruments and glue which are expensive. SFIOL serves the same purpose but is more time consuming.

5. FINAL VITRECTOMY AND CLOSURE

It is very important to ensure that there is no vitreous in the wound or AC. After putting the IOL constrict the pupil with preservative-free intracameral pilocarpine and inject diluted Tricort in the AC. Final vitrectomy is done by removing each and every strand of the vitreous. At this time a small iridectomy can also be performed with vitrectomy cutter.

Closure

It is absolutely important to have watertight wound in case of PCT. The incidence of endophthalmitis is higher in patients with PCT. Not only one should suture the main incisions but also large, distorted and leaking side port.

Management by Posterior Segment Surgeon

The experienced cataract surgeon may be competent to continue with surgery in the presence of a posterior capsular tear. However, once it has been identified that a nuclear fragment has dropped into the vitreous cavity, it should be accepted that referral to a vitreoretinal surgeon will be necessary.

ROLE OF CATARACT SURGEON

The pre-operative management of eyes with posteriorly dislocated lens matter begins in the hands of the cataract surgeon. The posterior segment surgeon would require corneal clarity and good visibility in order to remove the posteriorly dislocated lens matter, and the anterior segment surgeon's initial management should facilitate this. A few basic guidelines for the cataract surgeon are:

- Do not chase after the falling nuclear fragments and avoid unnecessary manipulations, in order to avoid vitreous traction and a consequent retinal detachment or CME. If retinal detachment occurs, a simple surgery will become unnecessarily complicated.
- Do an anterior vitrectomy and ensure that there is no vitreous in the wound. If the required instrumentation to do a good anterior vitrectomy is not available then it should be left for the posterior segment surgeon to do it.
- If soft lens matter is present in the anterior chamber it should be carefully removed with the suction mode of the cutter after doing anterior vitrectomy. It is important to retain good capsular support, and in case it is difficult to clear the residual lens matter in the anterior chamber it should be left for the posterior segment surgeon who would be able to remove it more easily from the posterior approach.
- Avoid unnecessary damage to the corneal endothelium and iris to prevent corneal haze and inflammation.
- IOL placement: In previous years, dropped nuclei had to be removed from the limbal route after bringing them to the anterior chamber. Now with the availability of the fragmatome it is possible to safely emulsify them within the vitreous cavity and removal through the anterior route is very rarely done except sometimes in case of an exceptionally rock hard black cataract. Therefore, the cataract surgeon should implant an IOL (in the sulcus with optic capture, scleral fixated, or glued), but only if it is stable. If the stability or centration of the lens is questionable, it should not be implanted. Insertion of an ACIOL should also be avoided before pars plana lensectomy to avoid the risk of its posterior dislocation and corneal damage.
- In case the intraocular lens dislocates into the vitreous after implantation, do not try to remove it, as traction on vitreous base may cause retinal tear/RD. Also, do not place a second IOL if the first one is in the vitreous.
- Suture the corneal wound with 10-0 nylon, even if it appears to be "self-sealing", to ensure a stable, non-leaky chamber for the posterior segment surgeon. If necessary suture the side port as well.
- Start frequent corticosteroid antibiotic drops and cycloplegic drops and make sure the intraocular pressure is well controlled.

Every cataract surgeon should have an **arrangement for referral**, with a vitreoretinal surgeon and establish a protocol regarding the initial management of the patient. In case a vitreoretinal surgeon is available in the same hospital, and provided there is adequate corneal clarity, the pars plana lensectomy can be done in the same sitting as the cataract surgery. In case a vitreoretinal surgeon is not available, or if the cornea is hazy the surgery can be deferred for as long as 3 weeks with no difference in the visual outcomes.

The information that would be helpful for the vitreoretinal surgeon includes the amount and type of retained lens matter, any manoeuvres performed while attempting to retrieve it, the hardness of the lens matter, the presence or absence of intraocular lens, the amount of capsular support and the calculated IOL power in case an IOL has not been implanted.

ROLE OF POSTERIOR SEGMENT SURGEON

The vitreoretinal surgeon first needs to assess the patient and make a judgement about the amount and hardness of lens matter present and the urgency with which intervention is required.

Initial examination

The cataract wound should be checked for any leak. The corneal clarity with particular reference to Descemet's fold is assessed and AC reaction and intraocular pressure evaluated. Indirect ophthalmoscopy will confirm the presence of lens matter in the vitreous cavity. Cortical matter will appear white and fluffy and nuclear matter will appear yellowish brown with well-defined borders, unless it is surrounded by cortical matter. The examination should also look for peripheral retinal tears, retinal detachment or choroidal detachment.

In case direct visualization of the fundus is not possible due to corneal haze, severe AC reaction, lens matter in the pupillary area or associated vitreous hemorrhage, a B Scan ultrasonography should be done. The lens matter would appear hyperechoic and may show acoustic shadowing and mobility with ocular movement.

Indications for surgery

The complications of a dropped nucleus may include raised intraocular pressure (IOP), uveitis, corneal edema, cystoid macular edema, and retinal detachment. Therefore, with improved instrumentation, in the present era, even the smallest nuclear fragment is preferably removed.

Sometimes, eyes with a small amount of cortical matter may be treated conservatively provided there is no inflammation and rise of intraocular pressure. However, they would need a close and prolonged follow up, as delayed uveitis, secondary glaucoma and CME may occur and require a late pars plana vitrectomy with removal of the lenticular matter.

Timing of surgery

In case adequate corneal clarity is present and a vitreo-retinal surgeon is available, the removal of lens fragments should not be delayed. If the cornea is hazy and would interfere with visualization, the surgery would have to be deferred till the cornea regains its clarity. Delaying it by 2 to 3 weeks will not cause any damage to the eye, as long as inflammation and IOP are controlled.

Eyes with retinal tears, retinal detachment, uncontrolled intraocular pressure or severe inflammation will need early intervention.

OPERATIVE TECHNIQUE

The management of posteriorly dislocated lens matter by the vitreoretinal surgeon entails –

1. Pars plana vitrectomy
2. Removal of retained lens matter
3. Intraocular lens management
4. Management of associated complications e.g. Dropped IOL, Retinal detachment.

1. Pars plana vitrectomy

A three port pars plana vitrectomy (PPV) is the procedure of choice in eyes with retained lens matter and the standard of care today is microincision vitreous surgery (23 G or 25 G). One of the ports has to be enlarged to 20 G in case a fragmatome needs to be used (23 G fragmatome is not easily available as yet).

Before starting vitrectomy, ensure a well-sealed cataract wound and a stable anterior chamber, so that there is no chamber collapse and iris prolapse during insertion of the cannula as well as during the surgery. In case the wound is leaky do not hesitate to give additional sutures.

Port creation – The 23 G microcannulae are inserted through the conjunctiva (3–4 mm posterior to the limbus) using a trocar, in a two-step entry. After insertion through the sclera, the microcannulae are held by the collar to stabilize them while withdrawing the trocar. The first microcannula is inserted into the inferotemporal quadrant, and the infusion cannula is inserted into the external opening of the microcannula. The infusion is turned on only after visualizing the tip of the microcannula in the vitreous cavity. Two other microcannulae are inserted in the superotemporal and superonasal quadrants for a three port vitrectomy.

If lens matter in the pupillary axis prevents visualization of the infusion cannula, a 23 G butterfly cannula connected to an infusion bottle can be introduced through one of the superior ports and the vitreous cutter used through the other port to clear the lens matter in the pupillary area. The infusion is opened once the infusion cannula can be visualized in the vitreous cavity.

Anterior vitrectomy

The vitrectomy probe is first advanced to the pupillary area to cut any bands of vitreous in the anterior chamber connecting with the posterior vitreous. The lens matter retained under the iris, within the residual lens capsule, is removed with suction mode of the probe. Care should be taken not to damage the capsule in order to facilitate future IOL implantation. If an IOL has already been implanted, the cortical matter surrounding it should be removed, and vitrectomy done just below the lens. Next focus on the posterior segment. Visualisation during surgery may be hampered by corneal edema or a small pupil. The pupil can be dilated using adrenaline, mechanical stretching, hooks or pupillary expansion devices. Wide angle viewing systems are used to give a proper view. First try to visualize the dropped lens fragments and their relation to the vitreous as well as the status of the posterior hyaloid, before starting vitrectomy.

Core vitrectomy

Start by removing the central vitreous (core vitrectomy). Also clear the vitreous immediately in front of the ports, and then assess whether a PVD is present or not.

PVD induction

If not present, a PVD should be induced at this stage, if possible, by positioning the cutter just in front of the optic disc and then increasing the suction to engage the posterior hyaloid. The cutter is then drawn up slowly, keeping the maximum suction. If PVD is induced a shiny reflex will be seen moving forward together with the vitreous cutter. This manoeuvre may have to be repeated several times before a PVD is induced. Triamcinolone acetonide can be used to stain the vitreous before PVD induction for better identification and a complete removal. A bulky nucleus sitting on the cortical vitreous may not allow PVD induction at this stage. In this case it can be done towards the end, after removing the nucleus.

2. Removal of retained lens matter

Removal of small or soft lens fragments
These can be removed with the cutter (approx 800 cuts/min). The light pipe can be used to crush the pieces and feed them into the cutter. For cortical matter suction alone may be used intermittently.

Removal of large / hard nuclear fragments or entire nucleus
A special phacofragmatome is used in these cases. A phacofragmatome is similar to a phaco probe without an infusion sleeve and has a longer needle length. As the fragmatome is 20 G (23 G fragmatome is not easily available), one of the superior sclerotomies has to be enlarged with a 20 G MVR blade, after making a localized peritomy.

Before the nucleus is tackled with the fragmatome it should be ensured that a complete vitrectomy has been done and the nucleus is completely free from any vitreous. This is to avoid any vitreous fibrils from being sucked into the fragmatome and causing vitreous traction. Following this the softer epinuclear matter present around the nucleus is aspirated with the cutter to uncover the hard centre.

The phacofragmatome is then introduced into the vitreous cavity. Aspiration alone is used to engage the nucleus/nuclear fragments and gently lift them from the posterior vitreous cavity. Once they are elevated into the mid vitreous cavity the ultrasound power is turned on to emulsify them.

Settings for phacofragmatome
- **Power:** 20% to 50% depending on the hardness of the nucleus. Use minimum power required to prevent chattering and flying of the nuclear pieces away from the fragmatome tip.
- **Vacuum:** 150–200 mm Hg. Increase the bottle height before starting phacofragmentation to prevent hypotony, as it has a large bore size.
- **Mode:** Pulse mode with 10–20 pulses/min. The pulse mode also prevents repulsion of the nuclear fragments. As there is no capsular bag to provide counter resistance the nuclear pieces tend to be repelled by the ultrasonic energy and repeatedly fall back.

The endoilluminator can be used to support the nucleus from behind while it is being emulsified. A good technique is to spike the nucleus on the endoilluminator and in a cartwheel manner use the fragmatome to emulsify the nucleus. Try to work towards the light pipe without dislodging it, so that there is minimal need for reengaging the nucleus. (A lighted pick can also be used to stabilize the nucleus instead of the endoilluminator.) If the fragmatome tip goes through and through into the nucleus, the endoilluminator can be used to push it off the nucleus. It can also be used to crush and feed smaller fragments into the port.

In case the fragments fall down, stop suction immediately to prevent hypotony, and activate it only when the tip is occluded by a fragment. If milky fluid is released during fragmentation then wait for a moment for the media to clear up before continuing.

Alternative technique – A fluid needle can be used to aspirate and hold the nuclear pieces in the mid vitreous cavity while it is emulsified by the fragmatome. A chandelier light is used for illumination.

Sometimes if a PVD has not been induced before, small lens pieces get stuck to the posterior hyaloid. A PVD should be induced at this stage. When these pieces are lifted up with the posterior hyaloid they can be removed with the cutter. Very small pieces stuck to the retinal surface can also be removed with the fluid needle. In the end a peripheral examination with scleral depression should be performed and a peripheral vitrectomy done to eliminate peripheral vitreous traction. Also check for small pieces that can get entrapped at the vitreous base. In case a break/tear is detected, endolaser should be done around it. After all the retained lens matter is removed, the anterior chamber should be irrigated to remove any fragments that may be trapped in the angle. It is important to remove all of the lens fragments to prevent post-op inflammation, phacolytic glaucoma or CME.

Role of Adjunctive Perfluorocarbon Liquid (PFCL)
Some surgeons prefer to inject a small amount of PFCL after vitrectomy and before using the fragmatome, for the following purposes:
1. It protects the macula from contusion injuries which may be caused by the impact of lens pieces that fall posteriorly during fragmentation.
2. It causes the lens pieces to float on its surface, reducing risk of retinal damage during manipulating these pieces off the retinal surface.

3. It forms a protective layer over the posterior pole and may reduce the risk of damage from the ultrasonic energy of the fragmatome.

Only a small amount of PFCL should be injected, to extend till the arcades. Overfill can hamper with removal, because the meniscus of the bubble tends to cause displacement of the lens fragments towards the retinal periphery and vitreous base, making their retrieval difficult. Care should be taken to remove all the PFCL at the end of the surgery.

Removal of Rock Hard Black cataracts

In case of a rock hard black cataract where a prolonged and difficult phacofragmentation is expected, or in cases where the fundal view is compromised due to a hazy cornea, the nucleus can be brought into the AC and then delivered from a limbal incision. An adequate sized limbal corneal incision is first made and then sutured with 10-0 nylon. After core vitrectomy and PVD induction, PFCL is injected upto the level of sclerotomies (two vials would be needed for this) so that the nucleus is pushed up to the level of the pupil. Viscoelastic is then injected into the AC and the nucleus is manoeuvred into the AC using a membrane pick introduced from the pars plana incision and another instrument from the paracentesis. Limbal sutures are then cut to deliver the nucleus. Surgery is completed with resuturing of limbus, completion of vitrectomy and removal of PFCL.

3. IOL Management

After closing the two superior ports, the infusion is left in place in case an IOL is to be implanted, and removed only after IOL implantation. If an IOL was inserted at the time of cataract surgery, it may require repositioning, if decentred. Sometimes, more than one IOL may be encountered in such eyes – these need to be removed through the limbus. If an IOL was not placed it can be inserted now into the sulcus. In case inadequate capsular support is present, a scleral fixated or glued IOL can be considered. ACIOL can also be inserted provided the pupil constricts well with pilocarpine.

If there is significant corneal edema, choroidal detachment or haemorrhage, the IOL placement should be deferred.

4. Management of Associated complications

Dislocated IOL with retained lens matter

Posteriorly dislocated IOL along with a dropped nucleus may occur due to improper identification of capsular damage or due to incorrect positioning of the lens. The IOL is tackled after removal of the dropped lens matter and is either repositioned or explanted.

The IOL can be lifted with a retinal pick forceps and brought into the anterior chamber. If a three-piece IOL is present, it can then be manipulated into the sulcus if adequate capsular support is present, or may be glued to the sclera if the capsule is inadequate. Single-piece IOL or IOLs with broken haptics or plate haptics are generally explanted and replaced with the appropriate IOL.

Retinal detachment

If the eye with the dislocated lens fragments also has an associated rhegmatogenous retinal detachment and/or choroidal detachment, PFCL is injected after doing a vitrectomy to flatten the retina. After doing a vitrectomy, perfluorocarbon liquid (PFCL) is injected to flatten the retina. The lens matter floats over the PFCL and can be removed in the anterior vitreous with the fragmatome. After removal of the lens, endolaser is performed around the break. PFCL air exchange is done followed by gas or silicone oil injection.

POST-OPERATIVE MONITORING

After removal of retained lens matter the patient should be closely followed for signs of inflammation, increase in IOP, CME and signs of peripheral retinal tears or detachment are managed appropriately.

PROGNOSIS

A good percentage of patients (44% to 68%) obtain 6/9 or better visual acuity after pars plana vitrectomy done for the management of retained lens matter. Improved surgical techniques and instrumentation have improved the safety and visual outcomes of this procedure.

CONVERSION TO SICS/ECCE

Many times during course of phacoemulsification, the beginner surgeon may find it difficult to continue and may have to convert to SICS/ECCE. Under no circumstances, should the surgical outcome of conversion be poorer than that of planned ECCE. Besides cosmesis, uveitis, keratitis, decentred IOL, the post-operative astigmatism has to be given due attention for good long-term results. To achieve this goal, one needs to have proper understanding of the steps of conversion. Besides, you will be less enthusiastic for learning phacoemulsification if you do not know how to convert properly.

REASONS TO CONVERT

Most common reason for conversion is PCT. However, beginners may need to convert for other reasons.

I. CCC related problems

1. Small CCC (< 4.5 mm) and large nucleus—All steps will be difficult to do so it is better to convert.
2. Too large CCC—Nucleus will prolapse in to the AC and phaco will be difficult.
3. Discontinuous CCC—Beginners MUST convert without doubt. A discontinuous CCC may be due to inability to make a CCC or RMT during any step.

II. Excessive use of phaco & fluids (Prolonged surgical time)

This leads to corneal edema, which will interfere with visibility and cause striate keratitis post-operatively. An effective phaco time (EPT) of more than 1½ minutes usually causes sufficient intraocular damage to merit conversion. Under no circumstances should EPT be **greater than 3 minutes**. Surgeon should convert at this stage, even if there are no other complications. Another indication of prolonged surgical time is use of more than one bottle of infusion fluid. You may like to convert. If the surgery has taken more than one hour— convert.

III. Wound related problems

Leaking wound, with repeated iris prolapse is an indication for conversion particularly for beginners. Corneoscleral burn if excessive may also be a cause for conversion.

IV. Corneal edema

Due to any cause, disturbing visibility, once the case has been started, is an indication to covert.

V. Intraoperative meosis

It is hazardous to do sphincterotomy after starting the surgery as you may unknowingly cut the capsule; better to convert.

VI. Improper case selection

In some cases like deep AC syndrome/cramped AC after starting the case you may realize that it is a tough case. In a very deep AC the approach is vertical and all the surgical steps are more difficult. In other cases, the shallow AC can hamper all movements. If the surgeon is feeling nervous during a particular case, it is better to convert.

HOW TO CONVERT?

All cataract surgeons should attempt to perform a CCC while doing ECCE. It is always possible to convert a CCC opening into an ECCE capsulotomy later without hampering the surgery.

1. Conversion of intact CCC to perform planned ECCE/small incision (non-phaco) cataract extraction (Figs. 15.66 to 15.68)

(a) *Incomplete CCC:* In the area where you are not able to complete the CCC convert to either can-opener or envelope technique, whatever you are comfortable with.

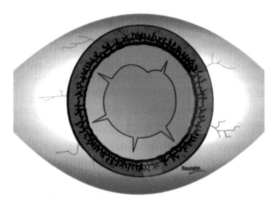

Fig. 15.66. Conversion of intact CCC. Multiple snips made in CCC to release it.

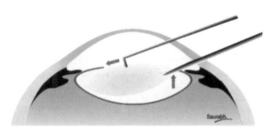

Fig. 15.67. Prolapse the superior pole out of the CCC margin by pushing down with one instrument and lift with the other.

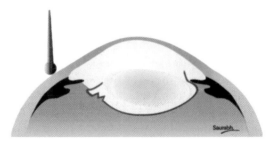

Fig. 15.68. Failure to deliver the superior pole first can lead to rupture of the zonules and the lens will get tumbled as in intracapsular extraction.

(b) *Complete CCC:* If the CCC is large enough (i.e. 1–3 mm less than delineation ring) then because of the stretchability of CCC margin it is possible to prolapse the nucleus into the AC without breaking the CCC. This can be done by nudging the nucleus down with a Sinskey hook (in a well-inflated eyeball) and trying to lift it up with a second instrument inserted below the nucleus. Prolapse the superior pole out of the CCC first. Injecting VES beneath the nucleus will further facilitate the nucleus delivery. The nucleus can now be totally prolapsed out of CCC. Once the nucleus is completely out of CCC, one can either do an ECCE or perform the Blumenthal technique.

If the CCC is very small (3 mm)—disregard this rhexis and continue as if the capsule is intact, i.e. one can perform can-opener/envelope capsulotomy. You must make at least two relaxing capsulotomies. Only one relaxing capsulotomy will cause loss of elasticity and extension into the posterior capsule at the time of nucleus delivery. Still better you should try to make at least three to four relaxing incisions in case one of the attempted cuts is inadequate or not radially placed. While delivering, you should try to prolapse the superior pole of the lens out of the CCC before depressing on the inferior pole with the lens hook and sliding it out. If the CCC is not released properly the superior pole may get trapped under the CCC margin inferior pole will then try to tumble out as in ICCE leading to zonular dialysis.

2. Conversion of superior scleral tunnel
(Photos 15.20 to 15.31)

Extend the conjunctival flap to the size of the ECCE incision along the limbus on both sides. Make a posterior limbal gutter on either side of scleral pocket. Now release the side walls of the pocket by cutting with a scissors upto the limbal incision. Lift the scleral flap and dissect into the corneal valve upto the internal lip. Dissect onto the sides with decreasing the length of the corneal valve as you move away from the centre. At the extreme ends you should be 0–0.5 mm into the cornea. Now cut with the scissors from the centre to both the sides to complete the internal wound. For closing the wound after removal of the lenticular matter (i.e. completion of the ECCE) put two sutures on the extremes of the scleral flap (like a trabeculectomy flap). Close both sides of the limbal wound with shoe lace/interrupted sutures.

3. Conversion in a superior clear corneal/limbal incision

The principle is to maintain the same plane all along the incision. The margin of the external wound is extended on either side upto the extent required. Dissection of the wound and formation of the internal lip is as described above for extension of scleral pocket.

4. Conversion in a temporal incision
(Photos 15.32 to 15.34)

Temporal incision/modified temporal incision are usually corneal or anterior limbal. A large ECCE incision is not acceptable temporally mainly because of the exposed sutures and subconjunctival haemorrhage being cosmetically unpleasant. Maximum acceptable temporal incision is 6.5 mm for putting in a larger optic IOL. For extension of the temporal incision, you can directly extend it with the 5.2 keratome maintaining the configuration of the valve. The movement should be outside in to maintain the corneal lip. It can later be closed with running sutures or even one central shoe lace suture if the incision is not ragged. If you need a larger incision, it is best to disregard the temporal incision, move to the superior side and make a fresh limbal incision ensuring that it is sufficiently far away from the temporal tunnel.

IMMEDIATE POST-OPERATIVE ENDOPHTHALMITIS / TASS

Endophthalmitis is the most dreaded complication of any intraocular surgery. The commonest cause is poor instrument sterilization technique.

There is a need to understand the simplest and safest method to manage endophthalmitis. Here we will only discuss the management of immediate post-operative endophthalmitis. *High level of suspicion and early detection are the key to successful management without having to resort to invasive procedures.*

The patients should be well informed and instructed to report immediately in case of any decrease in vision. If it does occur, the surgeon must examine the patient at the earliest, i.e. within 6 to 12 hours. Examination should rule out keratitis as the cause of the drop in vision. Attempt should be made to differentiate TASS from early endophthalmitis and though pain, redness and watering are supposed to be pointers towards a septic inflammation, these are not pathognomic features of endophthalmitis. ***However, it is safer to presume and treat as endophthalmitis if there is any doubt.***

In case of suspected endophthalmitis, six to twelve hourly monitoring of visual acuity, red-reflex, direct, indirect ophthalmoscopic and slit lamp examination should be done. The patient should be instructed to perform monitoring of his own vision. As monitoring is difficult at night, the treatment needs to be more aggressive if the patient presents at night. Patient should be informed that at early stage it is difficult to differentiate reaction from infection. As the latter is potentially vision threatening, it is safer to treat all such cases by periocular injection of antibiotic steroid combination.

Based on slit lamp examination and clinical features, the following situations may be observed as potential/aseptic/septic endophthalmitis and should be managed as given in Table 15.1.

We recommend the following regime for presumed or frank early endophthalmitis:

• 500 mg Vancomycin is reconstituted with 2 ml of Amikacin and 2 ml of Decadron. 1 ml of this fluid is withdrawn and put in a bottle of Atropine eye drops. This is used topically as half hourly drops.

• 1 ml of 2% Xylocaine is then added to the remaining 3 ml of mixture. 1 ml of this fluid is withdrawn and administered as periocular injection.

TECHNIQUE OF PERIOCULAR ANTIBIOTIC-STEROID INJECTION

Skin is cleaned with Betadine and the conjunctival sac is anaesthetized with 4% Xylocaine drops. 0.5 ml of Xylocaine is injected in the periocular space through the skin. Leave the 26 G needle in place and remove the syringe. Wait for 3 minutes and now inject the prepared antibiotic steroid mixture through the same needle. Apply a pressure patch to the eye. Pad is removed after 4 hours and the patient starts putting drops. If delivered subconjunctivally this injection is very painful.

Any time after 24 hours if there is no improvement or worsening then it is better to give an intravitreal injection. In our experience, most patients respond to 2–3 periocular injections with hardly ever needing to give an intravitreal injection. This should not be taken lightly and if you are not comfortable with the procedure, it is better to refer the case.

Table 15.1. Differential diagnosis: TASS or Endophthalmitis?

	TASS	**Endophthalmitis**
Cause	Non-infectious reaction to toxic agent present in: • BSS solution • Antibiotic injection • Endotoxin • Residue • VES such as methyl cellulose	Bacterial, fungal, or viral infection
Onset	12–24 hours	2–7 days
Signs/symptoms	Blurry vision Pain: None, or mild to moderate Corneal oedema: Diffuse, limbus to limbus* Pupil: Dilated, irregular, non-reactive* Increased IOP* Anterior chamber: Mild to severe reaction with cells, flare, hypopyon, fibrin Signs and symptoms are limited to anterior chamber Gram stain and culture negative	Decreased VA Pain (25% have no pain) Lid swelling with edema Conjunctival injection Hyperaemia Anterior chamber: Marked inflammatory response with hypopyon Vitreous involvement
Treatment	Rule out infection Culture anterior chamber Intensive corticosteroids Monitor IOP closely for signs of damage to trabecular meshwork and side effects of steroids Watch closely over next few hours for signs of bacterial infection	Inflammation in entire ocular cavity* Culture anterior chamber and vitreous Intravitreal and topical antibiotics Vitrectomy

* Distinguishing feature (if severe)

CORNEAL COMPLICATIONS

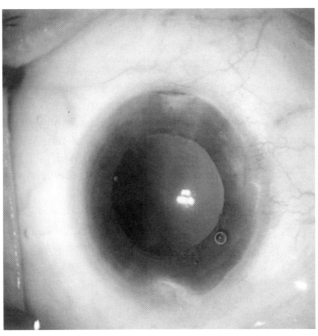

Photo 15.1. Corneal burn.

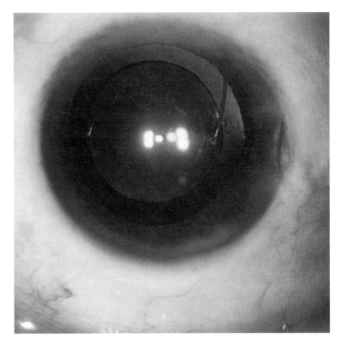

Photo 15.2. Inversion of outer lip in thin flap.

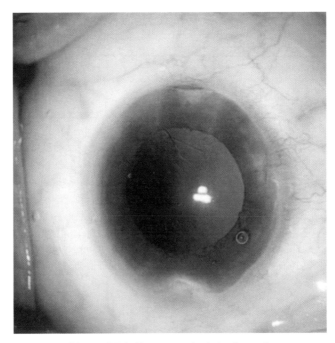

Photo 15.3. Descemet's detachment.

MANAGEMENT OF PCT WITH IMPENDING NUCLEAR DROP

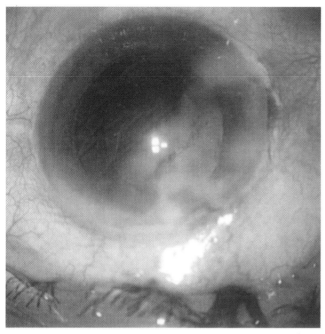

Photo 15.4. PCT with impending nucleus drop. Nucleus partly hanging in vitreous cavity.

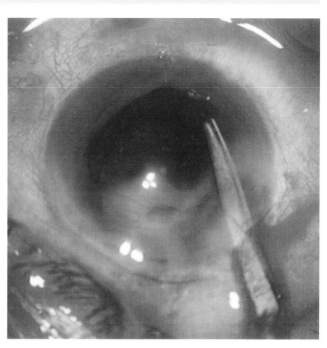

Photo 15.5. Releasing the CCC. Repeat on other side.

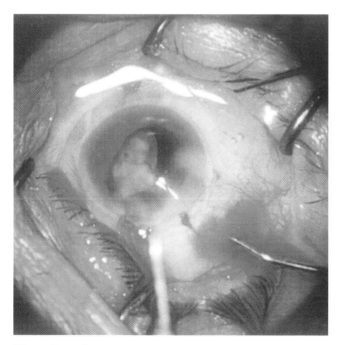

Photo 15.6. Stab incision made in pars plana. Sinskey hook introduced under the nucleus to stabilize it.

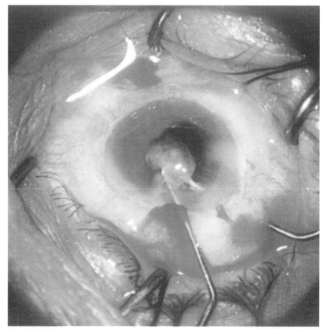

Photo 15.7. Second instrument passed through side port. Nucleus gripped by chop stick method.

MANAGEMENT OF PCT WITH IMPENDING NUCLEAR DROP (Contd.)

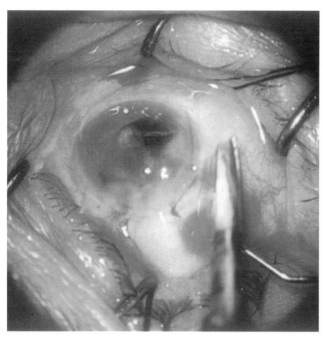

Photo 15.8. Nucleus brought anteriorly keeping the pars plana instrument in place. Section enlarged.

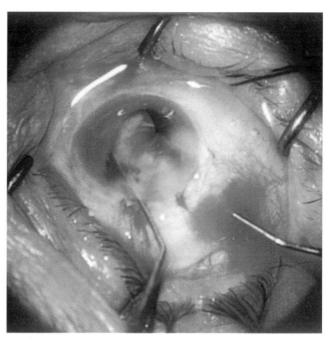

Photo 15.9. Use of second instrument to bring the nucleus closer to the section.

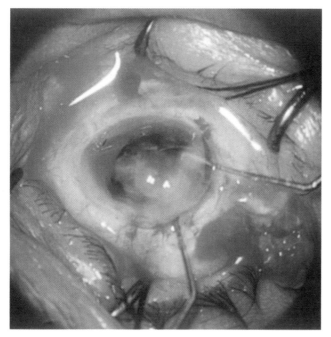

Photo 15.10. Once the nucleus is reasonably stabilized, remove the pars plana instrument and bring it into the AC to grip the nucleus.

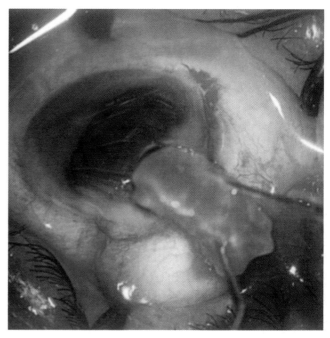

Photo 15.11. Use both instruments to deliver the nucleus out.

MANAGEMENT OF PCT WITH IMPENDING NUCLEAR DROP (Contd.)

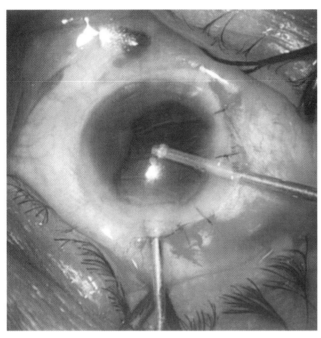

Photo 15.12. Application of interrupted sutures to do closed chamber vitrectomy.

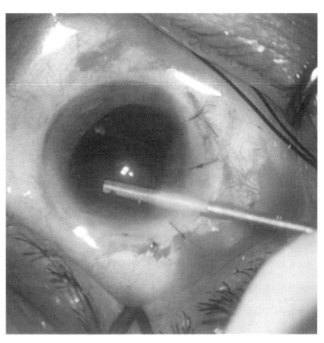

Photo 15.13. Removal of debris and blood with automated vitrectomy.

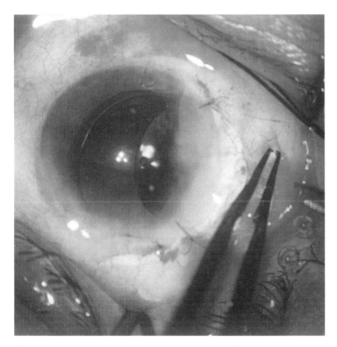

Photo 15.14. Insertion of 6.5 mm optic IOL. Lens inserted close to the corneal dome to press down any vitreous. Leading haptic is placed on top of the iris and then slipped under so as to lie in the sulcus, i.e. on top of the CCC.

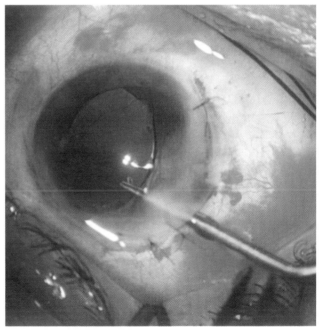

Photo 15.15. Trailing haptic held with McPherson forceps and slipped under the iris in the sulcus over the CCC.

MANAGEMENT OF PCT WITH IMPENDING NUCLEAR DROP (Contd.)

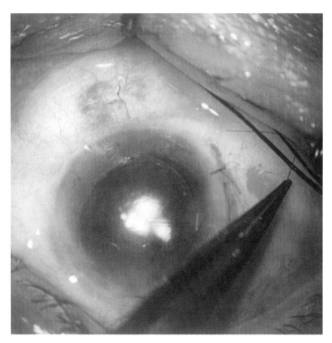

Photo 15.16. Pars plana wound sutured with 10-0 nylon.

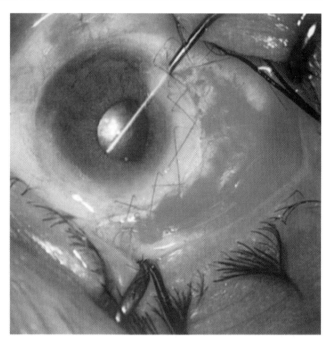

Photo 15.17. Suture the limbal section and put the rounded repositor to remove vitreous fibres in the section. Note the 'D' shaped pupil.

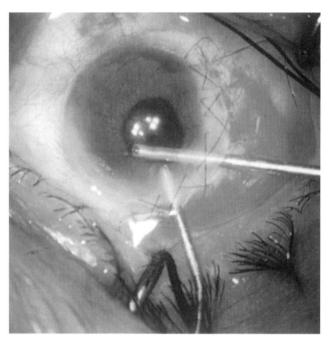

Photo 15.18. Repeat automated vitrectomy.

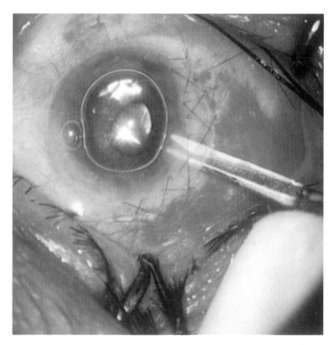

Photo 15.19. Air and pilocarpine injected in the AC to constrict the pupil. Look for peaking. Vannas scissors may be used for cutting any remaining vitreous fibres.

CONVERSION OF SCLERAL POCKET

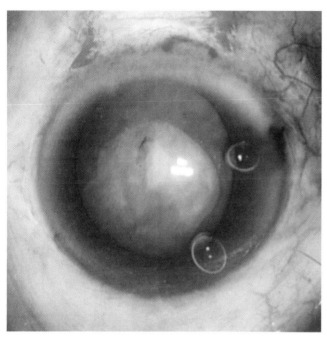

Photo 15.20. Posterior extension of CCC (incomplete CCC). Phaco may cause extension posteriorly.

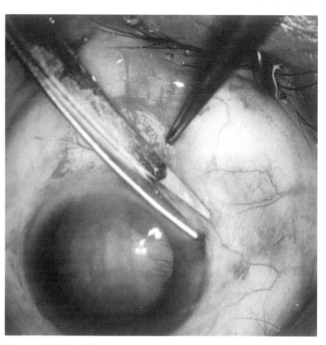

Photo 15.21. Detachment of conjunctiva and Tenon's as for ECCE section.

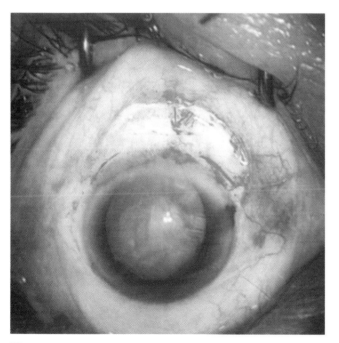

Photo 15.22. After light cautery, limbal groove made on both sides of the scleral pocket.

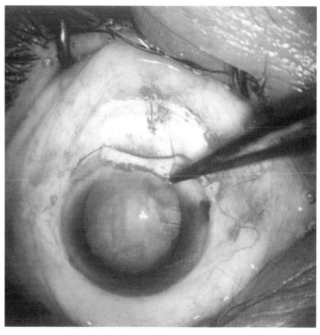

Photo 15.23. Releasing the scleral pocket.

CONVERSION OF SCLERAL POCKET (Contd.)

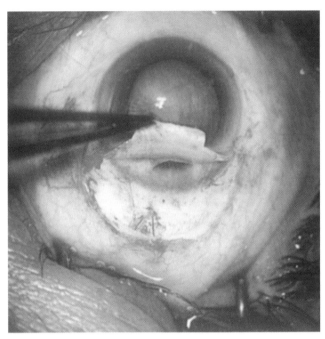

Photo 15.24. Dissection of limbal groove upto the internal wound on both sides.

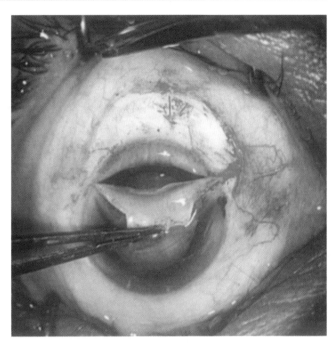

Photo 15.25. Enlarging the internal incision on both sides. Note that the corneal shelf keeps on decreasing as we go to the periphery.

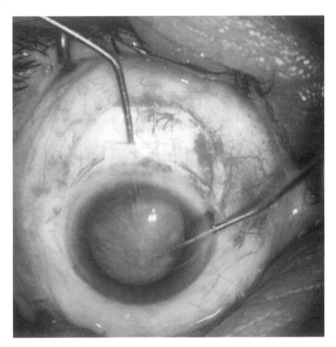

Photo 15.26. One Sinskey hook nudges the nucleus down while rounded repositor is passed or embedded into the upper edge of the nucleus to prolapse the upper edge out of the CCC margin.

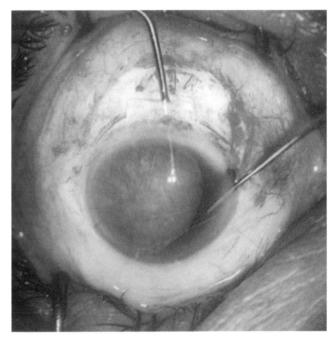

Photo 15.27. Prolapse of the whole nucleus into AC.

CONVERSION OF SCLERAL POCKET (Contd.)

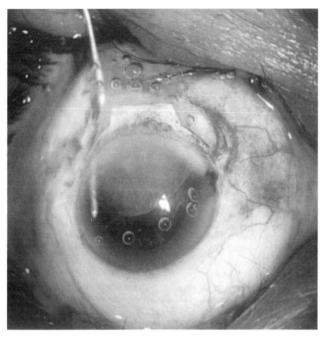

Photo 15.28. Viscoexpression of the nucleus.

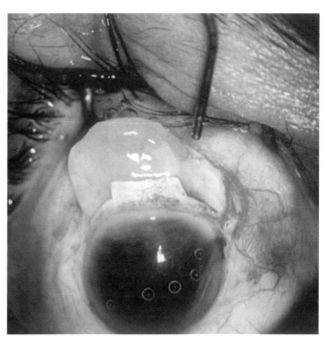

Photo 15.29. Nucleus delivered from the section.

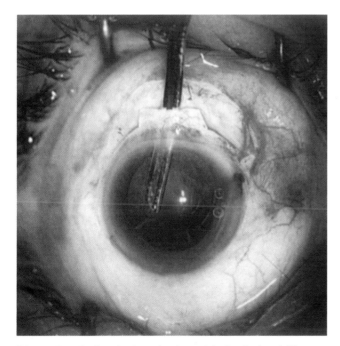

Photo 15.30. Cortical aspiration with the help of Simcoe cannula.

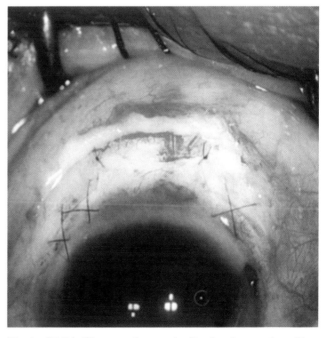

Photo 15.31. Closure of wound with shoelace suture. Two interrupted sutures at the corners of scleral flap (as in trabeculectomy). Limbal section closed by shoelace stitch.

6.5 MM CONVERSION

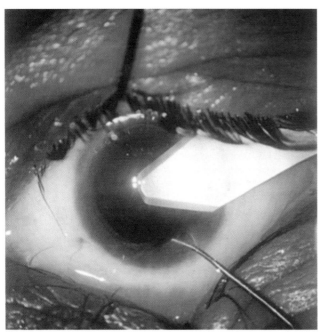

Photo 15.32. Enlarge the incision using a 5.5 mm keratome. Note the enlargement from outside-in.

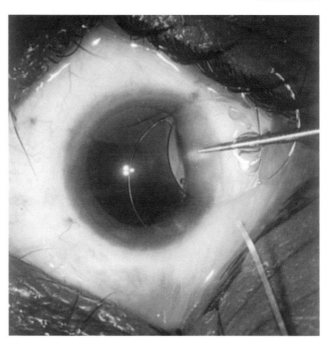

Photo 15.33. Insertion of 6.5 mm optic over the CCC in the sulcus.

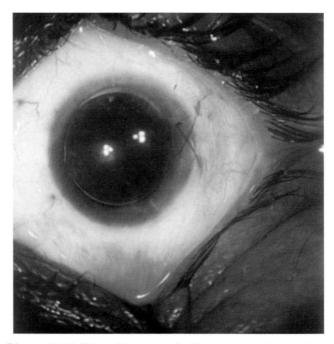

Photo 15.34. Wound is secured with single shoelace suture.

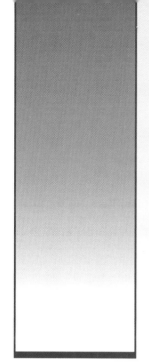

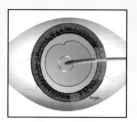

Index

Note: Numbers in **bold** indicate pages showing a particular step of phaco technique in colour pictures along with their captions.

45° coaxial irrigation-aspiration hand-piece with metallic sleeve, 22
6.5 mm conversion, **250**

A

A-scan biometer features, 33
Acoustic wave, 9
AMO phaco tip with Ellips technology, 27
Amount of astigmatism, 200
Anaesthesia, 191
Anterior chamber maintainer (ACM), 13
Anterior continuous curvilinear capsulorrhexis (CCC), 212
Area of highest followability, 15
Area of no followability, 15
Area of poor followability, 15
Aspiration cannula without handle for bimanual irrigation-aspiration, 23
Aspiration phaco, 113
Aspiration system, 13
Assessment of depth, 105
Assessment of the patient, 191
Astigmatic keratotomy, 197
Astigmatic neutral funnel, 43
Auditory feedback, 7
Autoclaving, 4
Avoiding errors in biometry, 33

B

Betadine cleaning, 191
Bimanual cortical aspiration, **164–166**

Bimanual irrigation and aspiration, 157
Bimanual irrigation-aspiration (IA) system, 155
Bimanual irrigation-aspiration infusion and aspiration cannulae, 23
Bimanual modified technique of irrigation and aspiration, 157
Biometry, 29
Biometry and IOL power calculation in
  Aphakic eye, 36
  Highly myopic eye with posterior staphyloma, 37
  Intumescent cataract, 36
  Pseudophakic eye, 35
  Silicone-filled eyes, 38
  Very short eye, 38
Biometry technique, 32
Biplanar corneal incision, 48, 49
Biplanar incision, 49, **60**, 199
Blunt chopper, 102
Box IOL folder, 23
Burst mode, 10

C

Calculation of true axial length (TAL), 37
'Cap vac' mode, 159
Capsular complications, 206
Capsular placement of accidentally opened IOL in AC, **187**
Capsular polishing, 158, 194
Cavitation phenomenon, 9

CCC in young patients, 75
Central chop, 112, 113, **128–133**
Central chop with partial trench with rotation, **137–138**
Central part, 7
Central PCC polishing, 158
Central safe zone (CSZ), 14, 209
Characteristics of a good A-scan, 33
Choosing the phacomachine, 21, 25
Choosing the instruments, 21
Choosing the viscoelastic substances, 21
Choppers, 102
Chopping, 109
Chopping and phacoaspiration, 193
Chopstick technique, 218
Cionni's ring fixation in cases of zonulo-dialysis, 206
Clear corneal incision, 48
Co-axial irrigation-aspiration, 155, **160–163**
Co-axial irrigation-aspiration system, 155
Cobra tip, 102
Cohesiveness, 24
Combination CCC, 73, **80–82**
Completion of CCC, 72
Compliance, 16, 210
  in a peristaltic system, 16
Complications of phacoemulsification, 205
Compression delineation, 96
Confirmation of PCT and hyaloid face rupture (HFR), 216

Console, 7
Continuation of CCC, 70, 71
Continuous curvilinear capsulorrhexis, 65
Control and delivery of power, 10
Control of surge, 18, 211
Conversion of scleral pocket, **247–249**
Conversion to SICS/ECCE, 238
Corneal complications, 206, **242**
Corneal transplantation combined with cataract surgery, 41
Corneal valve, 45
Correction of pre-existing astigmatism, 197
Cortical aspiration, 155, 194
Cortical cleaving hydrodissection, 95
Creating a platform, 109
Creation of vacuum seal and vacuum hold, 110
Critical limit, 16
Cystitome, 67, 68

D

Delay in start of the motor following occlusion break, 18
Descemet's detachment, 205
Design of OT, 3
Dialing the trailing haptic, 172
Differential diagnosis: TASS or endophthalmitis?, 241
Differential FR/vacuum settings before and after occlusion, 18
Difficulties in trenching, 106
Difficulty score for phacoemulsification, 192
Dimensions of the trench, 103
Direct chop, 113, **140–141**
Direction of shearing force, 66
Divide & Conquer, 18, 108, **118–122**
Modified technique, 108
Do I need to change IOL power?, 201
Donnenfeld nomogram, 198
Dos and Don'ts of hydroprocedures, 98
Double autoclaving, 4
Downward displacement method, 4
Draping, 191
Dry heat, 4
Dumbbell dialer, 22
Dyes in CCC, 74
Dyes in CCC (Controlled method), **88–89**
Dyes in CCC (Usual method), **90**

E

Echograph, 32
Echography principles, 31

Endothelial damage, 206
Enlargement of CCC, 74
Epinuclear plate removal, 145, 194
Problems, 146
Epinuclear plate removal (Flip & Chip technique), **149–153**
Epinuclear plate settings, 194
Estimation of IOL power, 29
Ethylene oxide (ETO), 5

F

Flip & Chip method, 146, 147
Flow rate (FR), 13
Fluidics, 12
Foldable IOLs, 171, 173
Foldable lens (Holder-folder method), **180–181**
Followability, 12, 14
Foot gradient, 8
Foot pedal, 7
in irrigation-aspiration mode, 8
Forceps, 68
Forceps CCC, 72, **76–80**
Formaldehyde fumigation, 4
Formalin chamber, 5
Friable capsule, 209

G

Glutaraldehyde 2% (Cidex), 4
Good followability, 15
Grades and density of the nucleus, 101

H

Halo test, 217
Handpiece, 7
High vacuum pump, 4
Hinged incision, 48, 49, 199
Holder with lock, 23
Holder-folder method, 173
Hydration of the wound, 194
Hydrodelineation, 96, **100**
Hydrodissection, 94, **99**, 214
Hydroprocedures, 93, 192
Hyperpulse, 10

I

I excursion, 8
IA excursion, 8
IAP excursion, 8
Immediate post-operative endophthalmitis/TASS, 240
Incidence of astigmatism, 197
Incision, 191
Incisions and wound construction, 43
Incomplete depth of trench, 105

Infusion system, 12
Initiation of CCC, 69
Injecting systems, 175
Injector system, **182–186**
Insertion of IOL, 171
Insertion of leading haptic under CCC, 172
Insertion of trailing haptic with forceps, **179**
Instruments, 21
IOL calculation formulas, 29
IOL folder, 23
IOL implantation, 224
IOL insertion, 194
IOL power calculation, 29
after radial keratotomy (RK), 41
in eyes after previous corneal refractive surgery, 38
in scarred corneas, keratoconus, 41
IOL power selection in children, 42
IOP at the time of leaving the eye, 194
Iridodialysis, 206
Iris chaffing, 206
Iris complications, 206
Irrigation-aspiration handpiece, 7

J

Jack-hammer effect, 9

K

Kelman flared tip, 102
Kelman tip, 102
Keratometry in eyes with corneal transplant, 35
Knives used for making incisions, 22

L

Length of the trench, 104
Lens, planes for hydrodissection and hydrodelineation, 93
Limbal incision, 50
Limbal/corneal relaxing incision, 197
Limitations of OCCI, 201
Loss of control, **83–84**
Loss of control of CCC, 73
How to regain control, 73
Why we lose control, 73
LRIs, 197

M

Management of PCT
by anterior segment surgeon, 217
by posterior segment surgeon, 234
with impending nuclear drop, **243–246**
Manual irrigation and aspiration, 157

Marking of the axis of astigmatism, 202
McPherson forceps, 22, 171
Measurement of axial length, 31
Measurement of corneal power, 35
Mechanism of PCT, 211
Mechanism of phaco, 9
Mini-delineation/mechanical delineation, 97
Modified bimanual cortical aspiration, **167**
Modified peripheral chop, 113, 114, **139**
Modified technique of Divide & Conquer, 108
Modified temporal incision (corneo-limbal/limboscleral), 50
Modified temporal limboscleral triplanar incision, **62–64**

N

Needle CCC, 69
Needle CCC in young patient, **90–91**
No followability, 15
Nomogram, 200
    Gills nomogram, 198
    Harbansh Lal nomogram, 200
    NAPA nomogram, 198
Nucleotomy, 101, 103, 193
Number of incisions, 200

O

OCCIs, 197
On axis cataract incision and opposite clear corneal incisions, 198
One-toothed forceps, 23
Ozil handpiece, 26

P

Partial coherence laser interferometry, 34
Partial delineation ring, 97
Parts of epinuclear plate, 145
Peripheral chop, 111, 112
Peripheral chop with partial trench without rotation, **134–136**
Peripheral unsafe zone (PUSZ), 14, 209
Peristaltic pump, 13
Peristaltic system, 13
Phaco chop, 111
Phaco handpiece, 7
Phaco profile IOLs, 171
Phaco tips, 11
Phacoaspiration, 115, **142–143**
Phacodynamics, 9
Phacomachine, 7, 21
Physics of capsulorrhexis, 66
Placement of folder, 174
PMMA lens, **176–178**

Polishing beyond the optical zone, 158
Polishing of anterior and equatorial zone, 159
Positive pressure pump, 12
Posterior capsular tear, 207
    during hydrodissection, 98
Posterior capsulorrhexis, 75
Power, 9
Pre-existing astigmatism (PEA), 197
Preferred technique for phaco-emulsification and settings in different situations, 191
Premature entry, 47
Preparing for phacoemulsification, 1
Pressurising the eye, **52**
Primary RMT, 212
Problems in initiation, 69
Problems with central chop, 112
Problems with co-axial IA, 156
Problems with peripheral chop, 111
Procedure for injecting IOL, **188–189**
Properties of an ideal viscoelastic substance, 24
Psuedoplasticity, 24
Pulse mode, 10
Putting the trailing haptic by forceps, 173

R

Recommended vacuum settings, 111
Regaining control, **85–87**
Relationship between vacuum, surge and flow rate, 17, 210
Relaxing nucleotomy, 104
Relocation of epinuclear plate, 223
Removal of already divided epinuclear plate, **154**
Removal of cortex by dialing the IOL, **169**
Removal of cortical matter after IOL insertion, 158
Replacement of BSS with VES before insertion of IOL, 172
Rhexis margin tear, 213
Ripping, 66
Ripping force, 66
Rise time (RT), 14
Role of cataract surgeon, 237
Role of posterior segment surgeon, 238
Role of vacuum and compliance in post-occlusion surge, 17
Rotation of the nucleus
    Bimanual rotation, 97
    Non-rotation of nucleus, 98
    Single-handed rotation, 97
Rounded repositor, 22

S

Scissors, angled Vannas, 22
Scleral/corneal burn, 205
Scleral disinsertion, 47
Scleral pocket, 45, **54–59**
Scleral tunnel, 45
Secondary RMT, 213
Selecting the appropriate IOL power, 41
Selection of the scan, 33
Self-sealing incision, 44
Setting the operation theatre, 3
Settings for phaco in various machines, 194
Settings for trenching, 103
Settings for vacuum seal, 111
Sharp tipped chopper, 102
Shaving action while trenching, 104
Shearing, 66
Shearing force, 66
Side port, **53**
Side port incision (SPI), 45
Sidekick functions of foot pedal, 9
Sidekicks, 7
Signs of a PC rupture during hydro-dissection, 214
Silicon IOLs, 175
Sinskey hook, 22
Site for hydrodissection, 95
Site of the incision, 200
Size of CCC, 66
Soft cataracts, 97
Splitting, 106, 193
Splitting and stretching forces, 107
Splitting the nucleus, 107
Sponge test, 217
Stabilization of the nucleus, 109
Standard or regular tip, 102
Starting the trench, 104
Steps in vacuum hold, 110
Sterilization by heat, 4
Sterilization techniques, 3
Stop and Chop (Splitting), **127**
Stop and Chop (V-Trench), **123–126**
Stop and Chop technique, 113
Sub-incisional cortex removal, 158
Suck & Spit (Sub-incisional cortex removal), **168**
Surface tension, 24
Surge, 16, 210
Surge and critical limit, 17
Surge and vacuum, 17
Surge prevention by the machine, 18, 211
Surgeon's control of surge, 19, 211
Surgical limbus, 44
Surgical pearls, 201

T

Tactile feedback, 7
Tangential force, 66, 67
Technique for single-piece PMMA
    lenses, 172
Technique of periocular antibiotic-steroid
    injection, 241
Techniques of CCC, 69
Techniques of correction, 202
Techniques of irrigation and aspiration,
    155
Thick cannula for modified bimanual
    irrigation-aspiration, 23
Thin and shredded flap, 48
Thin flap, 48
Tips, 11
Too long corneal valve, 48
Toric intraocular lens (Toric IOLs), 197,
    201
Torn edges, 47
Trenching, 103, 193

Triangle of surge (TOS), 18
Triplanar incision, 48, 49, 199
Types of
    Choppers, 22
    Corneal incision, 48, 49
    Fold, 173
    Force, 66
    Grips, 114
    Incisions, 199
    RMT, 213

U

Uniplanar clear corneal incision, 50
Uniplanar incision, 49, **61**, 199
Utilization of power, 11
Utrata capsulorrhexis forceps, 22

V

V-trench or victory trench, 106, 107
Vacuum, 13

Various tips of the choppers, 102
Venting, 18, 19
Venturi effect, 13
Venturi system, 13
Viscoelastic substances (VES), 21
Viscoelasticity, 23
Viscopressurized eyeball, 171
Viscosity, 24

W

Width of the trench, 104
Wire speculum, 22
Wound construction, 200, 211
Wound gape in different types of
    incision, 44
Wound-related complications, 205

Z

Zone of safety, 14
Zones of followability, 15
Zonulodialysis, 206

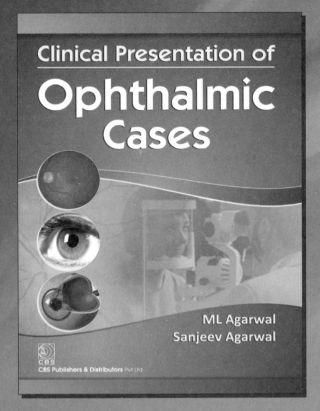

Clinical Presentation of
Ophthalmic Cases

ML Agarwal
Sanjeev Agarwal

CBS
CBS Publishers & Distributors Pvt Ltd

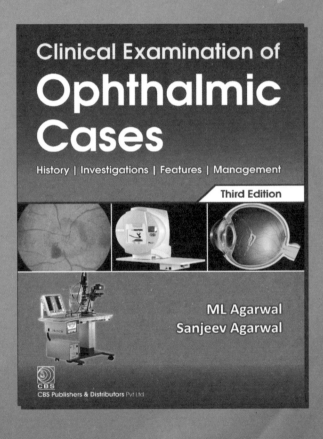

Clinical Examination of
Ophthalmic Cases

History | Investigations | Features | Management

Third Edition

ML Agarwal
Sanjeev Agarwal

CBS
CBS Publishers & Distributors Pvt Ltd

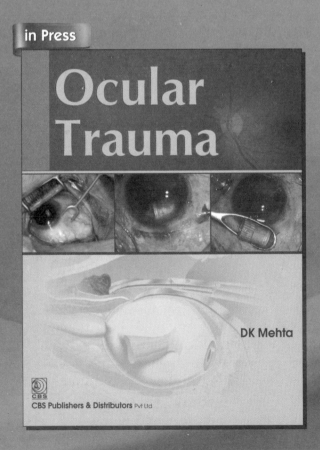

in Press

Ocular Trauma

DK Mehta

CBS
CBS Publishers & Distributors Pvt Ltd